Needs of Children and Young People Living with Complex Mental Health Difficulties

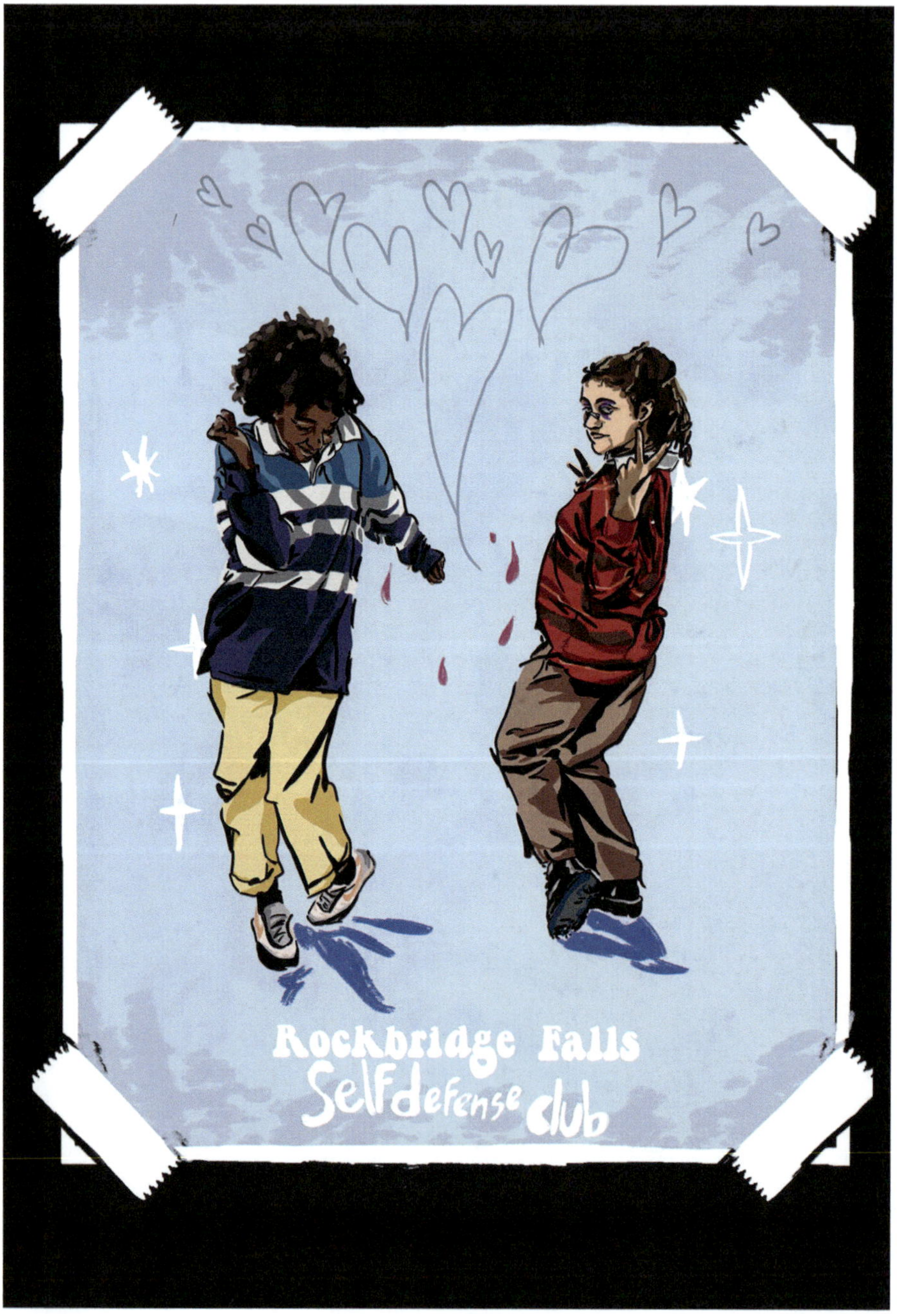
Rockbridge Falls
Self defense club

Gemma Trainor • Vanessa Heaslip
Editors

Needs of Children and Young People Living with Complex Mental Health Difficulties

Why it's Everyone's Business

Springer

Editors
Gemma Trainor
Mental Health Nursing, Directorate of Nursing and Midwifery
University of Salford
Salford, UK

Vanessa Heaslip
Directorate of Nursing and Midwifery
University of Salford
Salford, UK

Editorial Contact: Marie-Elia Come-Garry

ISBN 978-3-031-84531-4 ISBN 978-3-031-84532-1 (eBook)
https://doi.org/10.1007/978-3-031-84532-1

This Springer imprint is published by the registered company Springer Nature Switzerland AG
The registered company address is: Gewerbestrasse 11, 6330 Cham, Switzerland

Foreword

The mental health of children young people in our society is fast emerging as the single, major public health concern in the UK and globally. The crisis of young people's mental health can significantly impact future generations. One in four young people are concerned about their mental health, but this need outstrips the services available. To support this resource gap, the authors have focused on how to work more creatively to help children cope with mental health adversity to reach their potential. Considering the direct burden on young people and their families and friends, and the workforce challenges, there is a need to diagnose problems earlier. Those in the front line are required to offer practical advice and be aware of how to advise and support the relevant service.

Poor mental health increases the risk of chronic physical conditions yet there remains little parity of esteem, with physical health. We know that the developing brain needs nurturing in the same way as our physical development. Chapters in this book provide good examples of where parity of esteem needs to be improved. But this alone will not reverse the trend of growing mental health issues in young people.

Young people themselves will often seek support by confiding in the people they feel the most comfortable talking to and this includes their peers who play a pivotal role in adolescence. The internet is part of a young person's daily routine and while it can be a place to find solace and support, it can also be a place where toxic messaging triggers harm. This dilemma is helpfully explored in the book.

This book provides many examples of young people with lived experience co-authoring chapters, giving their views and insights into what support they need. One of the strengths of the book is the wide range and diverse nature of the contributors who demonstrate a wealth of knowledge and skills about how best to support children, young people and their families. Significantly, many of the young contributors to this book have made an impact nationally by advising the appropriate Royal Colleges, speaking at conferences and contributing to future research activities.

Overall, the authors have produced a clear description of the importance of young people's mental health, the prevalence of mental health issues, how to develop resilience and how to support all those involved in what is a challenging and complex world. The book explores the complex mental health disorders and how mental health problems develop and what is helpful to young people. It makes a timely and important contribution to assist all those involved in the mental health care of young people. It has been written by a multi-disciplinary team of passionate and experienced clinicians and experts by experience; for example, one of the young authors is also an ambassador for BEAT, a leading charity for eating disorder. The final words of the book are from a mother who tragically lost her son to suicide.

I commend this book to you as a practical guide to a set of inspiring interventions used to tackle one of the most challenging health and educational issues of our time.

Dame Anne Marie Rafferty

Professor of Nursing Policy,
King's College London and
Past President Royal College of Nursing
London, UK

Illustrator

My name is Robyn Heaslip, I am a transgender and neurodiverse amateur illustrator, with a diploma in animation. My art is often centred around portraiture, my affinity for film, queer identity, and my relationship through the modern world via individualist nurture and the divets remaindered from my adolescence. As such, my art strives to capture the interplay of a filmic lens, movements in under-loved and overshadowed communities, and visual poetry related to the theses of existence. I believe my work is fitting for this publication due to my personal experience with many of the segments mentioned, and the fact I have previously created art either tangentially related, or directly inspired by these narratives and worldviews.

Robyn Heaslip

Contents

About the Authors

Miriam Collett is a Lecturer in Children and Young People's Nursing at the University of Salford. She is a Specialist Community Public Health Nurse – School Nurse with over 17 years clinical experience working with a diverse range of people and communities across Greater Manchester. Miriam is passionate about reducing weight stigma and is a weight-neutral practitioner. Her doctoral study focuses on children with bigger bodies, inclusive school nursing practice and education.

Trudy Cowan is a CYP Nurse and Head of CYP Nursing at Salford University. Her research interests include inequalities that children face across society, namely not having their voices heard.

Nicola Curran is a Consultant Clinical Psychologist and Managing Director of Meadows Psychology Service with over 20 years' experience in leadership, service development, and trauma-informed practice. As a founder of Meadows Psychology Service, she leads a national team delivering psychological assessments, consultations, and training for systems supporting care-experienced individuals. Nicola is passionate about continuous improvement, governance, and embedding evidence-based therapeutic models across multi-agency systems.

Alicia Proton de la Chapelle is a French Masters graduate in intercultural studies. She suffered from anorexia when she was 18 and did her recovery between France and England which has given her an insight in the different treatments and methods in the two countries. She now lives in Denmark where she deepens her understanding of cultural differences and interculturality.

Lisa Fairclough is a specialist mental health nurse, at Bupa mental health clinical services customer facing support. She works with young people, families, and adults providing support, advice, and clinical guidance on a range of mental health conditions and is a level 5 safeguarding lead for BUPA clinical services. Lisa also has 29 years' experience working in the National Health Service (NHS) in specialist mental health services, including an Early Intervention in Psychosis team.

Jasmin Flynn is a teaching and learning fellow in Occupational Therapy at the University of Salford. Her clinical experience includes Paediatrics, Oncology and Palliative Care.

Celeste Foster is a senior adolescent mental health nurse, registered adolescent psychotherapist, and academic who has been working in Child and Adolescent Mental Health, since 1995. Celeste is an Associate Professor in mental health nursing at the University of Salford. She has published in the subjects of psychoanalytic approaches to working with adolescents and their professional networks in relation to self-harm, complex psychosomatic presentations, and developmental trauma. Celeste has been selected as the Eileen Skellern Memorial Lecturer for 2025, which is awarded in recognition of significant contribution to the advancement of mental health nursing practice, education, and research.

Laura Hales is an Associate Psychological Practitioner at Manchester University NHS Foundation Trust, Manchester, Greater Manchester.

Rebecca Hall is a Lecturer in Mental Health Nursing and has worked at the University of Salford for three years. She has worked in Higher Education since 2007 and maintained a part-time role in clinical practice until 2022. Rebecca is also a qualified Public Health Nurse and has over 20 years' experience of working with children, young people, and adults with mental health difficulties. Her specialist interests are in preventative and early interventions for mental health in school age populations, and also in drug use and addictions.

Elizabeth Harlow is an Assistant Clinical Psychologist at Manchester University NHS Foundation Trust, Manchester, Greater Manchester.

Corey Hartley is a dedicated advocate for trans* education and a leading voice in the promotion of inclusivity across various sectors. With a PhD from the University of Leeds, Corey has spent years working within academic institutions across the UK, empowering professionals with the knowledge and tools to better support trans* individuals in their environments. Corey's published research has contributed significantly to the field, and she is widely recognised as a passionate trans* advocate and queer ambassador. Her commitment to fostering understanding and championing trans* rights remains at the forefront of her work.

Robyn Heaslip is a transgender and neurodiverse BSc Illustration student who has a diploma in animation. Robyn's art is often centred around portraiture, film, queer identity, and their relationship with the modern world via individualist nurture, influenced by experiences of adolescence. As such, Robyn's art strives to capture the interplay of a filmic lens, movements in under-loved and overshadowed communities, and visual poetry related to the theses of existence.

Vanessa Heaslip is a Professor of Nursing and Healthcare Equity at Salford University. Her research interests are in communities who experience health inequity and social exclusion and whose voices are not traditionally heard in the academic and professional discourse. She has researched with a variety of individuals, groups, and communities including Gypsy, Roma, Travellers, people living with mental health issues, people living on the street, and those in the criminal justice system. Professor Heaslip has numerous publications including book contributions, journal articles (professional and peer reviewed), editorials, and discussion papers.

Lorraine Henshaw is an Associate Professor in Children and Young Peoples Nursing at the University of Salford with over 30 years nursing experience in a variety of clinical and educational settings. Lorraine's research interest lie in patient empowerment and the hearing of CYP voices and in the readiness and development of the workforce to meet future health and social care needs.

George Horwood has worked in childhood and adolescent mental health services for over 10 years, and currently works in preventive mental health and well-being support in a school-based services in England. He is qualified to provide clinical supervision to his team members and is currently in training to become a senior well-being practitioner.

Valerie Houghton is a qualified learning disability nurse, specialist practitioner, and nurse lecturer at Edinburgh Napier University. She has worked with children and young people with learning disabilities and their families, before moving into higher education teaching student learning disability nurses and social workers. She is passionate about social justice, and researching societal devaluation, disablist hate crime, stigma, and culture in care facilities.

Catriona Jones is a Lecturer in Children and Young Peoples Nursing at the University of Salford. Her background is mainly in paediatric Emergency Medicine with experience in paediatric hospice care.

Sarah Kennedy is a Senior Lecturer at the University of Bolton. She is qualified as a learning disabilities nurse and social worker and has worked with children, adults, and older adults during her career. Sarah is passionate about person-centred practice, and also practice learning and support and supervision of students whilst they are on placement.

Isobel McMillan is a researcher at the University of Salford within the school of Health and Society. Isobel holds a BSc and PhD in Psychology from the University of Manchester. Following doctoral study Isobel has worked in the field of health research both inside and outside of academia. Her research has focused on a wide range of health and mental health conditions with the unifying theme of improving care and outcomes.

Shelley O'Connor is a Senior Lecturer within the School of Nursing and Advanced Practice at Liverpool John Moores University (LJMU), UK. Shelley is a registered nurse in mental health, with experience in acute services, rehabilitation, forensics, prison service, and community drug and alcohol. She teaches both pre- and post-registration and is currently undertaking her PhD candidate exploring the student experience of the doctoral journey. Recently she authored a chapter about young people in the "Mental Health Interventions for the Emergency Services" handbook, and she also serves as a regular peer reviewer for a global academic publisher and for the *Journal of Medical Education and Curricular Development*.

Moyosore Opebiyi is a Lecturer on the Integrated Practice Learning Disabilities Programme at the University of Salford. She is a qualified nurse and a qualified social worker, and she has worked in Mental Health Hospitals, supporting people with enduring mental health problems by offering them medical and therapeutic interventions whilst building effective relationship with them and their families/carers.

Ben Robinson is a police officer who spends the majority of his time supporting children and adults with mental health problems. Ben has lived experience of anorexia nervosa and is passionate about the plight of young men. He is an ambassador for BEAT (a UK eating disorder charity) and is an advisor to the Royal College of Psychiatrists and to the Quality Care Commission. Ben has presented and published his work nationally. He supports families and young people with eating disorders by promoting recovery and instillation of hope.

Justine Rothwell is Head of Therapy at Meadows Care, leading a team providing therapeutic services for children and young people who have experienced trauma. An accredited CBT therapist with 19 years' experience, she specialises in psychological assessment, intervention, and clinical leadership, with a focus on self-harm and child sexual exploitation. Dr. Rothwell has contributed to research on adolescent self-harm and developed training modules for psychiatrists, advancing trauma-informed care.

Andrew Sweetmore is a Specialist Nurse Practitioner in a Tier 4 Community CAMHS team and a postgraduate researcher at Bournemouth University. His PhD research focuses on identifying early interventions for children and young people who self-harm. He has worked in mental health services since 2009 and has held positions such as Ward Manager of a psychiatric intensive care unit and Clinical Site Manager.

Gemma Trainor is Associate Professor in Mental Health Nursing at the University of Salford. Previously she held the post of Senior Lecturer in Mental Health Nursing at Liverpool John Moores University (2020–2023) having earlier spent over 3 years as a lecturer and researcher at Kings College, London (2016–2020). Clinically, she has over 30 years direct experience of working with young people and adults with complex mental health difficulties. Up to Summer 2016, Gemma was Nurse Consultant for a Tier 4 CAMHS day service and outpatient service with GMW NHS Foundation Mental Health Trust in Manchester. Here she specialised in working with young people who self-harm and was a member of the NICE guideline development committee on self-harm which was published in 2022.

Patience Udonsi is a Lecturer in Learning Disabilities Nursing and Social Work at the University of Salford, England, United Kingdom. Patience has an extensive background in professional practice, as a Community Learning Disability Nurse and a Mental Health Social Worker. Her research interests include promoting equity for individuals with intellectual disabilities who are neurodivergent and anti-racist practice within the context of Health and Social Care practice. Patience delivers training to Health and Social Care Provider services to support diversity and inclusion within staff teams. She is also a national senior Positive Behaviour Management Trainer.

Samita Wilson is an Associate Professor of Child Welfare at Norwegian University of Science & Technology (NTNU). Her primary research focuses on the complexities of children's rights and citizenship, especially highlight their right to protection and elevating the voices of marginalised children and families.

1 Picture of Mental Illness in Young People, Globally and in the United Kingdom

Gemma Trainor and Vanessa Heaslip

G. Trainor (✉)
Mental Health Nursing, Directorate of Nursing and Midwifery, University of Salford, Salford, UK

V. Heaslip
Directorate of Nursing and Midwifery, University of Salford, Salford, UK
e-mail: V.A.Heaslip@salford.ac.uk

G. Trainor, V. Heaslip (eds.), *Needs of Children and Young People Living with Complex Mental Health Difficulties*,
https://doi.org/10.1007/978-3-031-84532-1_1

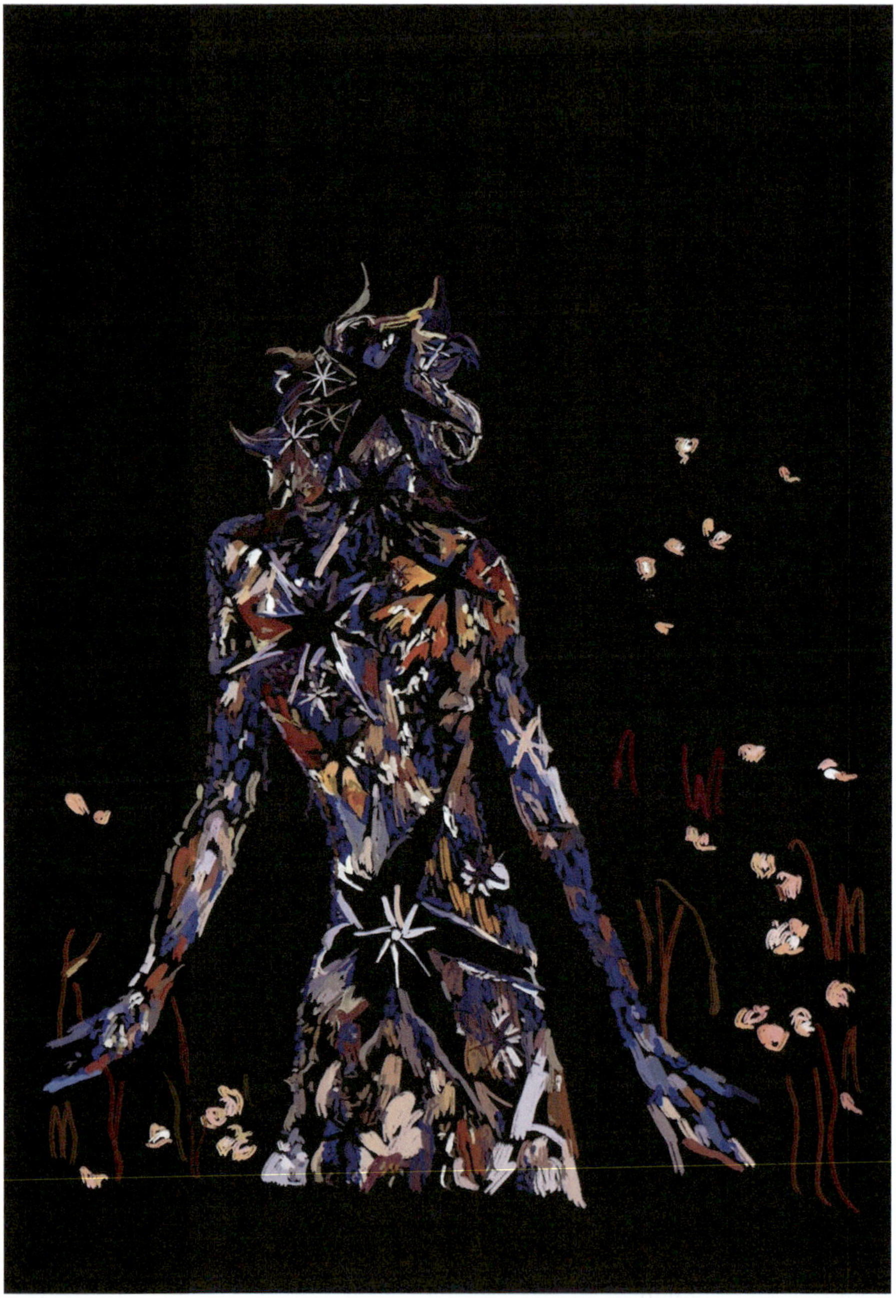

1.1 Global Prevalence of Mental Illness

The global impact of mental illness is significant in terms of human and economic costs. Human costs are estimated by identifying disability-adjusted life years referred to as DALYs, which are the total years of life lost (YLLs) and years lived with disability (YLDs), where one DALY equals one lost year of a healthy life (Global Burden of Disease Study 2020). The global DALYs due to mental illness are thought to be around 418 million (Arias et al. 2022), equating to 418 million lost years of a healthy life. The financial cost of mental illness globally is estimated to be around 5 trillion USD (Arias et al. 2022). In terms of children and young people (CYP), the World Health Organization (WHO 2021a) estimates that one in seven 10–19-year-olds experiences a mental disorder, accounting for 13% of the global burden of disease in this age group. Depression, anxiety and behavioural disorders are among the leading causes of illness and disability among adolescents. Suicide is the fourth leading cause of death among 15–29-year-olds (WHO 2021b). The consequences of failing to address adolescent mental health conditions extend to adulthood, impairing both physical and mental health and limiting opportunities to lead fulfilling lives as adults.

1.1.1 Overview of Prevalence and Service Provision for Children and Young People's Mental Health in the United Kingdom

Across the United Kingdom, there is a consistent picture of the percentage of children with a probable mental health disorder, which is a diagnosable condition recognised as such by the World Health Organization. These conditions include anxiety, depression, disruptive and/or hyperactive behaviours (e.g. ADHD) and other less common disorders such as autism.

In **England**, there has been a marked increase in these conditions over recent years. Among those aged 7–16, there was a rise in probable mental health disorders from 12.1% in 2017 to 18% in 2020, and similarly, for those aged 17–19, the prevalence over the same time period rose from 10.1% to 17.7% (NHS Digital 2018, 2022). This means that about one in six children aged 7–19 in England has a probable mental health disorder, a huge number of children, estimated to be 14 million in England alone (Office of the Children's Commissioner 2023). Also, the NHS Digital (2018) study for the first time provided statistics for pre-schoolchildren aged 2–4 where 1 in 18 (5.5%) had a disorder, and, of these, half were behavioural disorders. Recent statistics show that in 2022–2023, more than a quarter of a million (270,300) children and young people were still waiting for mental health support after being referred to Children and Young People's Mental Health Services (CYPMHS). Over the same time period, nearly 1 million children and young people (949,200) were referred to CYPMHS, equivalent to 8% of the 11.9 million children in England (Children's Commissioner 2024).

The picture in **Scotland** is very similar with increases in mental health difficulties observed over time. A literature review undertaken by the Scottish government in 2018 identified a decline in the mental wellbeing of adolescents across a number of indicators, particularly among teenage girls (Scottish Government 2019). The *Scottish Schools Adolescent Lifestyle and Substance Use Survey* (SALSUS 2019) found an increase in the proportion of 15-year-old girls reporting high levels of emotional and behavioural difficulties in the last decade. In 2015, 39% of 15-year-old girls had a borderline or abnormal total difficulties score, compared to 31% in 2006. Among the 15-year-old boys, 22% had a borderline or abnormal total difficulties score in 2006, compared to 28% in 2015.

Wales is no different. "Time to Change Wales", an alliance of leading Welsh mental health charities, reports that one in ten young people will experience a mental health problem and nearly three in four young people fear the reaction of friends when they talk about it (National Assembly for Wales 2018). The "Action for Children" report (Children in Wales 2020) highlighted that the proportion of 15–16-year-olds self-reporting anxiety or depression has doubled in recent years; that one in ten 5–16-year-olds has a diagnosable mental health disorder; and between 10% and 15% of teenagers have some symptoms of depression at any one time. The National Assembly for Wales report "Mind Over Matter" (2018) identified a step change was needed in emotional and mental health support for children and young people in Wales. Subsequently, the Strategic Programme for Mental Health was established in October 2023 (NHS Wales Executive 2023) with specific topic areas relevant to CYP covering eating disorders, child and adolescent mental health services (CAMHS), perinatal mental health and suicide and self-harm prevention.

In **Northern Ireland**, the Youth Wellbeing Prevalence Survey provided data on more than 3000 children and young people and more than 2800 parents and found that 1 in 8 children and young people in Northern Ireland (NI) experiences common mood disorders such as anxiety and depression, and this is around 25% higher than in other UK nations, reflecting similar trends seen in adults across Northern Ireland (HSCNI 2020). The results indicate elevated prevalence rates of mood and anxiety disorders in children and young people in Northern Ireland compared to England and other international countries. Indicators for poor mental health include disproportionately higher rates of suicide in NI among those under 18 s compared to other parts of the United Kingdom, increasing antidepressant prescription rates for 0–19-year-olds, increasing self-harm rates for 0–18-year-olds and self-reported poor emotional wellbeing (Bunting et al. 2022).

Reasons for the increases in mental illness in children and young people over the past 15 years are multifactorial and require further investigation; however, the explosive increase in the use of social media and peer group influence over this time scale are likely to be particularly important factors. Furthermore, young people appear more willing to destigmatise mental health issues and as such are more willing to identify and speak about their problems. Celebrities and other role models are also coming forward to publicise and raise awareness of mental health issues, and "parity of esteem" within the health system has rightly provided an opportunity for appropriate attention to be given to mental health issues. All these factors may have contributed to the rise in reported numbers of young people with mental health difficulties. The recent COVID-19 pandemic also had a negative effect on young people's mental health (Heaslip et al. 2022), with a doubling in the number of young people reporting poor mental health (OECD 2021).

However, one needs to be mindful that any process that categorises CYP as having a mental illness, while helpful in many ways, also requires caution as these classifications are oversimplifications of the vast continuum of human behaviours. In particular, a young person's behaviour and emotions change rapidly, and their presentation may simply reflect a normal phase of growing up. Additionally, there are a range of different kinds of social experiences linked to health, particularly those in childhood years (known as ACEs—adverse childhood experiences). The task is to recognise that each young person is unique and likely to have individual, family and community determinants that can affect their development.

1.1.2 Current Service Provision Arrangements in the United Kingdom

Specialist services for CYP are provided through a network of services organised in four tiers and the roles of the different tiers in England (see Table 1.1). Similar arrangements exist in Wales, Scotland and Northern Ireland (NHS 2023).

Most young people are supported in the lower Tier 1 and Tier 2 services, which are delivered by third sector organisations including schools and local authority children's services. Additionally, there are a lot of young people who could be managed at a lower tier attending Tier 4 services particularly attending out of hours and over the weekends when there is significantly less child and adolescent mental health service (CAMHS) professionals. There is also often a cross-over between health and social services where the young person's difficulties are rarely due to just their psychological needs alone but rather both psychological and social care needs, for example, young people who need an alternative residential placement, which can result in them having a protracted stay in a Tier 4 inpatient facility.

1.1.3 Service Provision

The 2023 report from the Children's Commissioner for England (2023) indicates that the CAMHS service provision falls well short of what is required to help CYP both in terms of the number of CYP receiving treatment and the amount of time elapsing between referral and receipt of treatment. For example, of the 1.4 million children estimated to have a mental health disorder, less than half (48%) received at least one contact with CAMHS. Furthermore, the average waiting time between a child being referred to CAMHS and starting treatment increased from 32 days in 2020–2021 to 40 days in 2021–2022. In terms of Tier 4 provision, there are limited numbers of places, for example, only around 1600 across the whole of England (Children's Commissioner 2023).

Table 1.1 Service arrangements for CYP mental health

Tier 1	Services provided by practitioners in universal services (such as early years services, primary care, health visitors, school nurses, teachers, youth workers, charities and voluntary care agencies) who are non-specialists and who can: Offer general advice and in certain cases Provide treatment for less severe problems Promote mental health Aid the early identification of problems Refer to specialist services
Tier 2	A service provided by specialist individuals such as youth offending teams, primary mental health workers and school and youth counselling (including social care and education) who offer: Training and consultation for other professionals Consultation for families and carers Outreach to families and children requiring more help and who are unwilling to use specialist services Assessment, which may trigger further treatment
Tier 3	A specialist multidisciplinary service for more severe, complex or persistent disorders, offering: Assessment and treatment Assessment for referrals to tier 4 Contributions to consultation and training at tiers 1 and 2 Participation in research and development projects
Tier 4	These are specialist tertiary services comprising: Day units Highly specialist inpatient and outpatient services

Over the recent years, the government has worked to increase the availability of mental health support in schools. A governmental proposal entitled "Transforming Children and Young People's Mental Health Provision" (DHSC 2017) set out three key proposals: to incentivise schools to identify and train a new senior lead for mental health, to establish mental health support teams (MHSTs) to work across schools and colleges and to pilot a 4-week waiting time for specialist services. As of May 2023, MHSTs covered 35% of pupils in schools and learners in further education (Department for Education 2023), and the government has since committed to expand MHSTs so that 50% of all pupils are covered by 2025.

1.1.4 Current and Future Needs and How These Are Being Addressed

As identified, mental health problems are central issues affecting many young people. Mental health problems among young people contribute to impaired physical and mental health, which can extend well into adulthood. Epidemiological data indicate that 50% of all major psychiatric conditions (excluding dementia) are clinically diagnosable by 15 years of age and an additional 25% by their early 20 s (Kessler et al. 2007). Despite significant improvement in national policies and legislation, services remain disjointed, underfunded and varied across the four countries. In 2015, a taskforce for young people's mental health and wellbeing released guidance, entitled *Future in Mind* (DoH 2015), on their vision to transform mental health services nationwide. This included five key principles (see Fig. 1.1).

To support these ambitions, the clinical commissioning teams (CCTs) were required to develop local comprehensive transformation plans for the next 5 years to ensure children and their families have early access to appropriate support. This report was followed up by several policy initiatives relevant to the mental health of children including the "The Five Year Forward View for Mental Health" in 2016 and a consultation on "Transforming Children and Young People's Mental Health Provision" in 2017 and culminated in "The NHS Long-Term Plan" in 2019 (House of Commons Library 2023). Among the commitments in "The Long-Term Plan" to be delivered by 2029 were:

- Funding for Children and Young People's Mental Health Services (CYPMHS) will grow faster than both overall NHS funding and total mental health spending.

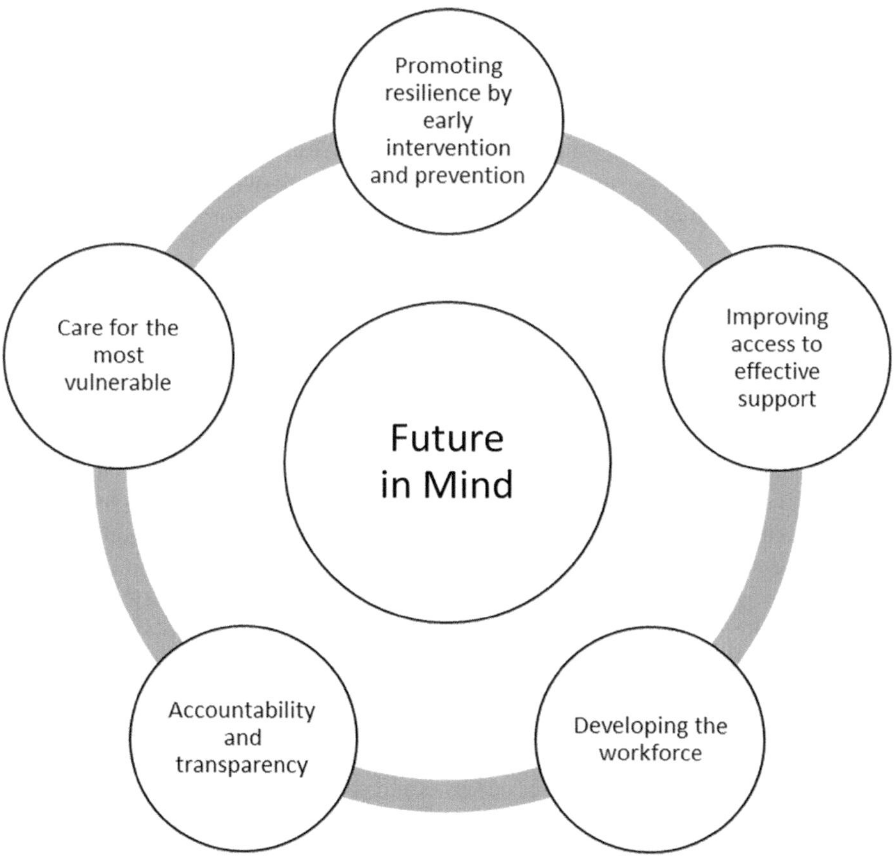

Fig. 1.1 Future in Mind principles created by the authors based on DoH (2015)

- At least 345,000 additional children and young people (up to age 25) will be able to access mental health support through NHS services or school- or college-based mental health support teams.
- Extra investment to meet waiting time standards for children and young people's eating disorder services.

Additionally, in 2023, the UK Government published a major conditions strategy that includes mental health, rather than having a standalone mental health strategy (House of Commons Library 2023), with the ambition that a joined-up strategy will ensure that mental health conditions are considered alongside physical health conditions, thereby acknowledging the ambitions of "parity of esteem".

1.1.5 Aetiology of Mental Health in Children and Young People

Childhood and adolescence are critical stages of rapid growth and development; therefore, there is a need to acquire important skills to mitigate the risk of developing psychiatric disorders. The risk factors for mental health disorders are well established, and substantial progress has been made in developing the workforce; however, this is a long way off meeting the complex needs of this population. The recent COVID-19 pandemic added to this, as young people had to navigate their way through schools going online, lack of physical contact, loss and bereavement, financial tensions, exposure to domestic violence and ongoing concerns about health and their future (Bellis et al. 2018).

1.1.6 Risk and Protective Factors

Mental health problems can have a wide range of causes and are likely to be a combination of factors including individual, family and community factors. The more risk factors adolescents are exposed to, the greater the potential for this to impact their mental health (WHO 2021a, 2022). However, protective factors can function as a buffer to risk factors. The presence and absence of protective and risk factors are contextual variables that contribute to the mental health of young people. Table 1.2 gives examples.

The presence and absence of protective and risk factors are contextual variables that contribute to the mental health of young people. The risk assessment should inform and influence the care of the young person and how to support them effectively. Additionally, it must be recognised that risk is constantly changing and not an exact science. Therefore, any risk assessment tools should not replace a thorough psychosocial assessment but should help shape the case formulation. Four key overarching strategies for helping to reduce risks and promote protective factors include:

- Developing and enforcing laws and policies that promote mental health globally.
- Implementing school-based programmes to include anti-bullying interventions.

Table 1.2 Risk and protective factors for children and young people's mental health

	Risk factors	Protective factors
Child	Genetic Low IQ Developmental delay Dysfunctional attachment style Communication difficulties Difficult temperament Physical illness Academic failure Low self-esteem Lack of emotional and behavioural control	Secure attachment experience Good communication skills Having a belief in control Positive attitude Intelligence and good problem-solving and coping skills Motivation and commitment to succeed Experience of success and achievement Capacity to reflect Good morality and sense of right and wrong
Family	Disharmony breakup Inconsistent disciplinary style Parents with MH illness/substance abuse Physical and sexual neglect of emotional abuse Parental criminality or alcoholism Death, abandonment and loss Intergenerational trauma	Family harmony and stability Supportive parenting Extended family supports Strong family values Affection Clear consistent disciplining/boundaries Support for education Absence of abuse High or low expressed emotion
School	Bullying Discrimination Breakdown or lack of family friendships Deviant peer influences Peer pressure Poor pupil-teacher relationships	Positive school climate, enhancing belonging and connectedness Clear policies on behaviour and bullying "Open door" policy for children to raise problems A whole-school approach to promoting good mental health Positive peers and adult role models
Community	Socioeconomic disadvantage Homelessness Disaster, accident, war or other overwhelming effects Discrimination and stigmatisation Other significant life events Lack of access to support services	Wider support network High rates of crime and poverty Easy access to drugs and alcohol Low community involvement among residents Good housing High standard of living Opportunities for valued social role Range of sport/leisure activities

Adapted from Public Health England (2016a)

- Supporting caregivers to provide nurturing care.
- Improving the quality of community environments and digital spaces for all young people in all countries at all income levels.

1.1.7 Adverse Childhood Experiences

Negative experiences in childhood and adolescence can result in chronic physical and mental ill health. These experiences are known as adverse childhood experiences (ACEs) and are often highly stressful and traumatic events or situations that occurred in childhood (Anda et al. 2010; Berens et al. 2017). There are multiple ACEs affecting children and young people (see Table 1.3).

There are many common risk and protective factors that apply to a range of different ACEs similar to those cited above. They can be a single event or prolonged threats to a young person's safety (CDC 2024). Kaiser Permanente and the Centers for Disease Control and Prevention (1998) study on ACEs identifies that these negative traumatic experiences are a root cause of many emotional cognitive and social impairments that can lead to unhealthy self-destructive behaviours (van der Kolk et al. 1991). Awareness around ACEs is growing, and this has influenced how front-line staff respond to these circumstances, leading to a growth in trauma-informed care. The general purpose behind a trauma-informed approach to care is to reduce any further trauma that young people may experience inadvertently from caregivers (see Chap. 7). There is evidence that the negative effects of ACEs can be mitigated through psychosocial and resilience-building interventions. A retrospective study by Bellis et al. (2018) examining ACEs and resilience identified that in those children with four or more ACEs, the presence of significant resilience assets (such as having supportive friends and enjoying community culture) reduced the prevalence of poor childhood health by a third (from 59.8% in those with no resilience assets to 21.3% for those with such assets).

1.1.8 Resilience

Resilience is defined as the process of being able to bounce back from adversity (Srivastava 2011). Resilience is also contested and critiqued due to a potential focus on the individuals coping alone, without addressing wider society's issues. While research in this area is in its infancy, studies that have been conducted are supportive

Table 1.3 Adverse childhood experiences

Adverse childhood experiences
These include growing up in families where there is:
Abuse (emotional, physical, sexual, neglect), including sibling abuse
Domestic violence
Alcohol and drug abuse
Ongoing experiences of mental illnesses
Relationship stress (such as separation, divorce or death)
Criminal activity
Organised violence
Forced marriage
Living in communities where there is:
Criminal and collective violence
Early conscription (e.g. child soldiers)
Bullying and other forms of peer-to-peer violence
Socioeconomic disadvantage (poverty)
Social exclusion (race, gender, immigration status, class and social inequities)

Adapted from Anda et al. (2010) and Berens et al. (2017)

Table 1.4 Strategies to build resilience

Strategies	Activities
Learning from the past	Think back over situations that have helped you deal with things, what skills did you use and then that you can use again. Having confidence in your ability to deal with things
Reach out to others for support	Build healthy relationships and get connected by joining groups Don't pursue relationships that bring you down
Recognise that you can't always change the past	Recognise that you can change your future
Be optimistic	It is important to be aware that you can be hopeful about things changing by developing your confidence in approaching situations differently
Set achievable goals	This is a good way to develop self-efficacy. Ensure you are not being overly ambitious and setting yourself up to fail
Understand and avoid negative self-talk	Promote positive self-talk and celebrate your achievements. Look for evidence for why you are thinking like that and consider what advice you might give someone else in that situation
Be kinder to yourself by looking after yourself	Ensure lots of exercise and a good healthy diet
Embrace change	Flexibility is essential; by being more adaptable, you will be better equipped to deal with things
Develop problem-solving skills	Come up with solutions to a problem by making list of potential ways to solve the problem and then experimenting with different strategies

of its modulating role in mental health. A review of 25 studies in children and adolescents by Mesman et al. (2021) showed unanimously that higher levels of resilience were related to fewer mental health problems. Over the life course, a person's resilience can adapt and change to allow coping mechanisms to develop that help young people to take control of stressful situations. Resilience can be developed and enhanced through focused activities (see Table 1.4).

Resilience and adversity interact; however, this does not mean that children who experience severe adversity have no resilience. Indeed, some young children who have experienced multiple adversities can have high levels of resilient factors such as having their own agency and being active contributors to society (Gladstone et al. 2006).

1.2 Future Directions and Developments

1.2.1 Increasing Capacity and Integrated Working

At the national conference on "Mental Health Is Everyone's Business" in May 2023, UNICEF opened the discussion on the need to strengthen the systems of mental health support for children and their families (UNICEF 2023). Mental health needs need to be considered on a continuum as people of all ages can experience mental health issues; however, we need to promote a supportive environment where children can grow and flourish. The "No health without mental health" strategy is over a decade old now, yet there remain disparities between access, availability and quality compared to the treatment of physical health conditions (Mitchell et al. 2017). Other initiatives like parity of esteem did go some way to ensure that mental health would be valued in the same way as physical health (Health Foundation 2014); however, as we have noted earlier in this chapter, there is still a way to go to ensure that all CYP who need access to CYPMHS can access it.

There remain many barriers to managing child and adolescence with mental health problems. Although effective treatments are available, only a minority of children who are affected access them (O'Brien et al. 2016). The transformation of children and young people's mental health is now being led locally, meaning that across local NHS services, public health, social service authorities, education, non-statutory services and youth justice are working together with children, young people and their families to design and provide the best possible services. These plans are living documents, and as such, the clinical commissioning groups are expected to republish them every year to ensure transparency of resources and investment. Those providing care need to address the shortfalls that have been addressed in several key documents such as improving waiting times, improving access to services by providing single point of access (SPA), improving care for the most vulnerable, promoting accountability and transparency and developing the workforce (DoH 2015). Mental health services have struggled to keep up with the demand, resulting in high levels of unmet need as identified by the Children and Young People's Mental Health and Wellbeing Taskforce (DHSC 2017). This has resulted in many services moving away from the tiered model of care mentioned previously in this chapter to a more integrated model of care. The ambitions align with the THRIVE model of care (Wolpert et al. 2016), which describes a more integrated model that may be less confusing for young people and their families/carers with an emphasis on all frontline agencies working together in a focused way (see Fig. 1.2).

Additionally transformational plans stress the importance of offering to deliver alternative supplementary mental health support, which may help in part with the long-standing concerns around staff retention around the world (Coates and Howe 2015). What has become increasingly clear is that specialist mental health services cannot in isolation meet the demands of young people's mental health needs. The soaring rates of mental health disorders were intensified by the pandemic, and it cannot be the responsibility of just one organisation or healthcare system; rather everyone must consider what they can do to provide the best possible support at the earliest opportunity.

"It takes a village to raise a child" is a well-known African proverb and perhaps is helpful when considering the importance of the entire community to provide positive interaction to ensure young people grow up in a safe and healthy environment. This proverb perhaps reflects the importance of the entire village/community's need to provide for and interact positively to ensure children grow up in a safe and healthy environment. It reminds us of the need to move past a siloed, professional-centric approach when not just working with the child but also families, schools and

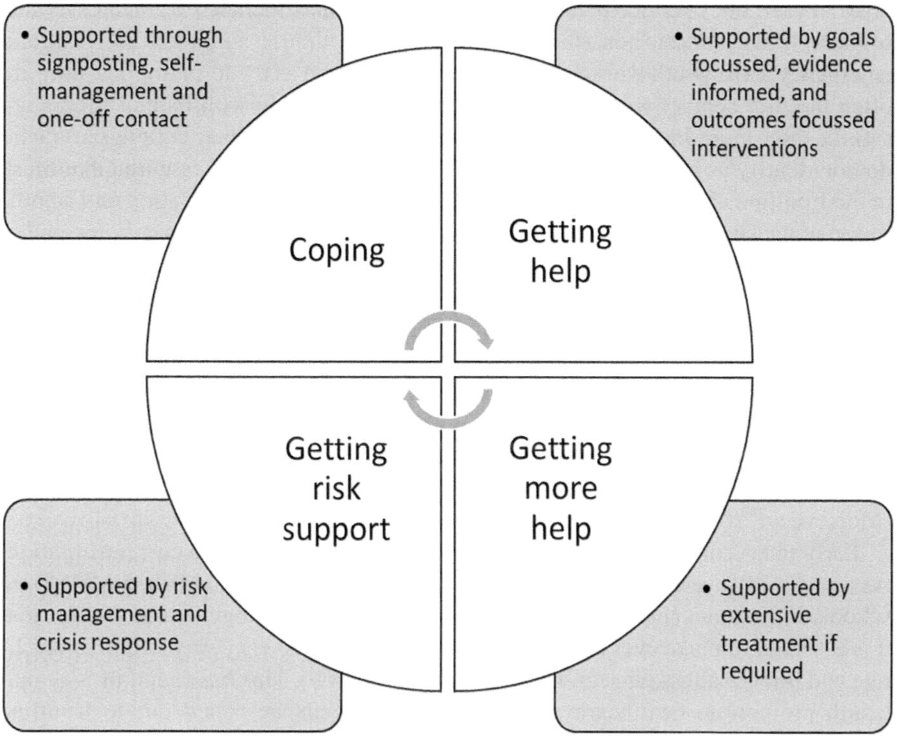

Fig. 1.2 THRIVE model. (Adapted from Wolpert et al. 2014)

communities. This book highlights the need to move beyond this approach when working with children and families.

Mental health disorders are as important as physical health problems, and good mental health is fundamental to good physical health and ensuring that young people can reach their potential. As such, everyone must consider what they can do to provide the best support for children/young people and their families. There is growing evidence through the mental health support teams (MHSTs) within schools providing low-intensity interventions and teachers training in mental health first aid of the importance of early interventions. Therefore, there needs to be a graded range of support from non-CAMHS specialists to identify how to intervene earlier in the young person's life to prevent deterioration by ignoring the problem or waiting for the young person to go into crisis. The "Mental Health Crisis Care Concordat" (HM Government 2014) is a national agreement between services and agencies in the care and support of people in crisis, which agrees the role of how police, ambulance professionals, social services and mental health services should work together to help people in mental health crisis, thereby acknowledging that mental health is everybody's business.

Mental health presentations of young people account for a significant and increasing share of the growing demand for emergency healthcare (Andrew et al.

2020). Emergency service personnel and first responders include paramedics, police officers, triage nurses, non-statutory personnel, paediatric and adult accident and emergency staff, youth workers and social workers, and as the term implies, they are often the first contact with a youth in crisis. Young people with mental illness are significantly more likely to encounter emergency staff than their counterparts who do not identify as having mental health problems. It is therefore essential that those in the frontline are suitably trained to respond and provide de-escalation and stabilisation of the situation ensuring where possible the child's safe return to home and to their community. To achieve this, the crisis response services should partner with other appropriate services who are or can be involved in the continuum of care.

Frontline responders such as police have a vital role to play in working and supporting young people with mental health problems ensuring their safety and that of the public. There is no need to be a mental health expert to respond to the emergency, and there are many good examples of best practice. For example, in some localities, there is a scheme known as "the Triage Car" where mental health nurses accompany police officers to incidents and give expert on-the-spot advice (MerseyCare 2024).

Early intervention and prevention are key issues to improve the current situation. As a result of several government initiatives, there are now established MHSTs in schools in England (DoH 2015). There is also a health strategy that advocates that it is essential to make every contact count as a simple and easy way to deliver accurate and brief health advice and screening (PHE 2016b). This has found its way into health promotion, healthcare and training, which can be rolled out to frontline responders. Emergency personnel such as paramedics and police officers often provide the pre-screening; therefore, they are required to be suitably trained in acute emergency mental healthcare. Analogous stories in the public arena suggest that children and young people with mental health problems are presenting to emergency services with much more frequency (Lo et al. 2020). This increased utilisation of acute emergencies in this population has generated considerable concern (Gonzalez et al. 2020). Emergency staff and those encountering young people in crisis need to be equipped as they play a critical role in the young person's journey as currently the demand is outstripping the needs of this vulnerable group. The goal is to provide optimal and equitable early intervention to any service.

1.2.2 Empowering and Upskilling Practitioners

Children and young people do not often access healthcare services; most of their access is through national immunisation and screening programmes delivered by health visitors and practice and school nurses or through accidents and attendance at emergency departments. Because of this, other professionals are of utmost importance to identify if a young person is struggling with their mental health such as teachers, police officers and youth workers.

It is estimated that between 20% and 40% of police time is spent dealing with mental health issues (West Midlands Police and Crime Commissioner 2020). For teachers, research by the Mental Health Foundation (2018) had identified that 71% of teachers feel they lack the right education and training to help pupils with mental health concerns and only 13% had received mental health first aid training. For community nurses (health visitors, school and practice nurses), Heaslip et al. (2022) argue that many of them feel unequipped to manage children and young people's mental health needs. Yet a systematic review assessing the existing literature on the effectiveness of mental health training courses for non-specialist health workers (Caulfield et al. 2019) identified that training non-specialist workers in mental healthcare is an effective strategy for improving knowledge, skills and confidence among the staff. This said young people themselves can take important steps to protect, improve and advocate for their mental health.

This book aims to re-address this by providing non-specialist mental health staff with guidance, understanding and tools to help them to support young people who are struggling with their mental health, as well as understanding the process for specialist referrals. This book will include appropriate case studies to help those professionals make links to their practice as well as a variety of reflective activities to enable them to critically examine their current practice and identify any future learning needs.

1.3 Summary of Chapters

Subsequent chapters in this book will provide straightforward guidance for professionals who interact with young people on how best to engage with them and provide the support and help that children and young people need.

Chapters 2, 3 and 4 will focus on three specific complex mental health difficulties experienced by young people, namely, **self-harm, eating disorders and psychosis/bipolar disorder**, respectively. A mixture of case studies with helpful advice on how to support these young people will be provided as well as describing up-to-date evidence on recommended treatments and interventions.

The focus in Chaps. 5 and 6 will be on young people who have **learning disabilities, are neurodivergent or who present with gender dysphoria** as mental health needs (often undiagnosed) are common for these groups of young people. Again, case studies and the voices of young people with lived experience will highlight how best to support these young people with regard to improving access to services and the issues around psychological and physical interventions.

Social and environmental factors such as **social exclusion and discrimination** (racial and economic) can have serious impacts on children and young people's mental health. Chapter 7 will examine how these issues contribute to the poor mental health of young people and will include information on wider support groups and evidence-based strategies which practitioners can use when working with these young people. In addition to these experiences, the impact and the effect on children and young people's access to and use of **social media** and attendant safeguarding issues will be explored in Chaps. 8 and 13. Chapter 8 focuses on issues related to child protection and safeguarding informing readers of their statutory requirements to keep children safe. Chapter 13 will provide practical guidance on how to engage with young people in supportive discussions about their Internet usage that will ultimately support their emotional wellbeing.

Strategies aimed at helping children and young people cope with their emotional and mental health difficulties will be covered in Chaps. 9, 10 and 11. Chapter 9 will cover **understanding emotional and behaviour control difficulties that can lead to aggression and relationship problems** by utilising dynamic developmental approach to understanding how young people see themselves and the world around them, how they perceive threat and how they understand and manage emotions and relationships. The chapter on **Trauma Informed Care** (Chap. 10) will present evidence-based therapeutic models along with strategies to support those working with children and young people who have experienced developmental trauma, while the chapter **Assessing, Formulating and Responding to Mental Health-Related Risks** (Chap. 11) will provide a straightforward guide to considering and making sense of some of the risks commonly associated with mental health needs (such as bullying, drug and alcohol abuse, violence and aggression and vulnerability to others). Consideration of the practitioners themselves is covered in Chap. 12, **Therapeutic Use of Self and Reflective Practice for Engaging Young People and Their Families**, which provides practical guidance on how to engage young people to enter into supportive discussions that enable individuals and their family members, promoting agency and openness to intervention. This, which will ultimately support their emotional wellbeing.

The Conclusion chapter (Chap. 14) will summarise the key chapters described above, synthesising the overall content and how professional bodies and international, national, regional and local healthcare and social care systems can contribute to the transformation of care pathways to ensure joined-up working. It will cover holistic care with parity of esteem and a discussion of system maturity by describing "what good looks like". Future research ambitions, access to training and education and a list of up-to-date relevant resources are also provided.

References

Anda RF, Butchart A, Felitti VJ, Brown DW. Building a framework for global surveillance of the public health implications of adverse childhood experiences. Am J Prev Med. 2010;39(1):93–8. https://doi.org/10.1016/j.amepre.2010.03.015.

Andrew E, Nehme Z, Cameron P, Smith K. Drivers of increasing emergency ambulance demand. Prehosp Emerg Care. 2020;24(3):385–93. https://doi.org/10.1080/10903127.2019.1635670.

Arias D, Saxena S, Verguet S. Quantifying the global burden of mental disorders and their economic value. eClin Med. 2022;54:101675. https://doi.org/10.1016/j.eclinm.2022.101675.

Bellis MA, Hughes K, Ford K, et al. Adverse childhood experiences and sources of childhood resilience: a retrospective study of their combined relationships with child health and educational attendance. BMC Public Health. 2018;18:792. https://doi.org/10.1186/s12889-018-5699-.

Berens A, Jensen SKG, Nelson CA. Biological embedding of childhood adversity: from physiological mechanisms to clinical implications. BMC Med. 2017;15(135):135. https://doi.org/10.1186/s12916-017-0895-4.

Bunting L, Nolan E, McCartan C, et al. Prevalence and risk factors of mood and anxiety disorders in children and young people: findings from the Northern Ireland youth wellbeing survey. Clin Child Psychol Psychiatry. 2022;27(3):686–700. https://doi.org/10.1177/13591045221089841.

Caulfield A, Vatansever D, Lambert G, Bortel TV. WHO guidance on mental health training: a systematic review of the progress for non-specialist health workers. BMJ Open. 2019;2019(9):e024059. https://doi.org/10.1136/bmjopen-2018-024059.

Centre for Disease Control. Adverse Childhood Experiences; 2024. Available from: https://www.cdc.gov/violenceprevention/aces/index.html. Accessed 25 Mar 2024

Children Commissioner for England. Children's Mental Health Services 2021–22; 2023. Available from: https://assets.childrenscommissioner.gov.uk/wpuploads/2023/03/Childrens-Mental-Health-Services-2021-2022-2.pdf. Accessed 12 Feb 2024

Children Commissioner for England. Children's Mental Health Services 2022–23; 2024. Available from: https://www.childrenscommissioner.gov.uk/resource/childrens-mental-health-services-2022-23/. Accessed 25 Mar 2024

Children in Wales. Annual report and accounts 2018–19; 2020. Available from: https://www.childreninwales.org.uk/application/files/8016/2512/7352/2018_-_19_Annual_Report_English.pdf. Accessed 12 Feb 2024

Coates D, Howe D. Combatting staff burnout in mental health: key managerial and leadership tasks that are fundamental to staff wellbeing and retention. Asia Pacific J Health Manag. 2015;10(2):24–32.

Department for Education. Transforming children and young people's mental health implementation programme data release; 2023. Available from: https://assets.publishing.service.gov.uk/media/646248cf427e41000cb437ab/Transforming_CYPMH_implementation_programme__data_release_May_2023.pdf. Accessed 12 Feb 2024.

Department of Health. Future in Mind, Promoting, protecting and improving our children and young people's mental health and wellbeing; 2015. Available from: https://assets.publishing.service.gov.uk/government/uploads/system/uploads/attachment_data/file/414024/Childrens_Mental_Health.pdf. Accessed 12 Feb 2024.

Department of Health and Social Care. Transforming children and young people's mental health provision: a Green Paper. Department of Health and Social Care; 2017. Available from: https://www.gov.uk/government/consultations/transforming-children-and-young-peoples-mental-health-provision-a-green-paper. Accessed 13 Feb 2024.

Gladstone B, Boydell K, McKeever P. Recasting research into children's experiences of parental mental illness: beyond risk and resilience. Soc Sci Med. 2006;62:2540–50. https://doi.org/10.1016/j.socscimed.2005.10.038.

Global Burden of Disease Collaborative Network. Global Burden of Disease Study Seattle, United States: Institute for Health Metrics and Evaluation (IHME); 2020.

Gonzalez K, Faisalmohemed Patel F, Cutchins L, Kodish I, Uspal N. Advocacy to address emergent pediatric mental health care. Clin Pediatr Emerg Med. 2020;21(2):100778. https://doi.org/10.1016/j.cpem.2020.100778.

Health Foundation. Mental health; 2014. Is policy moving towards parity? Available from: https://www.health.org.uk/blogs/mental-health-is-policy-moving-towards-parity. Accessed 12 Feb 2024.

Heaslip V, Glendening N, Snowden J. Promoting young people's mental health: the role of community nurses. Nurs Stand. 2022;38:43. https://doi.org/10.7748/ns.2022.e11967.

HM Government. Department of Health, No health without mental health: a cross-government mental health outcomes strategy for people of all ages; 2011. Available from: https://assets.publishing.service.gov.uk/media/5a7c348ae5274a25a914129d/dh_124058.pdf. Accessed 12 Feb 2024.

HM Government. Mental Health Crisis Care Concordat. Improving outcomes for people experiencing mental health crisis; 2014. Available from: https://assets.publishing.service.gov.uk/media/5a7c1ff0e5274a1f5cc75f09/36353_Mental_Health_Crisis_accessible.pdf. Accessed 12 Feb 2024.

House of Commons Library. Policy paper. Major conditions strategy: case for change and our strategic framework Updated 21 August 2023 https://www.gov.uk/government/publications/major-conditions-strategy-case-for-change-and-our-strategic-framework/major-conditions-strategy-case-for-change-and-our-strategic-framework-2. Accessed 9 April 2025.

HSCNI. Youth Wellbeing Prevalence Survey 2020 Health and Social Care Northern Ireland; 2020. Available from: https://online.hscni.net/our-work/social-care-and-children/children-and-young-people/youth-wellbeing-prevalence-survey-2020/. Accessed 12 Feb 2024.

Kessler RC, Amminger GP, Aguilar-Gaxiola S, Alonso J, Lee S, Ustün TB. Age of onset of mental disorders: a review of recent literature. Curr Opin Psychiatry. 2007;20(4):359–64. https://doi.org/10.1097/YCO.0b013e32816ebc8c.

Lo CB, Bridge JA, Shi J, Ludwig L, Stanley RM. Children's mental health emergency department visits: 2007-2016. Pediatrics. 2020;145(6) https://doi.org/10.1542/peds.2019-1536.

Mental Health Foundation. Shocking research reveals half of teachers affected by mental ill health due to work pressure; 2018. Available from: Shocking research reveals half of teachers affected by mental ill health due to work pressure | Mental Health Foundation. Accessed 6 Mar 2024.

MerseyCare. MerseyCare NHS Trust. Mental Health Triage Cars; 2024. Available from: https://www.merseycare.nhs.uk/our-services/liverpool/mental-health-triage-cars. Accessed 3 Apr 2024.

Mesman E, Vreeker A, Hillegers M. Resilience and mental health in children and adolescents: an update of the recent literature and future directions. Curr Opin Psychiatry. 2021;34(6):586–92.

Mitchell AJ, Hardy S, Shiers D. Parity of esteem: addressing the inequalities between mental health and physical healthcare. BJPsych Adv. 2017;23(30):196–205. https://doi.org/10.1192/apt.bp.114.014266.

National Assembly for Wales Children. Young People and Education Committee s Mind over matter A report on the step change needed in emotional and mental health support for children and young people in Wales; 2018. Available from: https://senedd.wales/laid%20documents/cr-ld11522/cr-ld11522-e.pdf. Accessed 12. Feb 2024.

NHS. Children and young people's mental health services; 2023. Available from: https://www.nhs.uk/mental-health/children-and-young-adults/mental-health-support/mental-health-services/. Accessed 18 Feb 2024.

NHS Digital. Mental Health of Children and Young People in England, 2017. Summary of key findings; 2018. Available from: https://dera.ioe.ac.uk/id/eprint/32622/1/MHCYP%202017%20Summary.pdf. Accessed 12 Feb 2024.

NHS Digital. Mental Health of Children and Young People in England 2022 – wave 3 follow up to the 2017 survey; 2022. Available from: https://digital.nhs.uk/data-and-information/publications/statistical/mental-health-of-children-and-young-people-in-england/2022-follow-up-to-the-2017-survey. Accessed 12 Feb 2024.

NHS Digital. Mental Health of Children and Young People in England 2023 – wave 4 follow up to the 2017 survey; 2023. Available from: https://digital.nhs.uk/data-and-information/publications/statistical/mental-health-of-children-and-young-people-in-england/2023-wave-4-follow-up/part-1-mental-health. Accessed 18 Nov 2024.

NHS Wales Executive. Strategic programme for Mental Health; 2023. Available from: https://executive.nhs.wales/functions/strategic-programme-for-mental-health/. Accessed 11 Feb 2024.

O'Brien D, Harvey K, Howse J, Reardon T, Creswell C. Barriers to managing child and adolescent mental health problems: a systematic review of primary care practitioners' perceptions. Br J Gen Pract. 2016;66(651):e693–707. https://doi.org/10.3399/bjgp16X687061.

Organisation for Economic Co-operation and Development (OECD). Supporting young people's mental health through the COVID-19 crisis. Tackling Coronavirus (COVID-19): Contributing to a global effort; 2021. Available from: https://read.oecd-ilibrary.org/view/?ref=1094_1094452-vvnq8dqm9u&title=Supporting-young-people-s-mental-health-through-the-COVID-19-crisis. Accessed 5 Mar 2024.

Public Health England. The mental health of children and young people in England; 2016a. Available from: https://assets.publishing.service.gov.uk/media/5a80c3e240f0b62305b8d06c/Mental_health_of_children_in_England.pdf. Accessed 25 Mar 2024.

Public Health England. NHS England and Health Education England. Making Every Contact Count (MECC) A consensus statement; 2016b. Available from: https://www.england.nhs.uk/wp-content/uploads/2016/04/making-every-contact-count.pdf. Accessed 29 Mar 2024.
SALSUS. Scottish Schools Adolescent Lifestyle and Substance Use Survey (SALSUS): mental wellbeing report 2018; 2019. Available from: https://www.gov.scot/publications/scottish-schools-adolescent-lifestyle-substance-use-survey-salsus-mental-wellbeing-report-2018/. Accessed 12 Feb 2024.
Scottish Government. Exploring the reported worsening of mental wellbeing among adolescent girls in Scotland; 2019. Available from: Exploring the reported worsening of mental wellbeing among adolescent girls in Scotland – gov.scot (www.gov.scot). Accessed 12 Feb 2024.
Srivastava K. Positive mental health and its relationship with resilience. Ind Psychiatry J. 2011;20(2):75–6. https://doi.org/10.4103/0972-6748.102469.
UNICEF. Mental health is everyone's business; 2023. Available from: https://www.unicef.org/northmacedonia/press-releases/mental-health-everyones-business#:~:text=Skopje%2C%203%20May%202023%3A%20At,response%20in%20the%20schools%20and. Accessed 18 Feb 2024.
van der Kolk BA, Perry JC, Herman JL. Childhood origins of self-destructive behavior. Am J Psychiatry. 1991;148(12):1665–71. https://doi.org/10.1176/ajp.148.12.1665.
West Midlands Police and Crime Commissioner. Predicting the Volume of Demand from Mental Health Related Police Incidents; 2020. Available from: 14122020-EC-Agenda-Item-5c-Mental-Health-Deman-Investigation.pdf (westmidlands-pcc.gov.uk). Accessed 6 Mar 2024.
Wolpert M, Harris R, Jones M, Hodges S, Fuggle P, James R, Wiener A, Mckenna C, Law D, Fonagy P. THRIVE; The AFC–Tavistock Model for CAMHS; 2014. Available from: Thrive.pdf (implementingthrive.org). Accessed 1 Apr 2024
Wolpert M, Harris R, Hodges S, Fuggle P, James R, Wiener A, McKenna C, Law D, York A, Jones M, Fonagy P, Fleming I, Munk S. THRIVE elaborated. 2nd ed. London: CAMHS Press; 2016. https://www.implementingthrive.org/wp-content/uploads/2016/09/THRIVE-elaborated-2nd-edition.pdf. Accessed 25 Mar 2024
World Health Organisation. Mental health of adolescents; 2021a. Available from: https://www.who.int/news-room/fact-sheets/detail/adolescent-mental-health. Accessed 18 Feb 2024.
World Health Organisation. Suicide worldwide in 2019; 2021b. Global Health Estimates. Available from: https://iris.who.int/bitstream/handle/10665/341728/9789240026643-eng.pdf?sequence=1. Accessed 3 Apr 2024.
World Health Organisation. World Mental Health Report Transforming mental health for all; 2022. Available from: https://www.who.int/publications/i/item/9789240049338. Accessed 25 Mar 2024.

Self-Harm

2

Gemma Trainor, Rebecca Hall, George Horwood, and Catriona Jones

G. Trainor (✉)
Mental Health Nursing, Directorate of Nursing and Midwifery, University of Salford, Salford, UK
e-mail: gemma.trainor@outlook.com

R. Hall · C. Jones
Directorate of Nursing and Midwifery, University of Salford, Salford, UK
e-mail: r.a.hall3@salford.ac.uk; c.jones53@salford.ac.uk

G. Horwood
Pennine Care NHS Foundation Trust, Manchester, UK
e-mail: George.horwood@nhs.net

G. Trainor, V. Heaslip (eds.), *Needs of Children and Young People Living with Complex Mental Health Difficulties*,
https://doi.org/10.1007/978-3-031-84532-1_2

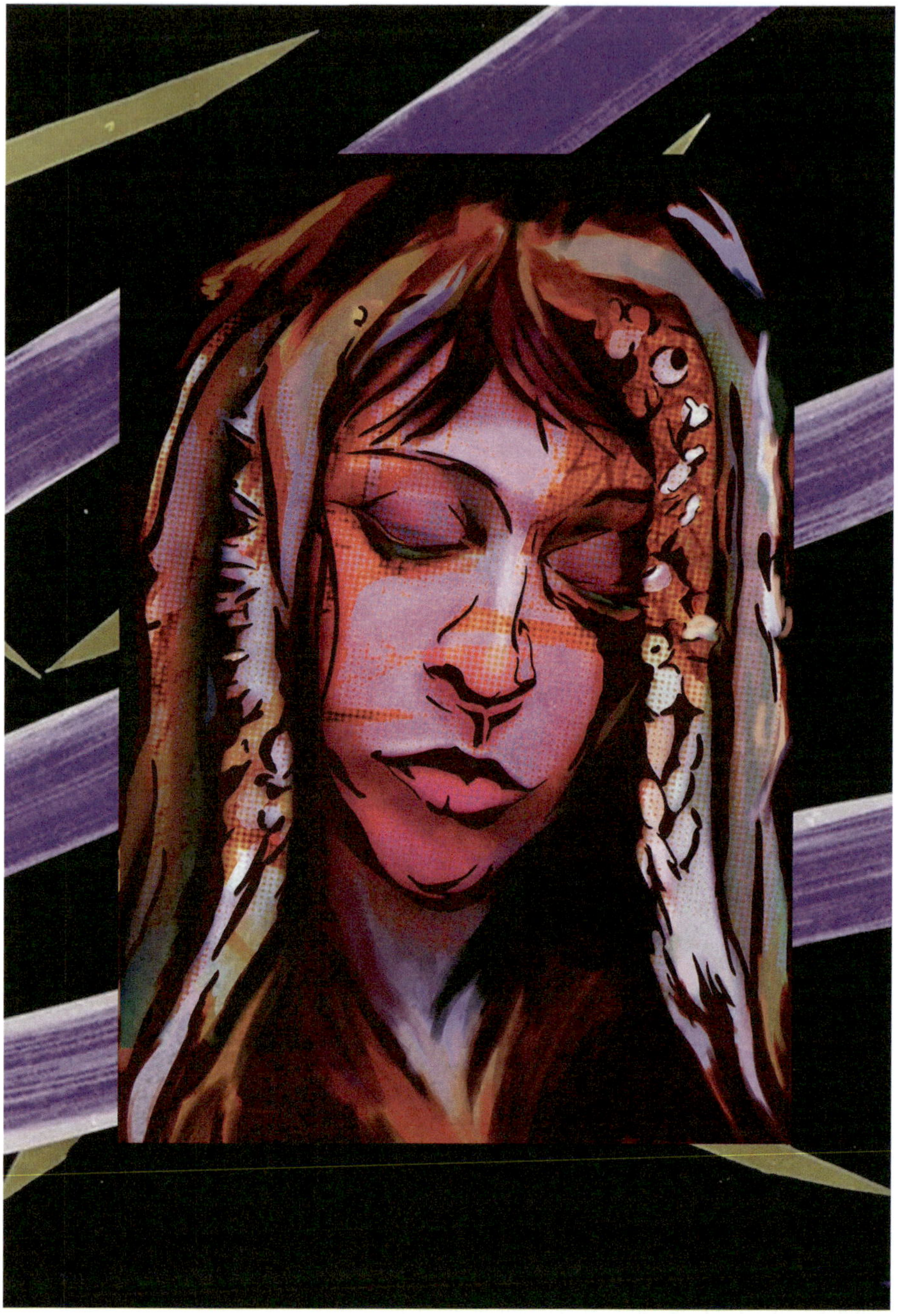

2.1 Introduction

Self-harm in young people is a growing public health problem that accounts for upward of 200,000 presentations to acute hospitals in England per annum (Hawton et al. 2007; Hawton et al. 2012). Having said that, many children and young people do not present to services, and therefore, self-harming in this population can be a hidden phenomenon, and the true prevalence remains unknown. Additionally, young people in institutionalised settings such as residential homes where self-harm can be a common problem are often excluded from the data. The recent NICE guideline (2022) was very clear about the need for those involved in the care of these young people seeing it as a collective responsibility. Self-harming young people can present to a variety of services including schools and accident and emergency and third sector organisations; therefore, it is essential for non-specialised staff to know how best they can support these uniquely challenging young people.

2.2 The Facts

Self-harm is an umbrella term used to describe any intentional self-poisoning or self-injury irrespective of the apparent purpose of the act (NICE 2022). Although the NICE guidance is across the lifespan, it is particularly problematic in young people. Prevalence estimates suggest that the average age of onset is around 12–13 years of age with a peak during middle adolescence and that about 17% of young people would have self-harmed in their lifetime (Gillies et al. 2018). It used to be a rare event for young people under 11. However, this is no longer the case. Community surveys indicate that between 3% and 10% report at least one episode of self-harm in the past year with lifetime prevalence rates being between 9% and 14%. Approximately half of adolescents who self-harm do so more than once, and methods such as cutting and overdosing are the main methods used (Madge et al. 2011).

Prevalence statistics are unreliable because it is a problem that is sometimes hidden and is not reported and reflected in collected statistics. Recent UK data reported by NICE (2022) indicate that:

- 7.3% of girls aged 11–16 and 3.6% of boys aged 11–16 had self-harmed or attempted suicide at some point.
- 21.5% of girls aged 17–19 and 9.7% for boys aged 17–19 had self-harmed or attempted suicide at some point.
- There is evidence that there has been a recent increase in self-harm among young people in England.

Only a minority of people who have self-harmed present to hospital services, but it remains one of the commonest reasons for hospital attendance. Self-harm may be one-off episode for some people, but repetition is also common, with 20% of people (both young people and adults) repeating self-harm within a year. People who have self-harmed are at a greater risk of suicide, with a 30- to 50-fold increase in risk in the year after hospital presentation. About half of the people who attend an emergency department after an episode of self-harm will have visited their GP in the previous month.

2.3 Worldwide Incidence of Self-Harm

Self-harm is not a UK exclusive concern. A systematic review by Lucena et al. (2022) explored incidence of self-harm globally and found the highest reported rates in China (23%) and Azores (29%); in comparison, England's reported incidence is 19%. These authors also explored global socioeconomic factors relating to self-harm. They found that higher population densities and urbanisation (communities with <10 k people) had higher reported rates of self-harm, whereas areas of low income and deprivation had less reported numbers.

As teenagers and adolescents are statistically more likely to self-harm, school environment was explored by Foster et al. (2017) who found people with positive connections to their school had lower reported numbers of depression, anxiety and suicidal ideation. Poor connection to school resulted in higher numbers of self-harm.

Globally, the utilisation of the Internet and social media is commonly thought to contribute to the incidence of self-harm (Patchin et al. 2023; Cheng et al. 2023; Lucena et al. 2022) with the suggestion that exposure to others harming and triggering stimuli is a contagion. Marchant et al. (2017) also highlight social media 'challenges' within self-harm and the glorification of self-harm that is seen across platforms. However, Lucena et al. (2022) offer the suggestion that social media can be a supportive factor for people, as there is a reduction in isolation, the ability to seek help and the option of online therapy. A UK study by Jones et al. (2011) reported that 98% of people who self-harmed found support online during the time of crisis.

During the COVID-19 pandemic, Cheng et al. (2023) reported that social media had a significant impact on the incidence of reported self-harm in the early stages of the pandemic. During this time, females in Asia were reported as more likely to self-harm. Similarly, Xiao et al. (2022) found that adolescents in China had the highest reported numbers of non-suicidal self-injury at this time. The limitation of this study was mainly related to Chinese and English studies and should be interpreted with caution. It is worth mentioning that there is a lack of evidence in the literature from Africa and Central and South America.

2.4 The Continuum of Self-Harm and Suicide

There is a need in clinical practice and research for clarity on the continuum of self-harm and suicide. Despite self-harm and suicide being and having distinctive features, the terms are often used interchangeably. Self-harm does not always reoccur, but those young people who repeatedly self-harm are a high-risk factor for attempting or completing suicide (Whitlock et al. 2013). More recent data from the UK indicated that those young people who present to hospital on at least one occasion were 30 times more likely to die by suicide within a year (Hawton et al. 2020). However, there is a lack of information regarding the features of self-harm, which may be a driver for suicide (O'Loughlin et al. 2020). Very worrying is that a meta-analysis estimated that adolescents and adults with a history of self-harm had a two-fold increased risk of subsequent suicide attempts and a 1.5-fold increased risk of dying by suicide (Ribeiro et al. 2016).

Conversely, a lot of young people who self-harm do not have active suicidal thoughts (Klonsky et al. 2013). An act of self-harm is not necessarily an attempt or even indicator of suicidal intent; conversely, it can be an act of self-preservation. Because of this conflicting picture and the fact that self-harm is complex with the motivation for the act varying between episodes, it is crucial to ascertain what was the young person's intention at each presentation. Self-harm can be a manifestation of emotional distress. An important rule of thumb is to be mindful that when a young person is out of control with their emotions, it is imperative that concerned adults remain in charge of theirs.

2.5 Definitions and Terminology

Self-harming behaviour covers a spectrum of behaviours, and a universally agreed definition is not easy to find; however, for the purpose of this chapter, we will adopt the definition in recent NICE guidelines, "Self-poisoning or injury irrespective of the apparent purpose of the act" (NICE 2022).

The terminologies are the subject of much debate globally with lots of controversies around using terms such as deliberate, intentional, non-fatal, non-suicidal and non-suicidal self-injurious behaviour. Some other terminologies used to describe self-harm are presented in Box 2.1.

Box 2.1: Other Definitions of Self-Harm

- Direct self-harm: suicide attempts, overdosing, hanging, jumping, self-injury, wrist and arm cutting.
- Indirect self-harm: substance abuse, eating disorders, risk-taking behaviour.
- Deliberate self-injury: perceived as a pejorative term by service users.
- Non-suicidal self-injury (NSSI): deliberate destruction of one's own body tissue in the absence of intent to die.
- Non-suicidal self-injurious behaviour (NSIB): without conscious suicidal intent.

No one term absolutely or accurately defines all acts. Therefore, "intent" needs to be ascertained. Young people are encouraged to describe the behaviour and their motivations in their own words.

2.6 Risk Assessment

All young people are likely to have a risk assessment, and the recent NICE guideline has indicated that this should, where possible, include parents and carers particularly in the case of young people. This assessment may take place in a variety of settings, and a lot of young people will be triaged in their local accident and emergency department. Additionally, there is often a crossover between mental health and social care needs. These episodes can arise when the level of distress cannot be managed within the young person's current circumstances. A central question for those assessing the young persons' risk is whether they can safely return home. Emergency services personnel although not necessarily tasked with completing a thorough psychosocial assessment are often required to respond and support young people in crisis.

> Today is my 1 year since my last and most serious suicide attempt. I am thankful to the stranger, the police and paramedics that saved my life that night. Because of you I have a future. (Twitter, 2021)

The assessing practitioner should follow NICE guidance on assessing risk in young people (NICE 2022). The assessment involves a comprehensive evaluation of the social, biological and psychosocial factors that may influence the self-harming behaviour. This assessment needs to be carried out by a suitably trained professional and will inform the plan for short- and long-term support and intervention. The use of risk assessment tools should not replace the psychosocial assessment and should not be used to predict future suicide risk (NICE 2022). See Box 2.2.

Box 2.2: Considerations for Assessment and Care by Healthcare Professionals and Social Care Practitioners Following an Episode of Self-Harm

- Treat the young person and their family/carers with dignity and respect ensuring cultural sensitivity by appreciating the cultural context of the young person's lives.
- Establish history of self-harm and accessibility of methods in their environment. Negotiate with young person and family/carer the removal of potential medication ligature or sharp objects.
- Assess any issues regarding capacity or consent and seek advice from relevant professional.
- Ask for consent to liaise with those supporting the young person including family/carers in gathering information.
- Discuss with all involved support network, and draw up a safety plan identifying ongoing coping strategies.
- Carry out concurrent physical and psychosocial assessment as soon as possible following episode of self-harm.
- Make referral to mental health professional a priority.

It was felt important in the NICE guideline (2022) to provide specific advice about assessment in different care settings. Consequently, there is an extensive section in the guidance around assessments in primary care by ambulance staff and paramedics, in general hospitals by non-mental health emergency department professionals and in social care and other sectors. It is imperative that all people supporting these young people adhere to the guidance set out in this helpful document (NICE 2022). There was clear consensus by the guideline development committee about self-harm being "everyone's business", and the guidance reflects this viewpoint. Due to a lack of robust published peer-reviewed evidence of best approaches, the recommendations in the guideline were based on the committee's own knowledge, expertise and experience.

2.7 Safety Planning

Safety planning is part of case management and follows the risk assessment. According to NICE (2022), it is a written prioritised list of coping strategies and/or sources of support for the person who has self-harmed. It is a tool that helps the young person navigate urges to self-harm or distract them from ongoing suicidal thoughts.

The safety plan is created with the young person who is at risk and can be reviewed as and when risk can be a constantly changing phenomenon. For it to be meaningful, it must be completed with the young person and include relevant adults who the young person feels could be helpful. Some services have their own template; however, to promote ownership, it is imperative to let the young person identify their own strategies, which can be shared with all those involved. An illustration of the typical content found within a safety plan is provided in Box 2.3.

Box 2.3: Typical Content of a Safety Plan

- Why and when you will use the plan.
- Reasons to stay alive.
- Personal warning signs.
- Things that help the young person feel calm and comforted.
- People they would like to talk to when they feel an urge to self-harm.
- How the young person and families/carers can make their environment safe, e.g. removal of sharp objects and locking up tablets.
- What parents/carers, schools, police, ambulance staff, emergency responders, peers and local communities can do to support the young person.

The plan should include a list of agencies and professionals including out of hours. Phone numbers of key people need to be included.

In order to understand these issues further, please explore the case study of Sarah.

Case Study of Sarah

Sarah (name has been changed) aged 15 presented to her local A and E department having taken an overdose of an unspecified amount of paracetamol. Sarah is agitated and irritable at interview saying she doesn't want her mother involved in the assessment. Sarah has a 2-year history of increasing oppositional behaviours and is hanging out with much older girls. She is close to one of these girls' mother and has an older boyfriend aged 19 years. She often spends time with her friend's mother instead of going to school. She is refusing to have her bloods taken and now wants to leave but not with her mother who has been sat in the reception area.

The Assessment

It is imperative that Sarah is persuaded to have her bloods taken and complete risk assessment. The practitioner needs to be suitably trained and should explain how the interview will be conducted and the rules of confidentiality explained, particularly if the young person is presenting significant risk to themselves or to others or from others. The process of the assessment should be explained to Sarah and that she will be seen on her own and then her mother, and then both parties will be seen together to provide outcome of risk assessment using a case formulation approach. This is important as often the young person or parent may not be as candid as they would be in front of each other. The assessing practitioner must follow the guidelines on self-harm for assessing risk and those on self-harm (NICE 2022). As well as identifying risks and needs, protective factors need also to be considered. It is essential to assess Sarah's capacity to consent and her understanding of being at risk of serious permanent injury should she refuse any required medical treatment. She is clearly at risk by not agreeing to the procedure; therefore, her mother would be involved as Sarah would be classified as a minor under the Mental Capacity Act (2005). In relation to the Mental Health Act 1983 (as amended 2007), there is no lower age limit. The mother would also be assessed to ensure she can make decisions that are in the best interest of her child for any procedure to be carried out. As Sarah is a minor and placing herself at risk, her mother will have parental responsibility, and the practitioner can break confidentiality under the zone of parental responsibility.

This type of assessment can be complex and difficult to manage, and should concerns around risk continue, Sarah may meet the criteria as a "child in need" where she may be referred to social services and other agencies to ensure safeguarding Sarah from ongoing harm. If required, social services would need to involve her mother in this discussion, and the whole team needs to work together regarding safe discharge home. If Sarah had absconded from A and E, the police would need to be alerted and alternative provision considered. This type of scenario is not uncommon and can involve a variety of professionals to contribute to the safety plan including school personnel. Tailored and sensitive care should be given to the young person and their family.

2.8 Risk and Protective Factors

Assessing risk in young people is not without its challenges. Self-harm is a complex and multifaceted phenomenon (McManus et al. 2019), and it is essential for professionals to actively listen to a young person's account and experience of their health and wellbeing (Children's Society 2023). Understanding the motivation to self-harm can improve engagement with services and promote an individualised approach to care. This, together with the identification of risk and protective factors, can assist in the prevention or formulation of an appropriate person-centred intervention.

Risk and protective factors can influence a young person's mental health trajectory. They can present in various combinations, but they can also exist or be absent. These individual variables can help or hinder a young person's progress as they navigate mental and emotional milestones. Protective factors are characteristics that can lower the likelihood of negative outcomes and reduce the impact of risk factors. Conversely, a risk factor is associated with an increased likelihood of negative outcomes (McEvoy et al. 2023). In an already significant period of change, risk factors associated with self-harm in young people can be in abundance. Although there may be a correlation between the three categories, risk factors can be better understood in the context of individual, family and social factors (Trainor et al. 2017).

2.8.1 Individual Factors

Individual factors such as mental ill health have a strong correlation with self-harm (McEvoy et al. 2023), and these are conditions such as depression, anxiety, psychosis and bipolar disorder. Childhood neglect and sexual abuse are also strongly associated with self-harm. Other psychological risk factors that can be a precursor to self-harm are emotional distress or where a young person struggles to manage intense feelings, personality disorders, ADHD and eating disorders. Low self-esteem, negative body image and alexithymia (emotional blindness) are also individual factors that may increase the use of self-harm to regulate emotions. There is also a relationship between the difficulty in expressing and recognising emotions and alcohol use (Greene et al. 2020) and a consistent association between risky substance use and self-harm (Moller et al. 2013).

2.8.2 Family Factors

Evidence suggests that family influences can predict self-harm in young people (Hamza and Willoughby 2014a, b). Factors such as a lack of attachment security or quality, domestic violence, parental divorce, separation or bereavement and poor family relationships, which can take the form of absent or harsh and controlling parenting, are positive indicators for self-harm. Interestingly, there is little association between family structure or composition and self-harm (Valencia-Agudo et al. 2018).

2.8.3 Social Factors

Social factors that have an association with self-harm are plentiful. Conduct problems; discrimination; racism; bullying, whether traditional or cyber bullying; unemployment; and anti-social behaviour can all increase the risk of self-harm. Other associations can be seen in relation to young people who have been exposed to adverse childhood experiences (Cleare et al. 2018) or who are in the care system, feel isolated or excluded and have limited or poor-quality friendships, poor attainment and truancy from school. Moreover, there is a growing body of evidence to indicate that young people who identify under the umbrella term LGBTQ+ (how one self-identifies with their sexuality, gender identity and expression) and experience psychological distress due to discrimination may also be at greater risk of self-harm (Williams et al. 2019: Batejan et al. 2015).

2.8.4 Protective Factors

Identifying protective factors is as important as understanding the risk factors when assessing self-harm in young people; however, the exploration of protective factors is limited, and often less is known about resilience and coping in young people (Khan and Ungar 2023). Protective factors can be subdivided into two groups, internal and external factors. Internal factors are personal attributes that act as a buffer to adversity; such as young people who have greater cognitive competency to engage in problem-solving behaviours and to be able to rationalise and seek help when required (Wu and Liu 2019); positive coping mechanisms and being able to maintain a positive outlook and recognise one's own talents are also protective factors. External buffers or protective factors can be present where a young person has a sense of autonomy and a positive experience of relationships with family and friends and is connected to a positive social environment and social groups (Klemera et al. 2017), which can be around culture or religion (Aggarwal et al. 2017).

2.9 Promising Interventions and Treatments

As self-harm is a symptom of unmet need and not a diagnosis, as such it is difficult to be prescriptive regarding treatments/interventions. The recent NICE guideline development committee was tasked with reviewing the peer-reviewed evidence base (NICE 2022). Although there were some treatments that showed promise, the overall evidence base from peer-reviewed randomised controlled trial (RCT) was limited, and from the systematic reviews of different potential treatments, only limited recommendations could be made (Witt et al. 2021).

Treating those who engage in self-harm has two core functions. The first of these is about maintaining the physical safety of the client through reducing suicidality and creating a decrease both in terms of severity and frequency of self-harm. The second related function is to address any deficits that may impact the client's ability to navigate life's challenges (psychological and social) improving their quality of life by creating "a life worth living" (Miller et al. 2006).

Overall NICE (2022) recommended that for CYP only dialectical behaviour therapy for adolescents (DBT-A) was recommended, but with limited confidence due to the limited quality of the evidence database. Other treatments were reviewed, but no firm recommendations for CYP could be made as there was low confidence in the evidence base. Such treatments included cognitive behavioural therapy (CBT), mentalisation-based therapy (MBT), therapeutic assessment (TA) and group therapy. While no firm recommendations could be made, these treatments are still widely used in CAMHS in the UK and in CYP services in other countries.

2.9.1 Dialectical Behaviour Therapy for Adolescents (DBT-A)

DBT-A is described in Box 2.4. For DBT-A, the systematic review (Witt et al. 2021) identified only four randomised controlled trials (RCTs) showing a positive effect on self-harm, and so there was limited confidence in the evidence base. These studies included one by Mehlum et al. (2007), an RCT involving 77 young people (83% female), which showed a significant reduction in self-harm (and also reductions in suicidal ideation and depression) for the group following DBT-A compared with the group receiving treatment as usual (TAU). Overall, NICE considered that DBT-A had a positive effect on repetition of self-harm at post-intervention for adolescents, but the evidence was limited by the fact that participants in studies had all self-harmed more than once and were all older than 12 years and most were female. However, there was no evidence of effect of DBT-A on repeated self-harm at the 12-month follow-up. Nevertheless, NICE considered that DBT-A is likely to be similarly effective in younger children and boys but was not confident that DBT-A would be similarly effective for children and young people who did not frequently self-harm. The current advice from NICE was to consider DBT-A for children and young people with significant emotional dysregulation difficulties who have frequent episodes of self-harm.

Box 2.4: DBT-A: What Is It?

It is developed by Marsha Linehan for patients (initially women) with borderline personality disorder where self-harm is one of a number of risk behaviours (Linehan 1993).

- It is a manualised, typically 16-week behavioural treatment, comprising weekly concurrent individual therapy, a multifamily skills training group, between-session skills coaching for young people and their families, family therapy as needed and a peer consultation group for therapists.
- Aims to equip young people and their parents and carers with the skills to reduce or stop self-harm and suicidal behaviours, effectively manage their emotions and improve their relationships.
- Should be considered for those who meet criteria for emotionally unstable personality disorder (EUPD).
- Pretreatment assessment and then weekly individual DBT sessions and invited to attend a DBT skills group.
- DBT-A is a mixture of individual 1:1 session (track progress, manage risk) and group skills sessions (addressing the skills deficit to allow for improved regulation).
- A key feature of these skills sessions and DBT as a whole is "mindfulness". There are five skills areas: mindfulness, interpersonal effectiveness, emotional regulation, distress tolerance and walking the middle path. Of these skills areas, "walking the middle path" is specific to DBT-A.
- Many Child and Adolescent Mental Health Services (CAMHS) in the UK now provide DBT skills groups, and there are practitioners who are familiar with the model and informed by this in their practice.

2.9.2 Cognitive Behavioural Therapy (CBT)

A description of CBT is provided in Box 2.5. NICE (2022) considered that there was "low certainty evidence" whether CBT has an effect on repetition of self-harm at post-intervention. In the UK, CAMHS practitioners are usually familiar with CBT, and it is considered a first-line therapy for young people meeting criteria for treatment and is available for young people up to 18 years of age from CAMH services. For some of the commonly co-occurring mental health difficulties that children and young people present with who self-harm, CBT is the recommended treatment by NICE for depression (NICE 2018), social anxiety (NICE 2013) and post-traumatic stress disorder (PTSD) (NICE 2019). CAHMS practitioners would conduct an initial assessment, and if indicated, young people could typically be offered around 12 sessions of CBT. CBT also involves parents/carers if this is indicated and can be delivered as a group intervention.

Box 2.5: CBT: What Is It?

The fundamental premise of CBT is that the therapist can help the client to change how they feel by helping them to challenge the way they think and/or behave as our thoughts, feeling and behaviour are all linked (Gega 2017).

- CBT relies on condition-specific models to help the client understand the role of their thoughts, feelings and behaviour such as self-harming but also behaviours such as social phobia or eating disorders.
- When conducting CBT, the therapist uses Socratic questioning to help the client in a process of guided discovery rather than providing answers for them.
- CBT is a structured therapy, which helps people tackle problems such as low mood or self-harming from the perspective of understanding the thoughts and beliefs underlying emotional states and behavioural responses.
- Helps people identify and critically evaluate their thoughts about emotional experiences and events and aims to help them change the ways in which they deal with problems.
- Used also for depression, post-traumatic stress disorders, obsessive compulsive disorder and eating disorders.
- If self-harm is a symptom of any of these mental disorders, CBT would address self-harm in the therapy.

2.9.3 Mentalisation-Based Therapy for Adolescents (MBT-A)

A description of MBT-A is provided in Box 2.6. NICE considered that for adolescents MBT-A, there was "low certainty evidence" that the intervention had an effect on repetition of self-harm post-intervention. In an RCT with adolescents, Rossouw and Fonagy (2012) found that the MBT-A group, when compared with the treatment as usual (TAU) group, had fewer self-harm episodes over the course of the 12-month treatment together with a higher recovery rate. A small single-blind trial of young people already attending NHS CAMHS who had recently self-harmed showed that a relatively brief MBT-A could be a promising intervention (Griffths et al. 2019).

Box 2.6: MBT-A: What Is It?
MBT is an integrated form of psychotherapy bringing together elements of psychodynamic psychotherapy, cognitive behavioural therapy and systemic and ecological approaches.

- Initially created for adults struggling with borderline personality disorder (BPD).
- The core premise of this treatment is that those who struggle with "mentalisation" (the ability to be aware of one's own mental state and that of others) or both regulate themselves and manage interpersonal relationships.
- It is a manualised psychotherapy, which aims to increase the mentalising ability of patients.
- MBT-A includes both individual and family sessions. It can be applied in both inpatient and outpatient settings, and the average duration of therapy is about 12 months.

2.9.4 Other Potential Treatments

Of the other potential treatments for repetition of self-harm, therapeutic assessment (TA) showed some promise. While Ougrin et al. (2011) in an RCT found no effect on repetition of self-harm in those presenting at emergency department, TA showed a benefit in that overall treatment engagement remained higher in the TA group with a better linkage to outpatient treatment. A description of TA is provided in Box 2.7.

Box 2.7: TA: What Is It?
TA is a psychological assessment procedure that aims to help adolescents gain "insight" and apply this new insight to problems in their life.

- The aim is that the person who has self-harmed learns about themselves and how to manage a similar situation differently in the future ("insight" being the ability to recognise one's mental condition). The assessment aims to build a therapeutic alliance with the person.
- TA can be considered the first phase of treatment or as a brief standalone treatment.
- TA differs from the usual information-gathering process of psychological assessment where the objective is to diagnose accurately and then plan treatments and thereafter evaluate their effectiveness in collaboration with the young person.

For other potential interventions such as group-based psychotherapy and remote contact intervention, NICE (2022) found no consistent evidence of an effect on repetition of self-harm. However, these approaches are still commonly used in CAMHS in the UK.

Other approaches include individual therapy (covering crisis intervention, brief problem-solving, supportive counselling and psychoanalytical therapy) and family therapy. Typically, family-based interventions are based on joint sessions with the young person and their family members. While there may be several different approaches to family therapy, the guiding principle is that maintenance and/or origin of the self-harm may lie in the family (Chitsabesan et al. 2003). Consequently, such interventions seek to find solutions in the family by improving family functioning (Fortune et al. 2016). This is usually done through a series of tasks looking to create transgression in the family "status quo" and create new learning.

2.9.5 Psychopharmacological Interventions

NICE (2022) concluded that there was uncertain evidence on pharmacological interventions for self-harm and that drug treatments usually offered for other co-morbidities should **NOT** be offered specifically for self-harm. Typical co-morbidity drug interventions include:

- Antidepressants.
- Selective serotonin reuptake inhibitors (SSRI).
- Antipsychotic medication.
- Anxiolytics.

However, the prescription of psychotropic drugs to those who engage in self-harm is not unusual. This is typically due to co-morbidity with other diagnosable psychiatric disorders or high levels of distress.

2.10 Conclusions About the Evidence Base for Interventions

It is hard to read any research into treatments regarding self-harm without coming across issues with the evidence base. One of the biggest issues with the research is the heterogeneity of the population who might engage in self-harm. This leads to the questions about how much one can extract from individual studies.

For example, in the systemic evidence review considered by NICE (Witt et al. 2021), all or most people of all age groups involved in the various studies self-harmed either consistently or predominately through self-poisoning, which is consistent with those attending hospital for self-harm. However, this is not typical of self-injury in adolescents where the most reported method of self-injury in frequency is through cutting. So, a more nuanced recommendation from NICE (2022) might therefore be that DBT-A would appear to be an effective treatment for those who engage in self-harm.

2.11 Final Thoughts

2.11.1 Considering the Young Person's Views

It is important to hear from young people themselves. When asked about sharing some insights as to what professionals needed to consider when talking with a young person, the following "do's" and "don'ts" were articulated (Table 2.1).

As stated previously, the recent NICE guideline (2022) is very clear in its overarching theme in that self-harm is everyone's business. All professionals working across the health and social care system have a role to play in supporting people who self-harm, and it is not seen as the responsibility of those with mental health expertise. The guideline committee's new recommendations provided guidance for those working in primary care settings as well as those in psychiatric services. Additionally, there is guidance for those working in education and for ambulance staff, paramedics and non-specialist staff who provide initial care and across the criminal justice system. With the difficulties these young people face in accessing

Table 2.1 Do's and Don'ts

"Do's"	"Don'ts"
Be kind and non-judgemental	Ask me how I am feeling on a scale of 1 to 10
Be honest even if I don't want to hear it	Pretend you know how I am feeling
Listen to what I am saying	Bring your own issues into things
Be honest but above all be fun	Diagnose me!
Respect my rights for privacy	Use jargon
Talk about other things besides my problem	Talk over me or about me when I am there
	Get frustrated when you cannot fix things
Give me a sense of hope	Don't say "superficial" or "cry for help"
Discuss achievements	Fake sympathy or use your own personal strategies
Allow me a safe place to be myself	Above all do not be scared of me

specialist mental health services combined with the stigma experienced by the individual, it is crucial that those supporting people who self-harm can recognise and address the behaviour using a compassionate and non-judgemental approach.

References

Aggarwal S, Patton G, Reavley N, Sreenivasan SA, Berk M. Youth self-harm in low- and middle-income countries: systematic review of the risk and protective factors. Int J Soc Psychiatry. 2017;63(4):359–75.

Batejan K, Jarvi S, Swenson L. Sexual orientation and non-suicidal self-injury: a meta-analytic review. Arch Suicide Res. 2015;19(2):131–50.

Cheng H, Wand D, Wand L, et al. Global prevalence of self-harm during the COVID-19 pandemic: a systematic review and meta-analysis. BMC Psychol. 2023;11:149.

Children's Society. The Good Childhood Report; 2023. Available from: https://www.childrens-society.org.uk/sites/default/files/2023-09/The%20Good%20Childhood%20Report%202023.pdf. Accessed 7 Oct 2024.

Chitsabesan P, Harrington R, Harrington V, Tomenson B. Predicting repeat self-harm in children: how accurate can we expect to be? Eur Child Adolesc Psychiatry. 2003;12:23–9.

Cleare S, Wetherall K, Clark A, Ryan C, Kirtley OJ, Smith M, O'Connor RC. Adverse childhood experiences and hospital-treated self-harm. Int J Environ Res Public Health. 2018;15(6):1235.

Fortune S, Cottrell D, Fife S. Family factors associated with adolescent self-harm: a review. J Fam Ther. 2016;38:226–56.

Foster CE, Horwitz A, Thomas A, Opperman K, Gipson P, Burnside A, Stone DM, King C. Connectedness to family, school, peers and community in socially vulnerable adolescents. Child Youth Serv Rev. 2017;81:321–31.

Gega L. Cognitive behaviour therapy (CBT). In: Psychiatric and mental health nursing. 3rd ed. Routledge; 2017.

Gillies D, Christou M, Dixon A, Featherston O, Rapti I, Garcia-Anguita A, Villasis-Keever M, Reebye P, Christou A, Kabir N, Christou P. Prevalence and characteristics of self-harm in adolescents: meta-analyses of community-based studies 1990–2015. J Am Acad Child Adolesc Psychiatry. 2018;57(10):733–41. https://doi.org/10.1016/j.jaac.2018.06.018.

Greene D, Boyes M, Hasking P. The associations between alexithymia and both non-suicidal self-injury and risky drinking: a systematic review and meta-analysis. J Affect Disord. 2020;260:140–66.

Griffths H, Duff F, Duff L, Brown S, Hockaday H, Eliasson E, et al. Efficacy of mentalization-based group therapy for adolescents: the results of a pilot randomised controlled trial. BMC Psychiatry. 2019;2019(19):167.

Hamza C, Willoughby T. A longitudinal person- centred examination of non-suicidal self-injury among university students. J Youth Adolescence. 2014a;43:671–85.

Hamza C, Willoughby T. A longitudinal person-centred examination of non-suicidal self-injury among university students. J Youth Adolesc. 2014b;43(4):671–85.

Hawton K, Bergen H, Casey D, Simkin S, Palmer B, Cooper J, et al. Self-harm in England: a tale of three cities. Multicentre study of self-harm. Soc Psychiatry Psychiatr Epidemiol. 2007;42:513–21.

Hawton K, Bergen H, Kapur N, Cooper J, Steeg S, Ness J, et al. Repetition of self-harm and suicide following self-harm in children and adolescents: findings from the multicentre study of self-harm in England. J Child Psychol Psychiatry. 2012;2012(53):1212–9.

Hawton K, Bale L, Brand F, Townsend E, Ness J, Waters K, Clements C, Kapur N, Geulayov G. Mortality in children and adolescents following presentation to hospital after non-fatal self-harm in the multicentre study of self-harm: a prospective observational cohort study. Lancet Child Adolescent Health. 2020;4(2):111–20. https://doi.org/10.1016/S2352-4642(19)30373-6.

Jones R, Sharkey S, Ford T, Emmens T, Hewis E, Smithson J, Sheaves B, Owens C. Online discussion forums for young people who self-harm: user views. Psychiatrist. 2011;35(10):364–8.
Khan A, Ungar M. Resilience to self-harm a scoping review. Crisis J Crisis Interv Suicide Prev. 2023;44(1):61–9.
Klemera E, Brooks FM, Chester KL, Magnusson J, Spencer N. Self-harm in adolescence: protective health assets in the family, school and community. Int J Public Health. 2017;62(6):631–8.
Klonsky ED, May AM, Glenn CR. The relationship between non suicidal self-injury and attempted suicide: converging evidence from four samples. J Abnorm Psychol. 2013;122(1):231–7. https://doi.org/10.1037/a0030278.
Linehan M. Cognitive behavioral treatment of borderline personality disorder. New York: Guilford Press; 1993.
Lucena NL, Rossi TA, Azeved LMG, Pereira M. Self-injury prevalence in adolescents: a global systematic review and meta-analysis. Child Youth Serv Rev. 2022;142:106634.
Madge N, Hawton K, McMahon EM, Corcoran P, De Leo D, de Wilde EJ, Fekete S, van Heeringen K, Ystgaard M, Arensman E. Psychological characteristics, stressful life events and deliberate self-harm: findings from the Child & Adolescent Self-harm in Europe (CASE) study. Eur Child Adolesc Psychiatry. 2011;20(10):499–508. https://doi.org/10.1007/s00787-011-0210-4.
Marchant A, Hawton K, Stewart A, Montgomomery P, Singaravelu V, Lloyd K, Purdy N, Daine K, John A. A systematic review of the relationship between internet use, self-harm and suicidal behaviour in young people: the good, the bad and the unknown. PLoS One. 2017;12:12.
McEvoy D, Brannigan R, Cooke L, Butler E, Walsh C, Arensman E, Clarke M. Risk and protective factors for self-harm in adolescents and young adults: an umbrella review of systematic review. J Psychiatr Res. 2023;168:353–80.
McManus S, Gunnell D, Cooper C, Bebbington P, Howard L, Brugha T, Jenkins R, Hassiotis A, Weich S, et al. Prevalence of non-suicidal self-harm and service contact in England, 2000–14: repeated cross-sectional surveys of the general population. Lancet Psychiatry. 2019;6:573–81.
Mehlum L, Tømoen AJ, Ramberg M, Haga E, Diep LM, Laberg S, et al. Dialectical behavior therapy for adolescents with repeated suicidal and self-harming behavior – a randomized trial. J Am Acad Child Adolesc Psychiatry. 2007;2014(53):1082–91.
Miller AL, Rathus JH, Linehan M. DBT for adolescents. New York: Guilford; 2006.
Moller C, Tait R, Byrne D. Deliberate self-harm, substance use, and negative affect in nonclinical samples: a systematic review. Subst Abus. 2013;34(2):188–207.
NICE. Social anxiety disorder: recognition, assessment and treatment Clinical guideline [CG159]; 2013. Available from: https://www.nice.org.uk/guidance/cg159/chapter/Recommendations
NICE. Post-traumatic stress disorder NICE guideline [NG116]; 2018. Available from: https://www.nice.org.uk/guidance/ng116/chapter/recommendations
NICE. Depression in children and young people: identification and management. NICE guideline [NG134]; 2019. Available from: https://www.nice.org.uk/guidance/ng134
NICE. Self-harm: assessment, management and preventing recurrence. NICE guideline [NG225]; 2022. Available from: https://www.nice.org.uk/guidance/ng225
O'Loughlin C, Gomer B, Ammerman B. The social context of non-suicidal self-injury: links to severity, suicide risk, and social factors. J Clin Psychol. 2020;77(4):1004–17. https://doi.org/10.1002/jclp.23073.
Ougrin D, Zundel T, Ng A, Banarsee R, Bottle A, Taylor E. Trial of therapeutic assessment in London: randomised controlled trial of therapeutic assessment versus standard psychosocial assessment in adolescents presenting with self-harm. Arch Dis Child. 2011;96:148–53.
Patchin JW, Hinduja S, Meldrum RC. Digital self-harm and suicidality among adolescents child and Adolescent Mental Health; 2023.
Ribeiro JD, Franklin JC, Fox KR, Bentley KH, Kleiman EM, Chang BP, Nock MK. Self-injurious thoughts and behaviors as risk factors for future suicide ideation, attempts, and death: a meta-analysis of longitudinal studies. Psychol Med. 2016;46(2):225–36. https://doi.org/10.1017/S0033291715001804.
Rossouw TI, Fonagy P. Mentalization-based treatment for self-harm in adolescents: a randomized controlled trial. J Am Acad Child Adolesc Psychiatry. 2012;51:304–13.

Trainor G, Rothwell J, Hales HL. Depression, self-harm and suicide. In: Bailey S, Chitsabesan P, Tarbuck P, editors. Forensic child and adolescent mental health: meeting the needs of young offenders. Cambridge: Cambridge University Press; 2017.

Valencia-Agudo F, Burcher GC, Ezpeleta L, Kramer T. Non suicidal self-injury in community adolescents: a systematic review of prospective predictors, mediators and moderators. J Adolesc. 2018;6(65):25–38.

Whitlock J, Muehlenkamp J, Eckenrode J, Purington A, Baral Abrams G, Barreira P, Kress V. Non suicidal self-injury as a gateway to suicide in young adults. J Adolesc Health. 2013;52(4):486–92. https://doi.org/10.1016/j.jadohealth.2012.09.010.

Williams A, Arcelus J, Townsend E, Michail M. Examining risk factors for self-harm and suicide in LGBTQ+ young people: a systematic review protocol. BMJ Open. 2019;9:e031541. https://doi.org/10.1136/bmjopen-2019-031541.

Witt KG, Hetrick SE, Rajaram G, Hazell P, et al. Interventions for self-harm in children and adolescents. Cochrane Database Syst Rev. 2021;3:CD013667.

Wu J, Liu H. Features of non-suicidal self-injury and relationships with coping methods among college students. Iran J Public Health. 2019;48(2):270–7. https://doi.org/10.18502/ijph.v48i2.825.

Xiao Q, Song X, Huang L, Hou D, Huang X. Global prevalence and characteristics of non-suicidal self-injury between 2010 and 2021 among a non-clinical sample of adolescents: a meta-analysis. Front Psych. 2022;13 https://doi.org/10.3389/fpsyt.2022.912441.

Eating Disorders

3

Gemma Trainor, Ben Robinson, Lorraine Henshaw, and Alicia Proton de la Chapelle

G. Trainor (✉)
Mental Health Nursing, Directorate of Nursing and Midwifery, University of Salford, Salford, UK
e-mail: gemma.trainor@outlook.com

B. Robinson
Greater Manchester Police, Greater Manchester, UK

L. Henshaw
Directorate of Nursing and Midwifery, University of Salford, Salford, UK
e-mail: l.henshaw@salford.ac.uk

A. P. de la Chapelle
Aarhus University, Aarhus, Denmark

G. Trainor, V. Heaslip (eds.), *Needs of Children and Young People Living with Complex Mental Health Difficulties*,
https://doi.org/10.1007/978-3-031-84532-1_3

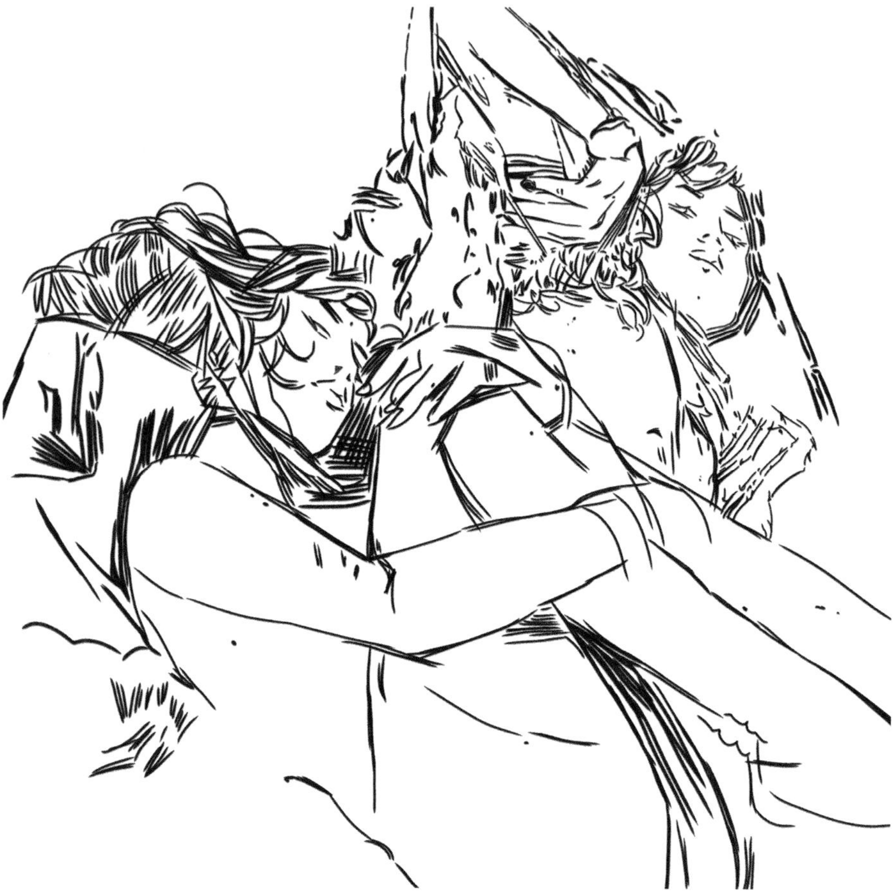

© Robyn Heaslip

3.1 Introduction and Diagnostic Criteria

The term "eating disorder" represents a group of complex physical and mental health difficulties that can seriously impair social functioning and has the highest mortality rate of any mental health disorder (Edakubo and Fushimi 2020). There are many types of feeding and eating disorders, and they come with their own defining features and characteristics. Because of this, it is essential that those working with children and young people understand these to be able to signpost young people at risk to relevant services. Improving diagnostic guidelines for feeding and eating disorders (FED) has significant implications for early intervention prevention and treatment.

There are two main diagnostic schedules that are recognised globally. They are the updated *Statistical Manual of Mental Disorders, fifth Edition* (DSM-5) (APA

2013, 2023) and the *International Classification of Diseases 11th Edition* (ICD-11) (WHO 2022), although there is no one diagnostic laboratory test to screen for the presence or absence of FED in young people or adults. Both of these take an nosological approach, but the major difference is the functional impairment, which is mandatory in DSM-5 but not in ICD-11. This chapter will focus on DSM-5 and the major changes to the way eating disorders are diagnosed; DSM-5 is the 2013 publication of the American Psychiatric Association (APA) of its assessment and classification tool. This tool is to assist clinicians in making effective diagnosis and assessment. The fifth edition underwent major changes and makes diagnosing easier. This edition of the DSM-5 now recognises binge eating disorder (BED). Additionally, DSM-5 has made two changes to the way anorexia nervosa (AN) is diagnosed by broadening its definition. These are the criteria around the person's weight, which is required to be at or under 85% of ideal body weight, and the body mass index (BMI) for a person who has reached a significantly low weight. Previous criteria excluded those who were suffering weight loss but have not yet lost enough weight to generate the diagnosis. The prior schedule also included a criterion of loss of menstruation three or more times. This too has been removed as not everyone loses their periods and being on contraceptive medication can create a false result. Eliminating it also allows males to meet the criteria. Despite some imperfections, DSM-5 is widely used in the literature, research and clinical practice.

The criteria for diagnosis of bulimia nervosa (BN) have also been amended from the fourth edition (DSM-4). Frequency of behaviours to generate diagnosis now requires the binge eating and compensatory actions to occur for at least once a week for at least 3 months. Three other significant changes are:

- The categories of purging and non-purging behaviours are now lumped together in the revised edition.
- Clinicians now recognise that people with eating disorder can engage in a variety of behaviours.
- The third change addresses phases of recovery, which can specify whether the person is on a partial or full remission from the disorder based on the frequency of bingeing and purging episodes and how debilitating the disorder is in their day-to-day life.

The DSM- 5 update (APA 2023) included two other forms of eating disorder to include:

1. Other specified feeding or eating disorders (OSFED). This broad category encompasses problems that don't fit into any current category. It relates to people who show clinical symptoms of ED but do not meet the criteria for AN, BN or BED. Previously, this was identified under the category EDNOS (eating disorder not otherwise specified).
2. Avoidant/restrictive food intake disorder (ARFID), which involves a restrictive food intake in the absence of body image disturbances.

- Orthorexia nervosa is currently not an official eating disorder recognised in DSM-5. However, it has attracted a great deal of attention and is described as an unhealthy obsession with healthy eating without the desire to lose weight.
- Diabulimia is an ED in which a person with type 1 diabetes restricts insulin in order to lose weight.
- Bigorexia, which is also known as muscle dysmorphia, where a person constantly thinks about muscle building.
- Pica is a behaviour of regular inappropriate consumption of substances, such as non-food items, and is listed in DSM-5 (APA 2023).

The DSM and ICD have always been works in progress due to ongoing debates and disagreements. Eating disorder is complicated and can be one of the most stigmatising mental health issues (Mulheim and Collins 2020).

3.2 Anorexia Nervosa (AN)

3.2.1 Prevalence

Anorexia or anorexia nervosa (AN) is a mental health disorder, which can cause an individual to limit and restrict how much they eat and drink (BEAT 2023a). While this disorder can affect all individuals regardless of age and gender, it is mostly prevalent among women and among adolescents and young adults (BEAT 2023b; NICE 2017). Worldwide, the prevalence of AN is reported to be 0.8–6.3% of women and 0.1–0.3% of men (Silén and Keski-Rahkonen 2022). In Europe, it is reported to be up to 4% in women and up to 0.7% in men. In the UK, it is estimated by BEAT (2023b) to be 0.3% for women aged 11–34 and 0.1% for men. Additionally, a report conducted by Just Like Us, a charity supporting LGBTQ+ rights, has shown that young LGBTQ+ people are three times more likely to have developed an eating disorder or to still be suffering from one (BEAT 2023a). AN has a higher mortality rate than any other mental health disorder with a weighted crude mortality of around 5.1 deaths per 1000 person-years. Additionally, 20% AN-related deaths are due to suicide (NICE 2017). In older adolescents, AN rates are higher than any serious chronic disease (Huang et al. 2014). An important thing to note is that evidence seems to show an increase in prevalence rates, both in the UK and worldwide, making AN and more generally eating disorders a concerning health issue to treat seriously.

3.2.2 Signs and Symptoms

AN manifests itself through a range of behavioural, psychological and physical signs and symptoms. Behavioural signs are usually characterised by a triggered behaviour around food. This can include excessive calorie counting, excluding certain groups of food such as fats or carbs, portioning food, skipping meals, lying about having eaten or how much has been eaten, avoiding eating with/around other people or hiding food. Other behavioural signs usually involve an impact on the individual's self-worth and image, for instance, checking one's appearance and body more often, avoiding mirrors and scales, body dysmorphia, lying about weight loss, excessive exercising, vomiting and avoiding situations of socialisation.

Psychological signs can include an obsessive attitude with thinness, spending more time thinking and planning around food, undermining the seriousness of the issue, low confidence and self-esteem and other mental health disorders such as depression, anxiety and obsessive-compulsive disorder (OCD).

Physically, AN manifests in various ways. Although rapid weight loss is a known and common symptom, some people suffering from AN may be considered a "normal" weight by health professionals. AN can therefore be an invisible disorder. Other physical symptoms include irregular periods or periods stopping altogether, tiredness, difficulty sleeping, concentration issues, low body temperature/being cold often, hair loss, constipation and bloating and muscle weakness (BEAT 2023a). These signs are non-exhaustive, and timely management of the disorder is key in the quality, effectiveness and long-lasting impact of the recovery. If not treated, AN can lead to serious long-term physical issues such as osteoporosis, heart conditions, fertility issues or damage to vital organs but also long-term psychological and emotional issues affecting the individual's relationship to food and social behaviour (BEAT 2023a).

Below is a personal reflection from one of the authors with lived experience:

> When I started developing my eating disorder, it was first seen as "watching my figure" and "working out more". It was rather easy to hide my triggered behaviour surrounding food (calorie counting, avoiding food groups etc.) and people's usual positive behaviour towards a person losing weight made it even easier. This shows how hard to see and detect AN can be, and how observant one must be, especially around young people.

3.2.3 Promising Treatments

Due to the effect all EDs have on a young person's body and mind, treatment options include a combination of psychological interventions, nutritional counselling and weight monitoring according to the National Eating Disorders Association (NEDA 2023b). EDs are treated in a variety of settings including inpatient, day patient, outpatient and community facilities. There is a commonly held myth that eating disordered behaviour is a personal choice, when conversely it is a very serious and, for some, often fatal illness that is associated with disturbances in eating behaviours, emotions and thoughts. There are high rates of co-morbidity; therefore, it is also important to treat co-morbid conditions such as depression, following the best possible evidence (NICE 2017).

Evidence-based treatment options include a range of psychotherapies and sometimes adjunctive pharmacological interventions. Antidepressants, small doses of antipsychotics and stimulants such as lisdexamfetamine are among the options. Sadly, a staggering 20–30% of people fail to respond to treatments and can go on to develop chronic refractory illness.

NICE guidelines agree that those suffering from an ED should be treated with structured psychological therapies divided into those that are for children and those for adults and based on developmental needs (Hilbert et al. 2017). Young people are often offered family-focused treatments where parents are provided with psychoeducation and strategies to support their child's recovery. This can be working with the whole family, the parents or multiple families.

Psychological treatments for anorexia nervosa in children and young people recommended by NICE (2017) include:

- Anorexia nervosa-focused family therapy for children and young people (FT-AN) delivered as single-family therapy or a combination of single- and multi-family therapy and typically consisting of 18–20 sessions over 1 year. If FT-AN is unacceptable, contraindicated or ineffective, consider adolescent-focused psychotherapy for anorexia nervosa (AFP-AN). This should typically consist of 32–40 individual sessions over 12–18 months, with more regular sessions early on, to help the person build a relationship with the practitioner and motivate them to change their behaviour.
- For those with anorexia who are not having treatment, because it has not helped or because they have declined it, and who do not have severe or complex problems, they should be discharged to primary care where they can ask their GP to refer them again for treatment at any time.
- NICE (2017) also urges that medication should NOT be offered as the sole treatment for anorexia nervosa. Dietary counselling should only be offered as part of a multidisciplinary approach. This can also include encouragement to take an age-appropriate oral multivitamin and multi-mineral supplement until their diet includes enough to meet their dietary reference values.
- Family therapy is usually a key element in recovery as AN can push a young individual to detach themself from their family, creating a lot of frustration and misunderstanding. In contexts where family played a significant role in the development of anorexia, it becomes even more relevant and essential to reconnect the young person with their family.

Below is a quote from one of the authors with lived experience:

> In my own recovery, family therapy was necessary to rebuild a link that had been broken by my disorder. Other forms of treatments also included group therapy through for instance artistic activities or yoga which helped focusing on something other than food but also to reconnect with my own body. The relationship I developed with some of the medical staff was also key in my recovery. Mealtimes were some of the hardest and having a nurse sitting next to me, talking to me about non-food related things and distracting me from obsessing over what was in my meal came to be extremely helpful.

3.3 Bulimia Nervosa

3.3.1 Prevalence

Bulimia nervosa (BN), often referred to simply as bulimia, is a significant mental health disorder (BEAT 2017). It can affect individuals of any age but is most commonly, first identified during late adolescence (NICE 2004). Prevalence does vary across the world, but clear patterns are found with an obvious weighting towards females who are more frequently affected than males (Galmiche et al. 2019). Worldwide the prevalence of the condition is reported as 1% in the general population, with a 0.3% prevalence in males and a 1.7% prevalence in females (Qian et al. 2022). In Europe, the prevalence is estimated as 1–2% with a 1.5% prevalence for females and 0.1% for males (Galmiche et al. 2019). In the UK, this is estimated to be 1% in females (aged 11–34) and 0.3% in males (BEAT 2023b). What is very noticeable from the evidence is that the prevalence rates are also rising worldwide (Qian et al. 2022). The DSM-5 (APA 2023) and ICD-11 (WHO 2022) classify the diagnosis of BN as the inclusion of recurrent binge eating, having no sense of control, overeating and inappropriate vomiting or other behaviours to inhibit weight gain.

3.3.2 Signs and Symptoms

The condition usually presents as a pattern of behavioural, emotional and physical symptoms. It is often characterised as a cyclical pattern of binge eating (eating large amounts over short periods), followed by self-induced vomiting, strenuous exercise, fasting and taking laxatives, diuretics or other medications. These are all used to compensate the binge eating behaviour, to prevent weight gain (called purging). Emotionally, there can be significant anxiety about gaining weight and a dissatisfaction with their body shape (NICE 2017). Eating can cause feelings of shame or guilt, and there can be mood instability, anxiety or depression (Levinson et al. 2017). Physically, bulimia can also cause serious complications. Teeth can become eroded due to frequent vomiting, and physical trauma can be caused by the mechanism used to make themselves vomit. Complications can affect the gastrointestinal tract, kidneys and heart, caused by excessive laxative use, and more general complaints include a lack of energy, abdominal pain, bloatedness, oedema/swelling in the hands and feet and irregular menstruation (NICE 2017; Mehler and Rylander 2015). It is important to recognise that people with bulimia are often of a normal weight and can be very effective at hiding the condition from the people around them, and they also do not often ask for help; it is thought this is driven by guilt and shame (Wade 2019). You may, however, notice mood swings, emotionality (such as anxiety and irritability), low self-worth and a reluctance to eat with others or being secretive or, conversely, fixated about food in general (Castillo and Weiselberg 2017; BEAT 2017; NICE 2017).

The binge/purge cycle of behaviours is commonly used as a mechanism of coping with negative or stressful situations and emotional difficulties, such as being angry, anxious or distressed and in some cases bored (Castillo and Weiselberg 2017). This pattern of behaviour can impact upon many aspects of daily life, including family relationships, friendships and social situations like school or college, as it becomes central to a person's way of controlling difficulties in their lives. Effective interventions and management of the condition are vital to prevent more serious complications, which include kidney failure, cardiac problems, dental issues and poor mental health (Castillo and Weiselberg 2017).

3.3.3 Promising Treatments

Treatment for bulimia nervosa involves various approaches, including psychological therapies, such as cognitive behavioural therapy (CBT). Psychological therapies focus on developing healthier thinking and behaviours and improving thoughts and feelings about food and body image. These may be alongside medications like antidepressants for underlying mental health conditions and improving mood, but this is usually only if other interventions are unsuccessful (Bould et al. 2017). Family-based therapy and nutritional counselling are also important parts of any treatment plan (Reiter and Graves 2010; NICE 2017; NEDA 2023b). Nutritional counselling educates individuals about nutrition and helps them establish a balanced diet. A multidisciplinary approach is important to effectively address the complex interplay of factors contributing to the disorder. Early intervention and individually tailored treatment plans are crucial for recovery and the prevention of serious complications, emphasising the need for awareness and education about this condition.

Psychological treatments for BN in children and young people recommended by NICE (2017) are as follows:

- NICE (2017) recommends bulimia nervosa-focused family therapy (FT-BN) to children and young people with bulimia nervosa. This should typically consist of 18–20 sessions over 6 months and relies on establishing a good therapeutic relationship with the person and their family members or carers without attaching blame. Also provide information about regulating body weight, dieting and the adverse effects of attempting to control weight with self-induced vomiting, laxatives or other compensatory behaviours.
- If FT-BN is unacceptable, contraindicated or ineffective, consider individual eating disorder-focused cognitive behavioural therapy (CBT-ED) typically consisting of 18 sessions over 6 months, with more frequent sessions early in treatment and including up to 4 additional sessions with parents or carers. The treatment begins with a case formulation with the person and setting goals and encouraging the person to address problematic thoughts, beliefs and behaviours with problem-solving.
- NICE (2017) also urges that medication should NOT be offered as the sole treatment for bulimia nervosa.

3.4 Binge Eating Disorder

3.4.1 Prevalence

The estimated lifetime prevalence of BED in young people and adults in Europe is 1.9% for females and 0.3% for males. BED is the most common ED in the USA with lifetime prevalence estimates in adolescents of 1.6% (Swanson et al. 2011). Although symptoms in young people may be transient, the highest past year prevalence in this population is 1.8–3.6% in girls, 1.5% in gender-diverse youths and 0.2–1.2% in boys (Olsen et al. 2021). Overall, the prevalence of eating disorders is highest among those with BED (5.5%), compared with 2% for BN and 1.2% for AN (Hudson et al. 2007). Hence, the treatment for BED should be prioritised in the same way as AN and BN. BED peaks in later adolescence and young adulthood.

3.4.2 Signs and Symptoms

BED is characterised by episodes where young people ingest large amounts of food and experience a loss of control. During such episodes, BED is often associated with obesity and mental health issues such as depression. This disorder can result in impairment in the quality of life of sufferers. BED was added as a diagnosis in 2013 to DSM-5 (APA 2013) and later to ICD-11 (WHO 2022). To fulfil these criteria for diagnosis, these episodes have occurred at least once a week for at least 3 months and have been associated with distress. Furthermore, DSM-5 (APA 2023) suggests that the binge eating episodes are required to experience at least three of the following:

- Eating despite not feeling physically hungry.
- Eating more rapidly than normal.
- Eating until feeling uncomfortably full.
- Eating alone because of associated guilt and/or embarrassment.
- Negative feeling after overeating.

It is important to note that people with BED do not regularly compensate for binge eating by exercising, which is common in those with AN or BN.

3.4.3 Promising Treatments

NICE (2017) advises that psychological treatments aimed at treating BED have a limited effect on body weight and that weight loss is not a therapy target in itself and that this should be made clear before treatment commences. The guideline recommends the following:

- Initially offer individual BED-focused guided self-help cognitive behavioural therapy (CBT) self-help materials, supplemented with brief supportive sessions (e.g. four to nine sessions lasting 20 min each over 16 weeks) and focus exclusively on helping the person follow the programme.
- If this proves ineffective, offer group eating disorder-focused cognitive behavioural therapy (CBT-ED). This typically consists of 16 weekly 90-min group sessions over 4 months. Alternatively, if this is not available or declined, consider individual CBT-ED, which should typically consist of 16–20 sessions.
- NICE (2017) also urges that medication should NOT be offered as the sole treatment for BED.

Currently, a broad range of novel treatments are being tested for BED. Some are amalgamated with established treatments such as those described above.

- Neurobiologically informed multicomponent psychological therapies that target inhibitory control/emotional regulation and compulsivity are being trialled for BED. However, whether these are more superior to conventional CBT for BED is less evident (Giel et al. 2017).
- Cognitive remediation therapy (CRT) and various computerised programmes are being used to help reduce overeating (Preuss et al. 2017). CRT is a form of psychotherapy that aims to improve neurocognitive functioning. Also, some models have focused on reducing food cue reactivity, overeating and body dissatisfaction.

3.4.4 Risk and Protective Factors for EDs

Risk factors for eating disorders are varied and include biological, psychological and social factors. Biological factors include having a family member or close relative suffering from an eating disorder or a history of mental illness (NEDA 2023a). In fact, genetic factors are significant in the development of EDs (Thornton et al. 2011). Having a parent with an ED increases the chance (×10 in the case of AN) of an individual also developing an ED (Bould et al. 2015). There are also clear genetic associations with specific co-morbidities including ADHD and ASD and mental health conditions (Barakat et al. 2023).

Psychological factors include personal mental health issues, as above, as well as a history of substance use disorder. Struggling with body image and perfectionism are also known to contribute to the development of the disorder (Barakat et al. 2023). Social factors vary depending on the individual's cultural background and environment. In the individual's close social environment, they can include bullying, for instance, at school, limited contact with others, isolation and a personal history of trauma. Broader social factors include weight stigma perpetrated by diet culture, social media and popular culture, which promote and glorify thinness while emphasising body shaming. Acculturation, where the individual might feel social pressure to conform to new cultural norms, can also be a determining factor (NEDA 2023a).

Below is a personal view from one of the chapter authors who has lived experience:

> In my own experience with anorexia, I have found that the disorder rarely manifests solely through one specific factor but rather through a combination of biological, psychological and social factors. I grew up in a family context where women always had a rather toxic behaviour around food and dieting and where comments would often be made on the bodies of the young women in the family. Additionally, I have multiple family members that have themselves struggled with eating disorders. However, it wasn't until a specific traumatic event occurred that my eating disorder developed.

The numerous risk and protective factors associated with EDs are listed in Table 3.1 (Barakat et al. 2023; Bould et al. 2017; NEDA 2023a).

As can be seen from Table 3.1, risk factors for eating disorders are multidimensional and include genetic and psychological factors and sociocultural influences. Mental wellbeing, societal and family expectations and influence and the impact of the media on acceptable body image all contribute to the risk factors for the

Table 3.1 Risk and protective factors for the three primary disorders (AN, BN and BED)

Risk factors	Protective factors
Biological risk factors Gender Genetic Timing/onset of puberty Psychological risk factors Low self-esteem Mood disorder 40% Depression Anxiety/OCD Personality traits (e.g. perfectionism, obsessive-compulsive) Stress Feeling out of control Overvaluation of weight/shape in defining self-worth Trauma Poor problem-solving skills	*Protective factors (individual)* Positive self-esteem and body image Good peer support networks Resilience Assertiveness Good social skills Good problem-solving and coping skills Body appreciation Good problem-solving skills Good level of insight Being self-directive and assertive High self-esteem
Social risk factors Cultural views of "ideal" weight and shape Involvement in a sport/industry where there is emphasis on body weight/shape (e.g. ballet, gymnastics, athletics, modelling) Pressure to achieve/succeed Peer pressure Teasing/bullying Problems in family/personal relationships Influence of media/social media Emphasis on dieting/weight/physical appearance in the family	*Protective factors (family)* Connectedness Eating regular family meals together Lack of emphasis on weight/physical appearance *Protective factors (social)* Positive role models, i.e. through social media Supportive peer and social groups (in schools/colleges, etc.)

disorder. In addition, participation in certain sport activities, such as swimming, dance and gymnastics, that have a focus on appearance, body shape and weight can add to the risks (Barakat et al. 2023). Complications from the disorder can be severe, even fatal, which underscores the importance of understanding and addressing these risk factors.

The protective factors against EDs include supportive relationships and environments, which encourage positive body image and body appreciation as well as general interventions to increase self-esteem and wellbeing alongside self-acceptance. The importance of a supportive family and wider network is clear, and there should be consideration of access to supportive sociocultural influences such as role models. Body acceptance involves developing an understanding of healthy eating habits without focusing on dieting and emphasising good balanced nutrition. This can help individuals develop a healthier relationship with food. Strengthening successful emotional regulation skills and helping in the management of difficult situations and negative emotions are crucial and will help to build resilience. It is important to provide supportive environments to enhance protective factors whether in family settings, schools or communities, to provide a solid foundation for preventing eating disorders.

3.4.5 Medical Emergency in Eating Disorder (MEED)

To tackle the serious health concerns relating to eating disorders, it is crucial that more is done to identify those at risk early on in their trajectory. The Royal College of Psychiatrists have developed guidelines on how to respond to medical emergencies in EDs (RCPsych 2022). It highlights the important role of frontline as well as healthcare professionals. It replaces previous guidance and has a risk assessment framework tool using a traffic light system assessing 11 of the likely risks to the health of young people adjusted for age and gender and how best to intervene in an emergency.

3.4.6 Consent and Compulsory Treatment

In some instances, a person's physical health is seriously compromised because of the severity of their eating disorder. Due to the denial some sufferers experience, they may not consent to treatment and may require inpatient admission. In these cases, professionals need to follow the legal framework for compulsory treatment under the Mental Health Act (MHA) 1983, as amended in 2007 (MHA 1983, 2007; NICE 2017). If the child lacks capacity and again their physical health is seriously compromised, their parents/carers can consent to treatment on their behalf, and again, it can require the use of compulsory treatment orders under MHA or the Children Act 1989. Having said that, one study has suggested that most families and patients accept that compulsory treatment may be required if the condition is life-threatening (Tan et al. 2010). For further information, see Sect. 3.4.8 of the MEED guidelines on compulsory admission and treatment (RCPsych 2022).

3.4.7 Case Scenario

The case scenario chosen below is focused on AN, given its seriousness in terms of morbidity, effects of starvation and the requirement to intervene early to prevent long-term consequences of the disorder. "Emma" is a hypothetical case, and her age was chosen to represent a common age of presentation, which according to NICE (2017) is between 13 and 17 years of age. Emma like a lot of youngsters is reluctant to acknowledge that she has a problem, and this can often be part of the disease process (RCPsych 2020). Concerns have been raised by Emma's peers, and she appears to have a short-term history of disordered eating. The aim would be to prevent a protracted stay in a Child and Adolescent Mental Health Service (CAMHS) Tier 4 inpatient facility and help Emma remain at home and within her school and wider community (see Box 3.1).

Box 3.1: Case Study: Emma

Emma is the second child of Mr. and Mrs. Douglas (not their real names). Her parents have successful careers. However, they are on the verge of splitting up.

Emma is 14 years of age and attends the local grammar school, where she is in the top sets for all subjects. She is a quiet, introverted child. She has two close friends who have spoken to the form tutor about their concerns about Emma stopping eating her lunch. She has started walking to school, even though it is about 5 kilometres from her home, and the girls feel that she has lost a lot of weight over the past 5 months.

Emma had never been overweight and has taken to having her evening meal on her own in her bedroom. One of the teachers spoke to Emma, but she denied having any problems with home, food, school or schoolwork. A few weeks later, Emma looked tired, and it was clear that her clothes no longer fitted her. The teacher referred Emma to the mental health support team (MHST), who invited Emma and her parents to discuss the situation. Her parents were candid about their personal issues and had noticed the weight loss and change in behaviour. However, they felt anxious about talking to her about it as she would become very angry and shut down any conversations.

3.4.8 Case Study Principles of Care

Regarding the case study in Box 3.1, below are some principles of care that should be applied for the identification of Emma' condition and to assess her needs (adapted from NICE 2017):

- Emma and her family need to receive assessment and treatment at the earliest opportunity.
- Although Emma has lost weight, she is not severely emaciated in that she requires urgent medical treatment. However, an explanation of the health risks she faces should be shared with Emma and her family.
- The assessment will involve a thorough physical examination (see MEED above).
- Assess for the presence of mental health problems including depression, anxiety, self-harm and OCD.
- Following assessment and diagnosis, Emma will be referred to a community eating disorder service (CEDS), and her treatment will commence.
- Those involved in Emma's ongoing care will be provided with psychoeducation about Emma's condition. CEDS will continue to monitor her weight, physical needs and mental health issues and any maintenance factors.
- The CEDS team around Emma will be from a variety of disciplines/multidisciplinary team (MDT).
- In conjunction with Emma and her family, a personalised treatment plan will be drawn up and with Emma's permission be shared with all involved.
- There will be clear guidance as to the roles and responsibilities of the MDT, the school, the MHST and the school nurse in Emma's recovery, e.g. discussion on meal plans and how to provide pre- and post-meal supervision at school and within the home.
- Address Emma's fears about weight gain and develop strategies for managing anxiety around eating.
- Address the impact of home situation, education and Emma's wider social environment, including Internet use.
- Offer her parents couples therapy separately to family sessions due to the breakdown in their relationship.
- Negotiate with Emma about how to involve extended family, teachers and peers about how best to support her during her recovery.

3.4.9 Do's and Don'ts: Reflections from a Service User

The statements below derive from the lived experiences of a male service user and one of the authors of this chapter:

- Don't let the person suffer in silence. Let the person know that you are there for them—Suffering from an eating disorder is a very lonely place to be in. I felt that people would judge me if I asked for help because "I am a 'man' and 'men' can't be seen as weak".
- Don't assume eating disorders always mean the person is low weight—I lost a drastic amount of weight over a short period of time, which inevitably meant me being hospitalised. However, after a re-feeding programme and being discharged, people automatically thought that I was "better" because I was now a healthy

weight. Even though this was the case, I was probably still just as unhealthy in the mind as I was prior to my hospital admission.

- Don't praise the person for the way they look—Through my hospital admission, at family visiting times, I would have a range of family or friends come visit me. I would always get comments such as "Wow Ben you're looking better now"—I automatically associated this comment with looking "fat". Better to me meant that I had put weight on, and when someone made this comment to me, the illness made me feel very guilty, and I would most probably refuse the next meal I was due because I didn't want to look "better", and I needed to put the illness's voice at bay.
- Speak to the person as you would've done before they became unwell—When I became unwell and was diagnosed with an eating disorder, people began to change the way they spoke to me. They talked to me almost as if I was a child and felt like they were doing this because they were scared to say the wrong thing or didn't want to upset me.
- Don't treat every eating disorder case as being the same—An eating disorder is not something you can learn inside and out through a textbook. Yes, you can learn a basic understanding from textbooks, research, etc., but the most valuable way you will learn to help someone suffering from an eating disorder is by sitting down with them and being honest with them. Ask them to help you understand what helps them/what doesn't help them because what works for someone else might not work for them. I found that the staff who helped me the most were the ones who spent that extra 5 min with me and constantly wanted to learn about my illness.
- Encouragement is key, not enforcement—When I was first hospitalised onto a paediatric ward, the nursing staff had very little knowledge around eating disorders. During the day, nurses would walk into my room with some chocolate, crisp, sweets, etc. and say "Go on Ben, you NEED to eat this", "You can't stay in here forever. If you make these little steps", etc. By trying to get my mind to focus on the positives ahead rather than the negative place that I was in at that time, then I think I would've made them steps sooner than I did.
- Don't make decisions without the person's involvement—There were times where decisions were made without my knowledge about my care and things were implemented without me even knowing. This sent my anxiety into overdrive and made me go into crisis causing restraints and distress to happen. Change is huge for someone when they're so low in mood and weight and have accompanying OCD.
- Never praise for weight gain—This was my biggest pet-hate! I used to be weighed twice a week in the unit—Mondays and Thursdays. My week evolved around these 2 days as weight gain was a massive fear of mine, no matter how big or small the gain was. A gain to me meant I was fat, so when it came to "weigh days", my anxiety would be through the roof. In my mind, any kind of praise for weight gain is not what the illness wanted. It felt vulnerable because, for one, I had put some weight on, but, for two, people were supporting me to put on weight and making me try to see the positives to this. Family therapy sessions

were great for issues like these because I was able to let my family and friends know that by them making these comments, how it made me feel.

- Keep them busy before/after mealtimes—This was a huge help for me. When I was in hospital to begin with, I used to eat my meal and then we would have a thing called “supervision”, which is where a staff member would sit with you for half an hour after your meal. I discussed this with the occupational therapist during a session, and we then devised a plan that staff would do an activity with me such as card games, board games, playing on the games console, etc., before a meal and after I had eaten. That hour before and after a meal can be torturous for some people like me, and by implementing something so simple to keep you distracted, it can make a huge amount of difference.
- Take the focus away from food around mealtimes—When I first moved home after leaving the unit, mealtimes were a very stressful time for my family as everyone was very anxious about it—NOT JUST ME. They would stare at me making the process feel weird. I ended up raising this with one of my family therapy sessions, and my parents were oblivious to what they were doing at mealtimes. So, we made a new “rule”, where at a mealtime, nobody would talk about food or anything to do with me eating it—we had to talk about anything but this.
- Include the person in social activities—I used to find social eating hard to do. When I was discharged, my friends would ask me if I wanted to go out for a meal with them, which was good of them to ask. However, eating out made me massively anxious! I spoke with my friends about this eventually, and after this, my friends began to arrange days out that would involve some kind of activity, which wasn’t based solely on eating out.
- Don’t let them push you away—If you are the person’s support network, the illness will try and make them push you away as much as possible, as it knows that you will fight against it and give the person some hope that they can beat the illness. My parents said to me “we are going to stay, whether your illness likes it or not”. The illness will try and isolate the person as much as possible.
- Don’t set a time limit on recovery—Never tell the person that they will be in treatment for 6 months, for example, or have eight therapy sessions and then they “will be better”. This was a huge setback for me when I was told this. I lost all trust due to them giving me a time limit on when I could leave the unit.

3.5 Conclusion

EDs are often complex and multifaceted. Because of this, the minimum treatment team would require a medical practitioner, a mental health professional and a dietician/nutritional expert. At the centre of the team would be the young person and their carers/families. Plans should be person-centred, family oriented, culturally sensitive and recovery focused (NEDC 2018). Although there should be a core team, other professionals and support staff could be co-opted into the team depending on the needs of the young person. Two of the authors of this chapter provide teaching, training and peer support to young people and their families and clinical and non-clinical staff, which are extremely well received and can provide helpful available insights to all concerned. This type of support involving connecting with others who have had similar experiences helps a young person understand their role in their recovery. Often, it is their peers, teaching staff and interested adults that notice that a young person is struggling; so, if they have the necessary information and understanding of referral routes and how best to provide a non-judgemental environment, it is more likely that the young person will engage with people they trust. Fitness professionals may also be vital for early intervention and signposting (NEDC 2018). The importance of seeking help early cannot be overstated. The earlier one intervenes, if this is done in a respectful way, the shorter the duration of the illness may be—especially for children and young people (Zipfel et al. 2015).

References

American Psychiatric Association (APA). Diagnostic and statistical manual of mental disorders fifth edition DSM -5™; 2013. Available from: https://repository.poltekkes-kaltim.ac.id/657/1/Diagnostic%20and%20statistical%20manual%20of%20mental%20disorders%20_%20DSM-5%20(%20PDFDrive.com%20).pdf. Accessed 7 Oct 204.

American Psychiatric Association (APA). Diagnostic and statistical manual of mental disorders. Updates to the Fifth edition DSM -5™; 2023. Available from: https://www.psychiatry.org/psychiatrists/practice/dsm/updates-to-dsm/updates-to-dsm-5-tr-criteria-text. Accessed 7 Oct 2024.

Barakat S, McLean SA, Bryant E, et al. Risk factors for eating disorders: findings from a rapid review. J Eat Disord. 2023;11:8. https://doi.org/10.1186/s40337-022-00717-4.

BEAT. Bulimia Nervosa. What is Bulimia? Last updated 2020; 2017. Available from: Bulimia Nervosa - Beat (beateatingdisorders.org.uk). Accessed 7 Oct 2024.

BEAT. Anorexia Nervosa; 2023a. Available from: https://www.beateatingdisorders.org.uk/get-information-and-support/about-eating-disorders/types/anorexia/. Accessed 7 Oct 2024.

BEAT. How many people have an eating disorder in the UK?; 2023b. Available from: https://www.beateatingdisorders.org.uk/get-information-and-support/about-eating-disorders/how-many-people-eating-disorder-uk/. Accessed 7 Oct 2024.

Bould H, Sovio U, Koupil I, Dalman C, Micali N, Lewis G, Magnusson C. Do eating disorders in parents predict eating disorders in children? Evidence from a Swedish cohort. Acta Psychiatr Scand. 2015;132(1):51–9. https://doi.org/10.1111/acps.12389.

Bould H, Newbegin C, Stewart A, Stein A, Fazel M. Eating disorders in children and young people. BMJ. 2017;359:j5245. https://doi.org/10.1136/bmj.j5245.

Castillo M, Weiselberg E. Bulimia nervosa/purging disorder. Curr Probl Pediatr Adolesc Health Care. 2017;47(4):85–94. https://doi.org/10.1016/j.cppeds.2017.02.004.

Children Act. https://www.legislation.gov.uk/ukpga/1989/41/contents; 1989.

Edakubo S, Fushimi K. Mortality and risk assessment for anorexia nervosa in acute-care hospitals: a nationwide administrative database analysis. BMC Psychiatry. 2020;20(1):19. https://doi.org/10.1186/s12888-020-2433-8.

Galmiche M, Déchelotte P, Lambert G, Tavolacci MP. Prevalence of eating disorders over the 2000-2018 period: a systematic literature review. Am J Clin Nutr. 2019;109(5):1402–13.

Giel KE, Teufel M, Junne F, Zipfel S, Schag K. Food-related impulsivity in obesity and binge eating disorder–a systematic update of the evidence. Nutrients. 2017;9:1170.

Hilbert A, Hoek HW, Schmidt R. Evidence-based clinical guidelines for eating disorders: international comparison. Curr Opin Psychiatry. 2017;30(6):423–37. https://doi.org/10.1097/YCO.0000000000000360.

Huang U, Goldacre M, James A. 2014. Mortality following hospital discharge with a diagnosis of eating disorder: national record linkage study, England, 2001-2009. Int J Eat Disord. 2014;47(5):507–15. https://doi.org/10.1002/eat.22249.
Hudson JI, Hiripi E, Pope HG Jr, Kessler RC. The prevalence and correlates of eating disorders in the National Comorbidity Survey Replication. Biol Psychiatry. 2007;61(3):348–58. https://doi.org/10.1016/j.biopsych.2006.03.040.
Levinson CA, Zerwas S, Calebs B, Forbush K, Kordy H, Watson H, Hofmeier S, Levine M, Crosby RD, Peat C, Runfola CD, Zimmer B, Moesner M, Marcus MD, Bulik CM. The core symptoms of bulimia nervosa, anxiety, and depression: a network analysis. J Abnorm Psychol. 2017;126(3):340–54. https://doi.org/10.1037/abn0000254.
Mehler PS, Rylander M. Bulimia Nervosa – medical complications. J Eat Disord. 2015;3:12.
Mental Health Act. 1983. Available from: https://www.legislation.gov.uk/ukpga/1983/20/contents. Accessed 7 Oct 2024.
Mental Health Act 2007. Available from: https://www.legislation.gov.uk/ukpga/2007/12/contents. Accessed 7 Oct 2024.
Mulheim L, Collins L. When your teen has an eating disorder: practical strategies to help your teen recover from anorexia, bulimia, and binge eating. New Harbinger Publications; 2020.
National Eating Disorder Association. Risk Factors; 2023a. Available from: https://www.nationaleatingdisorders.org/risk-factors/. Accessed 7 Oct 2024.
National Eating Disorder Association. Treatment; 2023b. Available from: https://www.nationaleatingdisorders.org/treatment/. Accessed 7 Oct 2024.
National Eating Disorders Collaboration. National practice standards for eating disorder; 2018. Available from: https://www.nedc.com.au/assets/Final-NEDC-PracticeStandards.pdf. Accessed 7 Oct 2024.
NICE. Clinical Knowledge Summary. Eating Disorders. How common is it? Last revised 2019; 2004. Available from: Prevalence | Background information | Eating disorders | CKS | NICE. Accessed 7 Oct 2024
NICE. Eating disorders: recognition and treatment. NICE guideline [NG69]; 2017. Last updated: 16 December 2020. Available from: https://www.nice.org.uk/guidance/ng69. Accessed 7 Oct 2024.
Olsen EM, Koch SV, Skovgaard AM, Strandberg-Larsen K. Self-reported symptoms of binge-eating disorder among adolescents in a community-based Danish cohort-A study of prevalence, correlates, and impact. Int J Eat Disord. 2021;54(4):492–505. https://doi.org/10.1002/eat.23458.
Preuss H, Pinnow M, Schnicker K, Legenbauer T. Improving inhibitory control Abilities (ImpulsE) – a promising approach to treat impulsive eating? Eur Eat Disord Rev. 2017;25(6):533–43. https://doi.org/10.1002/erv.2544.
Qian J, Wu Y, Liu F, et al. An update on the prevalence of eating disorders in the general population: a systematic review and meta-analysis. Eat Weight Disord. 2022;27:415–28.
Reiter CS, Graves L. Nutrition therapy for eating disorders. Nutr Clin Pract. 2010;25(2):122–36.
Royal College of Psychiatrists. 2020PS04/20 Improving core skills and competence in risk assessment and management of people with eating disorders: What all doctors need to know. Position Statement; 2020. Available from: https://www.rcpsych.ac.uk/docs/default-source/improving-care/better-mh-policy/position-statements/ps04_20.pdf?sfvrsn=6c927307_4. Accessed 7 Oct 2024.
Royal College of Psychiatrists. Medical emergencies in eating disorders (MEED) Guidance on recognition and management. R233; 2022. Available from: https://www.rcpsych.ac.uk/improving-care/campaigning-for-better-mental-health-policy/college-reports/2022-college-reports/cr233. Accessed 7 Oct 2024.
Silén Y, Keski-Rahkonen A. Worldwide prevalence of DSM-5 eating disorders among young people. Curr Opin Psychiatry. 2022;35(6):362–71. https://doi.org/10.1097/YCO.0000000000000818.
Swanson SA, Crow SJ, Le Grange D, Swendsen J, Merikangas KR. Prevalence and correlates of eating disorders in adolescents. Results from the national comorbidity survey replication

adolescent supplement. Arch Gen Psychiatry. 2011;68(7):714–23. https://doi.org/10.1001/archgenpsychiatry.2011.22.

Tan JOA, Stewart A, Fitzpatrick R, Hope T. Attitudes of patients with anorexia nervosa to compulsory treatment and coercion. Int J Law Psychiatry. 2010;33(1):13–9. https://doi.org/10.1016/j.ijlp.2009.10.003.

Thornton LM, Mazzeo SE, Bulik CM. The heritability of eating disorders: methods and current findings. In: Behavioral neurobiology of eating disorders, vol. 6; 2011. p. 141–56. https://doi.org/10.1007/7854_2010_91.

Wade S. The transdiagnostic theory of eating disorders: Investigation of maintaining mechanisms and clinical utility. 2019. [Doctoral Thesis, The University of Western Australia].

World Health Organisation. ICD-11 International Classification of Diseases 11th Revision The global standard for diagnostic health information; 2022. Available from: https://www.who.int/news/item/11-02-2022-icd-11-2022-release. Accessed 7 Oct 2024.

Zipfel S, Giel K, Bulik C, Hay P, Schmidt U. Anorexia nervosa: aetiology, assessment, and treatment, Lancet. Psychiatry. 2015;2(12):1099–111. https://doi.org/10.1016/S2215-0366(15)00356-9.

Psychosis and Bipolar Disorder

4

Lisa Fairclough and Celeste Foster

L. Fairclough (✉)
BUPA, Manchester, UK
e-mail: Lisa.fairclough@bupa.com

C. Foster
Directorate of Nursing and Midwifery, University of Salford, Salford, UK
e-mail: c.m.foster@salford.ac.uk

G. Trainor, V. Heaslip (eds.), *Needs of Children and Young People Living with Complex Mental Health Difficulties*,
https://doi.org/10.1007/978-3-031-84532-1_4

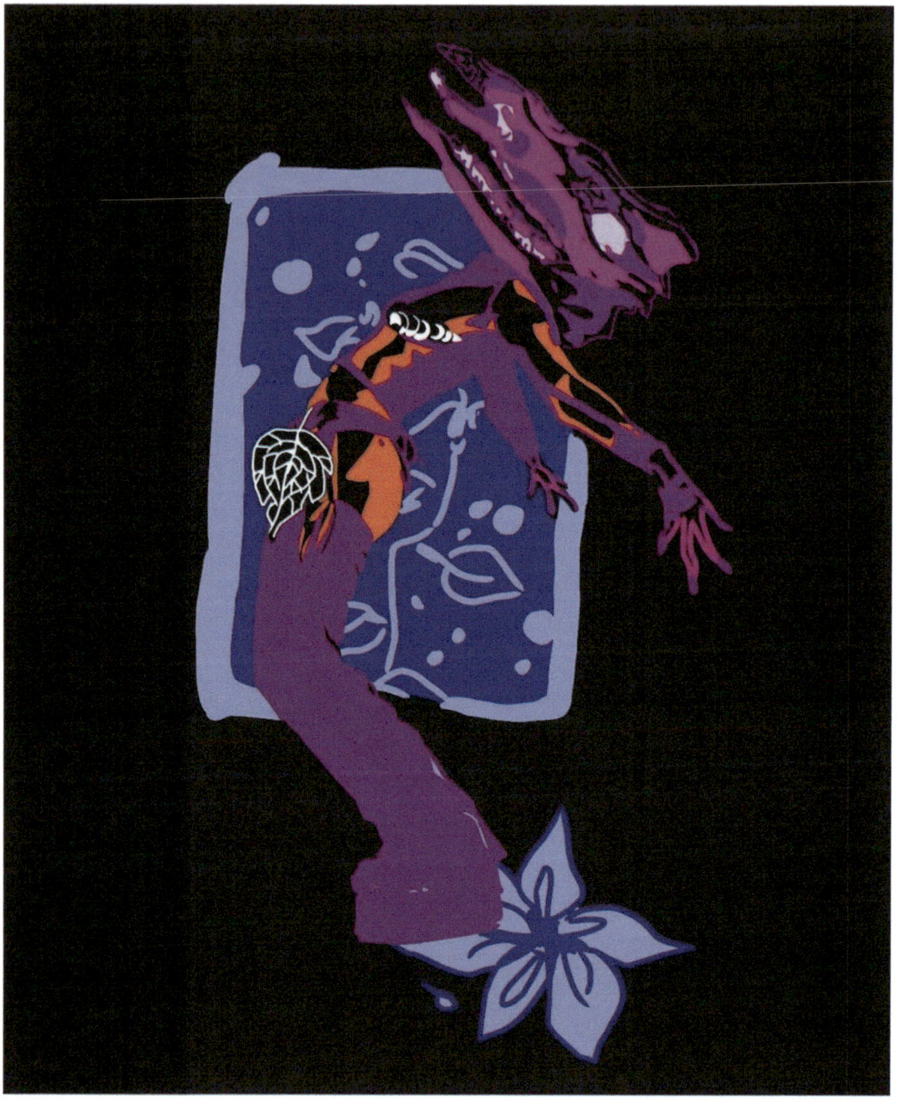

4.1 What Is Psychosis and How Common Is It?

Psychosis describes symptoms of a mental health condition that impacts on a person's thoughts and perceptions and cognitive experiences. It can lead to the person seeing the world very differently to others, or in an altered way, and losing touch with reality as other people see it (Young Minds 2024a, b). These experiences often change the way young people feel, as they cause anxiety and distress, and they can make young people behave differently, for example, avoiding people due to believing they are in danger. This is often very frightening for the young people who are experiencing these symptoms, as they can feel like their own minds and the responses of others are no longer trustworthy. For parents, having a child who is experiencing psychosis or psychotic-like experiences (PLE) is also often very frightening, as they may struggle to understand what is happening to their child, not know what to do, worry about whether their child is developing a serious mental illness and not know where to get help (Royal College of Psychiatry 2015).

As a professional who comes into contact with children and young people on a day-to-day basis, having foundational knowledge and understanding about psychotic experiences and symptoms, as a non-mental health specialist, can make a big difference to young people's trajectories and to their families, by helping reduce stigma and anxiety and helping to identify young people who may need specialist help and getting them to the right help, in the right place, at the right time (Northover 2022).

Hearing the word 'psychosis' can generate a lot of concern and unease. It gets linked with discriminatory terms such as 'psycho', 'schizo' and 'psychopath'. These are all unhelpful terms that can create fear and perpetuate stigma and shame, which then get in the way of young people seeking help. Psychosis is often also linked in people's minds with the medical term schizophrenia, which conjures up ideas of long-lasting and serious mental illness and myths about 'split personalities'. In fact, the term psychosis describes a collection of presenting symptoms, which can happen to any of us, given enough stress and/or coupled with any underlying vulnerabilities, and which can often resolve completely, on their own or with timely help and support. Even when young people have all of the symptoms needed to receive a diagnosis of schizophrenia, which denotes a more serious form of psychosis, it is important to understand that this condition is highly treatable (NICE 2016).

Psychosis is categorised by three main symptoms: hallucination, delusions and a diminished sense of what's real and what's not real, which can also include disruptions to usual thinking patterns, sometimes referred to as thought disorder (Royal College of Psychiatry 2015). Having psychosis doesn't mean you have to have all these symptoms. But regardless of how the young person's psychotic symptoms present themselves, it can be highly disturbing, frightening and debilitating for the young person.

Research has shown that psychotic experiences are influenced by social and psychological factors as well as biological ones. When psychological, social and biological factors interact, especially when acute life stressors occur, psychotic experiences can be the result, as people's usual apparatus for thinking gets overwhelmed. This is termed the stress vulnerability model (Patel et al. 2021). Hearing voices in particular seems to be a very common response to stress and anxiety in the general population. Ten to twenty per cent of the general population have heard voices at least once, and at least a third of the general population reported hearing a voice speaking their thoughts aloud, and research shows that 70% of people who hear voices do so following a traumatic event, e.g. sexual abuse, bereavement, sleep deprivation, experience of racism or discrimination of the grounds of a protected characteristics or being acutely physically unwell (Staines et al. 2022).

Psychotic experiences fall along a continuum, from having just one distinct symptom, which might only occur once or disappear spontaneously (usually an acute stress response), to having a cluster of symptoms that impact on the young person's overall wellbeing, don't go away on their own and indicate that the young person needs mental health assessment and support. Psychotic experiences can also occur as part of other emotional health difficulties and conditions. It is not uncommon for children and young people with acute anxiety to experience their own anxious thoughts as a voice that feels separate from the rest of their mind. Psychosis can be a symptom of depression or bipolar disorder, which are serious but treatable mood disorders (Young Minds 2024a, b). People who have experienced childhood abuse or discrimination with complex post-traumatic stress disorder can also experience the voice of their perpetrator and fragments of memory as auditory and visual hallucination-like phenomena (Longden et al. 2012).

The prevalence of psychotic illness in the general population (all ages) is estimated to be around 7%. The prevalence rates of psychosis and psychotic-like experiences in children and young people fall into two distinct categories (Staines et al. 2022):

- Seventeen per cent of 9–12-year-olds can experience unusual and psychotic-like symptoms.
- Eight per cent of 13–18-year-olds can experience unusual and psychotic-like symptoms.

Out of the 7.5% of adolescents that experience a first episode of psychosis, only an estimated 10–20% of those go on to have lasting or relapsing symptoms.

What is important to understand is that psychotic experiences and symptoms always have context and meaning. They often emerge as a natural human psychological response to stress or perceived threat (Johnstone and Boyle 2018). Remembering this can help engage young people; help them feel less stigma, shame and fear; and help them make sense of their experiences and access help. See Table 4.1 for a reflective activity to help you with this process.

4.1.1 What Is Bipolar Disorder and How Does It Relate to Psychosis?

Bipolar disorder is a diagnostic term used to describe a serious mood disorder that is characterised by a cycle of movement between extreme states of low mood or depression and very high or elated mood states, often referred to as mania (Royal College of Psychiatry 2015). When a person experiences extremes of low or high mood, they can often also experience psychotic-like symptoms alongside the mood disturbance; this most often presents as unusual or delusional ideas. The prevalence

Table 4.1 Reflective activity 1

Reflective activity 1: Contextualising and normalising psychotic experiences
How might we empathise with what a young person with psychosis is going through? The first thing is to recognise that nearly everyone has had a perceptual disturbance or psychotic-like experience at some point in their life. It is often helpful to young people to learn that psychotic-like experiences are quite common and can usually be explained
Think of a time when you have had unusual experiences or disturbance of perception. Perhaps you were overly tired, were jetlagged, had experienced bereavement, had a very high temperature due to being unwell and had a little more alcohol than you expected on a night out.
What was the experience that happened to you (e.g. auditory and visual disturbances, changes to your thoughts or how the environment around you looked)?
What did it feel like in the moment of having this experience?
What would have made these feelings worse?
What would have made them better?
Reflecting on this experience and the things that would help you, write down three things you could do to support a young person who is having psychotic experiences and to reduce their distress?

of bipolar disorder in the general population is estimated to be around 2% (Young Minds 2024a, b). The prevalence in children and young people is much lower than experiencing psychotic symptoms alone. It is extremely rare in children, and if a young person does develop bipolar disorder, onset is usually in late adolescence or young adulthood (16–24 years). The risk factors for developing bipolar disorder are very similar to those we have already explained for psychosis. Bipolar disorder is a major mood disorder that usually requires specialist multidisciplinary care, it is also highly treatable, and with early detection and help, young people and the adults can live well with long periods of remission. There are no standalone NICE clinical guidelines for the assessment and treatment of bipolar disorder in children and young people; instead, the guidelines and standards for identification, assessment and intervention for psychosis are used to guide care (NICE 2015). Therefore, the information in the rest of this chapter will help you understand how and why young people may be vulnerable to experiencing psychotic-like experiences and what to do if you suspect a child or young person you are working with to be experiencing either psychosis or extreme or rapid changes in their mood.

4.2 Developmental Factors That Might Make Young People More Vulnerable to Psychosis

Everybody has his or her own level of vulnerability or proneness to developing psychosis. This level is set by things we have inherited from our parents through our genes and by experiences we have had growing up. Evidence tells us that stressful life events very often happen to a person just before a psychotic episode. One way to think about the stress-vulnerability model is to use the stress bucket analogy, illustrated in Fig. 4.1 (Brabban and Turkington 2002). Some people will have quite a high level of vulnerability, and so only a small amount of stressful experience will

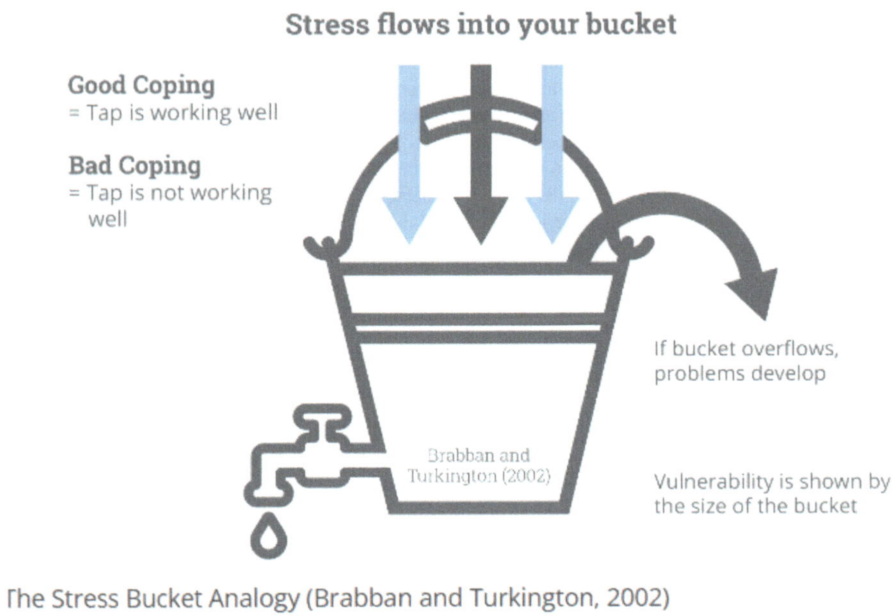

Fig. 4.1 Stress bucket analogy of the stress-vulnerability model

lead to psychosis. On the other hand, some people will have a low level of vulnerability, but if they experience a massive amount of stress, they will experience psychosis.

Imagine a bucket of water. The bucket might be small, so only a small amount of water is needed to make it overflow. On the other hand, it might be large, but pouring in lots of water will still make it overflow. Having a range of good coping skills and resources acts like a tap and can keep the bucket from overflowing.

For children and young people, normal developmental phenomena add to this mix, making it more complicated. Using the stress bucket analogy, their buckets are by definition smaller as they are still developing, and their coping skills tap is less well developed, and for teenagers in particular, the amount of water they have to hold in them is bigger.

You may have noticed that the prevalence of psychotic-like experiences in children aged 9–12 years is actually higher than in teenagers or adults. If you think about it, children in this age range are naturally wired to think in a very black and white way and to accept what they see, even if it doesn't quite add up (e.g. the story of Father Christmas). In child development terms, this is referred to as the concrete operational stage of thinking (Piaget 1976). It is usual for children to have magical thinking and vivid imaginations, essential to help them play, create and learn. You may even remember having an imaginary friend yourself at that stage of life and feeling as though they were absolutely real. At this age, children also do not have very developed capacities to cope with strong emotion and stress and have very little power to help them get away from stressful things. In good-enough circumstances, they rely on adults to help them with this, until they can learn to do it themselves. However, if a child's mind has to cope with something that is too big for their mental coping bucket, and they can't get away, then it becomes overwhelmed, and the unconscious survival strategy of dissociation kicks in (zoning out, feeling unreal or out of body). Psychotic-like experiences in young children are quite common and not usually an indicator of the onset of a psychotic illness, but more often a sign that a child may be feeling overwhelmed or worried by something.

In adolescence, there are additional physical, psychological and emotional burdens that are part of normal teenage development, but which can also add an extra layer of stress and which make adolescents more vulnerable than people in other life stages to experiencing psychotic symptoms and illness. These include significant changes in several domains, including brain structure and function, puberty and hormones, psychosexual development and social and environmental changes (Patel et al. 2021). To provide context, it is important to understand a little bit about young people's brain development and how this can bring about changes in brain functioning processing, emotional development and thinking and how a young person manages what life throws at them. Maturation of brain development ready for adulthood starts in the early to mid-teen and is known scientifically to be one of the most significant biological and psychological upheavals (Dumontheil 2016). In this life stage, teenage brains go through a protracted period of 'pruning'. Pruning is the term for the period of physical brain growth and refinement, where unused neural pathways and connections within the brain are either kept or pruned away. Pruning is a process that sets a young person's intrinsic thinking and processing, impacting on how the young person sees and responds to the world around them (Dumontheil 2016).

It is still relatively unknown among parents and people who work with teenagers, but not unsurprising given our new understandings of the brain, that even during a period of 'normal' brain development, a young person can experience transient unusual psychological phenomena such as psychotic-'like' symptoms. This can come in the form of hearing sounds, seeing objects and having unusual thoughts and beliefs. It can be precipitated by common life stressors, such as loss of a significant other, i.e. a grandparent, moving home or school, away from friends and subject to bullying. It is important to note that unusual symptoms as part of normal brain development doesn't mean a young person will go on to have a psychosis illness.

However, young people that are having to grow their new upgraded brains while being subject to trauma, abuse or other adverse childhood experiences (ACEs) are at much higher risk of developing a psychotic illness, due to the negative effects ACES are known to have on child neurodevelopment (Foster and Gardner 2023), especially if early help is not sought. Adolescence is also a time of higher likelihood of experimentation and exposure to recreational drug and alcohol use, which is known to have a unique interaction with the process of pruning and teenage neurodevelopment (Patel et al. 2021), making some young people much more susceptible to drug- and alcohol-induced psychotic symptoms, compared to adult counterparts.

As much as these additional stress factors can increase a teenager's vulnerability, the available positive growth-promoting relationships with reliable, thoughtful and supportive adults serve to offset the risks and act as protective factors, helping young people to increase the size of their stress bucket over time.

4.3 Identifying Signs and Symptoms of Psychosis

Clinicians describe the symptoms of psychosis as positive and negative symptoms, i.e. things that are 'added' and things that are 'taken away'. This refers to the symptoms and the impact of symptoms of psychosis. Table 4.2 summarises some of the main signs and symptoms of psychosis.

Table 4.2 Common signs, symptoms and impacts of psychosis

Positive symptoms	**Auditory hallucinations**	Hearing voices or sounds that cannot be heard by others. Visual hallucinations can vary in intensity, they can range between: hallucination, they can range from a clear voice or sounds to undistinguishable muttering, catching the odd word, whispers or sounds
	Visual hallucinations	Seeing people, shapes and forms that cannot be seen by others. Visual hallucinations can vary in there intensity, they can range between: A clear form, shape or person with distinguishable characteristics, i.e. male, female, eyes, nose and mouth Blurred form, shapes or person with undistinguishable features Forms, shapes or person out of the corner of the eye
	Delusions	Strong beliefs felt to be absolutely true that diverge from what is commonly believed by most people, for example: Beliefs that they have special gifts and powers that other do not have Ideas of reference—Making links with numbers or signs, believing messages are especially for them Beliefs that they are seriously ill despite medical evidence Beliefs that people are trying to harm them.
Negative symptoms	**Deterioration in global functions**	Presenting a more isolative, not seeing friends Not engaging the things they enjoy Refusing to go to school or playing truant Decline in self-care Sleep disturbance
	Deterioration in mood	Anxiety and low mood as a result of having unusual and frightening experiences and due to feeling of shame and stigma
	Disturbed cognitive processes	Feeling thoughts are blocked or can't be accessed Difficulties expressing oneself fluently (unusual speech patterns) Memory problems Problems with concentration

NICE (2015, 2016), Royal College of Psychiatry (2015), Staines et al. (2022)

Sometimes unusual fixed or delusional beliefs come without hallucinations, as young people misinterpret normal events that have happened to them (often through the lens of acute stress), leading them to come to incorrect or distorted conclusions. Sometimes delusional beliefs actually emerge later, in response to experiencing auditory and visual hallucinations, as the mind's way of trying to make sense of these strange experiences.

An important part of how mental health professionals assess the impact and severity of the symptoms the young person is experiencing is to understand the degree to which they believe that what they are seeing, hearing or thinking is real or absolutely true. This is referred to as the degree of conviction. When levels of conviction are high, it is more likely that the young person's behaviour will change as they respond to what the experience is telling them, for example, refusing food due to fear that it is contaminated or someone wants to poison them.

As adults, it is easier for us to recognise that our thoughts are not always 100% true or trustworthy and that they can change and be influenced by what is happening around us and by our mood. This allows us to recognise that something unusual is going on in our mind but also know that it is not all of our mind and to test the idea against what the rest of our experience tells us is reality. It can help us be less distressed or worried by transient psychotic-like experiences and also help us refrain from acting on unusual thoughts. Young people often find this harder and so are more likely to present in acute crisis, due to the distress caused by the symptoms and the behaviour changes and coping responses they produce. For example, young people may be more likely to present with agitation, aggression, suspicion or paranoia, if they are concerned others may want to harm them. They also may experience suicidal impulses and use alcohol or self-injury to cope, if the changes in their mind overwhelm them, and are more than they feel able to bear (Power and Robinson 2009).

This means whenever a young person shows up somewhere in crisis, even if, at first glance, their behaviour looks to be oppositional or 'usual teenage challenging/rebellious behaviour', all professionals should hold in mind the possibility that there may be more to it than meets the eye and take time to talk with the young person to understand their perspective and concerns.

4.4 At-Risk Mental State

Often, before young people develop very clear symptoms, there can be a run-up period, during which the young person's psychosocial and cognitive functioning deteriorates and people that know them or have contact with them on a day-to-day basis have a feeling that things are not quite right. This may include problems with memory and concentration, unusual behaviour and ideas, disturbed communication and affect, social withdrawal and loss of motivation. This is called an 'at-risk mental state' (Yung et al. 2005), or you may also sometimes hear professionals refer to the idea of a 'prodromal period', although this is something that can only be identified in hindsight, once a young person has received a diagnosis of a psychotic illness.

Identifying young people with at-risk mental states is a really important part of successful prevention and early intervention, and there is strong evidence that specialist assessment and access to education, CBT and family support can prevent at-risk mental states from developing into first-episode psychotic illness (NHS England 2023). Non-mental health specialists who know the young person well, such as teachers, support workers and youth workers, are usually in the best place to spot the early signs and signpost them and their families to get help.

4.5 Case Example

The case study in Table 4.3 highlights the challenges that young people face and how this can impact on their mental health, vulnerability and susceptibility to developing psychotic symptoms. It also highlights the importance of identifying early warning signs and of acting quickly to support young people to help avert them becoming unwell.

4.5.1 Identifying Challenges and Missed Opportunities for Ben

As we have already identified earlier in the chapter, adolescence is a time of significant change and psychological turmoil. The transition from school into further education and the change of peer group and environment are in itself psychological stressors and make young people more vulnerable to mental distress. While it is absolutely true that many young people who develop psychosis have a history of experiencing trauma or childhood adversity (Longden et al. 2012), this can also make professionals less alert to the needs of young people where there is no such history, meaning that important risk factors and early warning signs can be missed. It is clear from the case study that Ben's studies were important to him and that he was a high achiever in school. This can mask underlying performance anxieties and lead to high levels of expectation and pressure from inside the young person and from education environments that can make them highly susceptible to psychotic-type experiences, especially if something goes wrong in that area, as it did in this case. School and college procedures for fair practice and investigation allegations of wrongdoing are of course there for a reason and to help all pupils feel safe. However, these kinds of formal investigations are also very stressful and can be felt by young people as a threat to their future, even before finding yourself wrongly accused (imagine the impact as an adult of being incorrectly accused of wrongdoing in the workplace and facing a formal investigation, without any support from HR or a union, and now imagine being a young person who has received messages since childhood that how they perform in school will set the tone for the rest of their life).

Ben should have received support throughout the process of investigation, from a trusted teacher or other member of staff, as it was known that it was having a significant impact on his mental health. After it was discovered that he was the victim of plagiarism, additional support from pastoral care or college counsellor may have

Table 4.3 Case study

Case study: Ben's story
This is an example based on a composite of a number of real-life cases. Specific details have been omitted and changed, and the name given is a pseudonym, in order to maintain anonymity and confidentiality. In this case study, we will explore the circumstances that led to ben, a 16 years old, with no history of mental health difficulties, from a background without adversity and with very supportive family and good friends, to develop psychotic symptoms.
Presenting difficulties
Ben's parents have been ringing his GP, terribly distressed because he is not taking part in family life, has stopped seeing his friends, is very suspicious of them and is expressing ideas that people want to cause him harm. ben has withdrawn to his bedroom and stopped with his studies. When he does have contact with his parents, he is irritable and aggressive with them. They report finding it hard to get ben to eat regular meals or to wash and change his clothes.
Background history
Ben has always been very focused in his studies and has always been keen to achieve good grades. After achieving excellent GCSE results, he is now attending college, working toward A-levels, so he can go on to attend university to study biological sciences. There was an incident that occurred at college where he was accused of plagiarising a fellow student's course work. Following an investigation at college, it was later found that ben had been in fact a victim of plagiarism. Ben was then expected to continue with his studies as though nothing had happened. he was not offered any supportive feedback, or pastoral care, or help to return to studies. By the time the investigation was completed, ben had already started developing mental health symptoms of anxiety, depression and poor self-confidence. His parents later started to notice that he had started to become more irritable and behaving strangely and becoming paranoid that his phone and laptop was hacked.
Ben's mental health deteriorated further, and he became aggressive when her parents tried to support him. This got progressively worse and eventually came to a head when there was an incident of physical aggression from ben towards his father. At this point, the police were called to the home. The police left the home after talking to ben, stating he appeared calm and rational. there was another incident where ben became acutely mentally distressed and paranoid. The parents managed to get him to agree to be taken to their local A&E department for a mental health assessment. When the mental health triage team assessed ben after a wait in A&E, he was seen alone and presented as calm and rational. he was later discharged with phone contacts for NHS services and organisations that could support him if he wanted to discuss his mental health.
Reflective activity
Thinking about what you have learnt in this chapter so far, what factors do you think might have contributed to ben going 'under the radar' and not getting help more quickly?
Review the background information and identify at least three points in the timeline when something different could have been done to intervene earlier

averted a significant episode of mental distress. Arranging supportive contact with Ben in this way has the potential to avert development of an at-risk mental state or may have brought concerns about his at-risk mental state to light earlier and enabled a referral for specialist assessment to be sought. When the police attended and interviewed Ben and his parents, information could have been provided at that point about how to access mental health support from local services. When Ben attended A&E, although it was appropriate to interview him alone because of his age, the team could also have sought consent from Ben to meet with his parents to take a history of their concerns and gain a fuller picture of the situation. The A&E team could also have requested the GP or the local crisis team to do a follow-up appointment with Ben.

4.6 Specialist Mental Health Services and the Care Pathway for Young People Suspected to Be Showing Signs of Psychosis

The National Institute for Health and Care Excellence (NICE) has published clinical guidelines about the best evidence-based assessment and treatment and care pathways that children and young people experiencing psychotic symptoms should receive (NICE 2016). In 2016, Implementing the Early Intervention in Psychosis Teams (EIT) Access and Waiting Time Standard guidance was first published, and it was last updated in 2023 (NHS England). This key guidance was developed from the best available research into understanding psychosis to improve treatment and reduce the risk of young people needing to be assessed and cared for in psychiatric hospitals, which can have a negative effect on young people's wellbeing and development (Hannigan et al. 2019).

It resulted in the implementation of national minimum standards and creation of specialist mental health multidisciplinary services, available in every locality, for people at risk of or experiencing first-episode psychosis from the age range from 14 to 65. The key messages from the guidance (NHS 2023) is that assessing and identifying at-risk mental states (ARMS) and the early phases of psychosis quickly and providing multidisciplinary packages of evidence-based care in the community can prevent onset of illness for some young people, improve recovery rates and clinical outcomes for those who develop psychosis and reduce the likelihood of relapse in the future.

Young people with suspected ARMS or psychosis should have access to specialist EIP services via self-referral, GPs and Child and Adolescent Mental Health Services (CAMHS) and should be assessed within 2 weeks of the referral being received (NHS 2023).

The care pathway is summarised in Fig. 4.2. Early intervention in psychosis (EIP) services provide two arms of treatment: the Early Detection and Intervention Team (EDIT) for young people with at-risk mental states, but who have not yet developed a first episode of psychotic illness, and the Early Intervention Team (EIT), who provide multidisciplinary evidence-based treatments for young people identified as experiencing a first psychotic episode or illness.

4.6.1 What Should NICE-Approved Packages of Care Look Like?

The NHS England guidance provides clear information of what young people and families should expect from their treatment. This is summarised in Table 4.4. Knowing about this can help you help families advocate for their children.

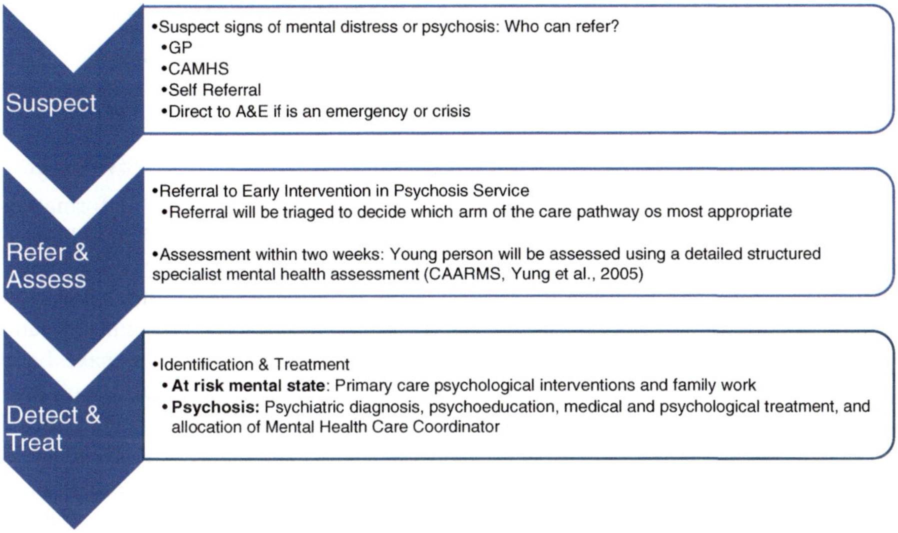

Fig. 4.2 Care pathway for young people suspected of ARMS or psychosis. (Adapted NHSE 2023)

Table 4.4 Evidence-based care packages

At-risk mental state	Early detection and intervention team (EDIT)	Assessment, diagnosis and commencement of antipsychotic medication (with consent), by a psychiatrist Psychological therapy/CBT for psychosis Psychoeducation: About psychosis Family work Care coordination and monitoring of physical and mental health Multi-agency review meetings Inpatient hospital care, only if needs and risks cannot be managed safely at home, even with extra support
Psychosis	Early intervention team (EIT)	Allocation of a primary care psychologist to deliver evidence-based CBT or other therapy for psychotic-like experiences Psychoeducation and information Family support
In all cases	Support to remain in, or reengage with, education or meaningful occupational and leisure activity	

Adapted from NHSE (2023)

4.7 What Can You Do to Support a Young Person You Suspect May Have Psychosis?

Equip yourself with information and provide parents/carers and young people with information

Reading this chapter is already a good start. Equipping yourself with information and knowledge so that you know how to spot the warning signs and know how to help a young person will make a big difference to the young people you work with. There are also some recommended online resources at the end of this chapter to help you build your knowledge further.

Don't be frightened to engage young people, to help reduce shame, stigma and fear

Listen, do not judge and seek to understand the young person's perspective, thoughts, feelings and concerns, even if these are different to yours. Validate their feelings and reassure where you can. Notice and be respectfully curious about changes in behaviours and thoughts, in order to try and get a better individual understanding of the young person's difficulties (Yung Yung et al. 2005). However, be sure to give the young person plenty of physical and interpersonal space. Respect their wishes and to go at their pace. Remember that young people may not be able to concentrate or take part for social interaction for very long, if they are experiencing symptoms of psychosis.

As many young people experiencing psychosis or psychotic-like experiences have a history of traumatic or adverse experiences, it is a good starting point to always adopt the principles of trauma-informed care (The Wave Trust 2024). These are things that anyone can do, and which help set the context, so frightened and traumatised young people feel safe, but they are also good for everyone. The key principle of trauma-informed care is to act in ways that promote:

- Safety.
- Trust.
- Choice.
- Collaboration.
- Empowerment.

You can learn more about how to implement these principles I practise via the online resources provided at the end of this chapter (Table 4.5).

Signpost and help with referrals to early intervention in psychosis services

Seek advice from your manager/senior member of staff. Arrange to talk with the young person to find out more. Talk to parents and carers and encourage self-referral or to contact the GP to ask for a referral. If the young person is in crisis or it is an

Table 4.5 Online resources

Information for young people
Young minds: Psychosis
https://www.youngminds.org.uk/young-person/mental-health-conditions/psychosis/
Information and guidance for concerned parents and family members
Royal College of psychiatry: Psychosis in children and young people a guide for parents and careers
https://www.rcpsych.ac.uk/mental-health/parents-and-young-people/psychosis-in-young-people
Understanding the way early childhood adversity and trauma can affect young people's cognitive development
Wave trust: 70/30 campaign
https://www.wavetrust.org/adverse-childhood-experiences-infographics
https://www.wavetrust.org/childhood-trauma-trauma-informed-care
Information about prevalence of common mental health disorders
Mental Health Foundation: Mental health statistics
https://www.mentalhealth.org.uk/explore-mental-health/statistics

emergency, advise the family to attend A&E, or if this is not possible (e.g. due to immediate risks to self or others), ring 999 and call an ambulance.

4.8 Conclusion

This chapter has explored how a young person's early influences, stressors, relationships, culture, access to education and leisure can shape their ongoing growth, development, coping, psychological wellbeing and resilience to developing significant mental health difficulties like psychosis. Through our new understanding of complex biological processes such as 'pruning' as a part of ordinary brain development and growth, we can see how a young person's formative years frames their thinking and how they see the world around them. In a good-enough circumstances, young people are equipped with a secure base of supportive relationships and developmental milestones such as education that serve as protective factors. However, the stress and strains of adolescent biopsychosocial development can still result in a struggle with their thoughts, perceptions and mental wellbeing. Understanding psychosis and psychotic-like experiences in an 'early development' and 'brain development' perspective can help you identify young people who need help early, including those who might otherwise 'go under the radar'. By being curious and knowing a little about a young person's experience and providing support in a timely way, you can contribute to averting significant mental distress. It is our role as adults to be flexible, responsive and mindful of potential challenges and appreciative of stressors that young people face. As a rule of thumb, if things don't look, sound or feel right, it usually follows that young person is not feeling alright; everything you notice about the changes they are presenting with is all important information.

Mental health services are now well developed to meet the needs of young people presenting with psychosis or psychotic experiences. Service frameworks for early intervention were implemented in understanding that psychosis is completely treatable with early identification and treatment. This is why it is absolutely imperative that early warning signs and symptoms are recognised at the earliest opportunity. In this way, all professionals can make an important contribution to prevention and recovery from psychosis, whether it be a teacher, a police officer or a social worker.

References

Brabban A, Turkington D. The search for meaning: detecting congruence between live events, underlying schema and psychotic symptoms. In: Morrison AP, editor. A casebook of cognitive therapy for psychosis. New York: Brunner-Routledge; 2002. p. 59–75.

Dumontheil I. Adolescent brain development. Curr Opin Behav Sci. 2016;10:39–44.

Foster C, Gardner L. Understanding the developmental impact of domestic violence and adverse experiences in childhood across the life-course. In: Roddy J, editor. Working with client experiences of domestic abuse. Taylor & Francis (Routledge); 2023. p. 117–32. https://doi.org/10.4324/9781003253266-9.

Hannigan B, Goold M, Maxwell E. Risks of admitting children and young people to mental health inpatient units. Nurs Manag. 2019;26(2):17–9.

Johnstone L, Boyle M. The power threat meaning framework: an alternative nondiagnostic conceptual system. J Humanist Psychol. 2018; https://doi.org/10.1177/0022167818793289.

Longden E, Madill A, Waterman MG. Dissociation, trauma, and the role of lived experience: toward a new conceptualization of voice hearing. Psychol Bull. 2012;138(1):28.

Mental Health Foundation. Mental health statistics; 2024. Available from: https://www.mentalhealth.org.uk/explore-mental-health/statistics. Accessed 7 Oct 2024.

NHS England. Implementing the Early Intervention in Psychosis Access and Waiting Time Standard; 2023. Available from: https://www.england.nhs.uk/wp-content/uploads/2023/03/B1954-implementing-the-early-intervention-in-psychosis-access-and-waiting-time-standard.pdf. Accessed 7 Oct 2024

NICE. Bipolar disorder, psychosis and schizophrenia in children and young people. Quality Standard 102; 2015. Available from: https://www.nice.org.uk/guidance/qs102. Accessed 7 Oct 2024

NICE. Psychosis and schizophrenia in children and young people: recognition and management. Clinical guideline 155; 2016. Available from: https://www.nice.org.uk/guidance/cg155/. Accessed 7 Oct 2024

Northover, G. GIRFT programme national specialty report for children and young people's mental health services. NHS England; 2022. Available from: https://gettingitrightfirsttime.co.uk/medical_specialties/mh-cyp/. Accessed 7 Oct 2024

Patel PK, Leathem LD, Currin DL, Karlsgodt KH. Adolescent neurodevelopment and vulnerability to psychosis. Biol Psychiatry. 2021;89(2):184–93. https://doi.org/10.1016/j.biopsych.2020.06.028.

Piaget J. Piaget's theory. In: Inhelder B, Chipman HH, Zwingmann C, editors. Piaget and his school. Berlin, Heidelberg: Springer Study Edition. Springer; 1976.

Power P, Robinson J. Suicide prevention in first-episode psychosis. In: McGorry P, Jackson H, editors. The recognition and management of early psychosis: a preventative approach. Cambridge University Press; 2009.

Royal College of Psychiatry. Psychosis in children and young people. A guide for parents and careers; 2015. Available from: https://www.rcpsych.ac.uk/mental-health/parents-and-young-people/information-for-parents-and-carers/psychosis-for-parents. Accessed 7 Oct 2024

Staines L, Healy C, Coughlan H, Clarke M, Kelleher I, Cotter D, Cannon M. Psychotic experiences in the general population, a review; definition, risk factors, outcomes and interventions. Psychol Med. 2022;52:1–12.

Wave Trust. Childhood trauma and trauma informed care; 2024. Available form: https://www.wavetrust.org/childhood-trauma-trauma-informed-care. Accessed 7 Oct 2024

Young Minds. Psychosis; 2024a. Available from: https://www.youngminds.org.uk/young-person/mental-health-conditions/psychosis/. Accessed 7 Oct 2024

Young Minds. Information for young people: Mental health conditions; 2024b. Available from: https://www.youngminds.org.uk/young-person/mental-health-conditions. Accessed 7 Oct 2024

Yung AR, Yuen HP, McGorry PD, et al. Mapping the onset of psychosis – the comprehensive assessment of at risk mental states (CAARMS). ANZJP. 2005;39:964–71.

Learning Disabilities and Neurodiversity

5

Valerie Houghton, Moyosore Opebiyi, Sarah Kennedy, and Vanessa Heaslip

V. Houghton (✉)
School of Health and Social Care, Edinburgh Napier University, Edinburgh, Scotland, UK
e-mail: v.houghton@napier.ac.uk

M. Opebiyi
Directorate of Social Sciences, University of Salford, Salford, UK
e-mail: m.opebiyi1@salford.ac.uk

S. Kennedy
Faculty of Health and Wellbeing, University of Bolton, Bolton, UK
e-mail: s.kennedy@bolton.ac.uk

V. Heaslip
Directorate of Nursing and Midwifery, University of Salford, Salford, UK
e-mail: V.A.Heaslip@salford.ac.uk

G. Trainor, V. Heaslip (eds.), *Needs of Children and Young People Living with Complex Mental Health Difficulties*,
https://doi.org/10.1007/978-3-031-84532-1_5

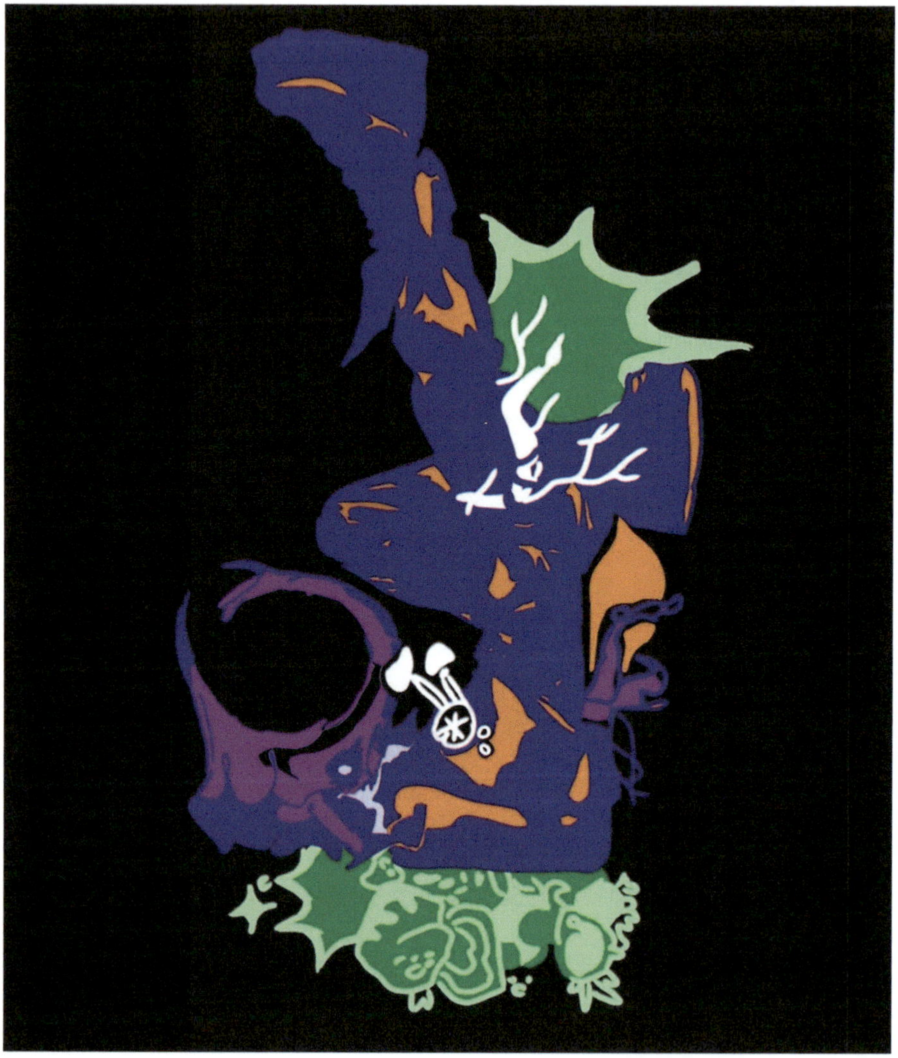

5.1 Background Context

It is estimated that 28.9 million (4.3%) of children aged 0–4 years, 207.4 million (12.5%) of children aged 5–17 years and 236.4 million (10.1%) of all children aged 0–17 years have moderate-to-severe disabilities globally (Olusanya et al. 2022). The life experiences of children living with disabilities are poor when compared to children without a disability. Children living with a disability are more likely to have poorer educational experience and attainment, have poorer physical health and mental health and are more likely to experience discrimination (UNICEF 2022). Furthermore, once they reach adulthood, they are more likely to be unemployed (United Nations undated) or in low-paid employment increasing their chances of living their lives in poverty (Chap. 7 discusses the links between poverty and mental health). However, 'disability' is somewhat a nebulous term as it collectively refers to individuals with different experiences, such as being born with a cognitive impairment or becoming disabled because of chronic illness or accident (Heaslip 2020). As such, it is difficult to identify prevalence of intellectual disability. Whilst there are a range of terms used globally, the most common is an intellectual disability or learning disability.

In terms of diagnosis of an intellectual disability, both the UK and international definitions (British Psychological Society 2015) identify three key criteria that must be met, including:

- Significant impairment of intellectual functioning
- Significant impairment of adaptive behaviour (social functioning)
- Both impairments arising before adulthood

Within this, it must be recognised that there is a continuum of needs, classified as mild, moderate, severe or profound, denoting the level of support the individual may need. Reasons for the development of an intellectual disability are varied and can include an inherited condition, abnormal chromosomes, exposure to environmental toxins or infections and illness during pregnancy, very premature birth or complication during birth or illness (Public Health England 2023).

Neurodiversity is the term used to describe a range of conditions including autism/autism spectrum condition (ASC)/autism spectrum disorder (ASD), attention deficit hyperactivity disorder (ADHD)/variable attention stimulus trait (VAST), dyspraxia, dyslexia, dysgraphia, dyscalculia and Tourette's syndrome (TS). It is estimated that one in seven people is neurodivergent (NHS England undated). Like intellectual disability, there can be a continuum of needs ranging from those who require minimal assistance to those who require significant support in day-to-day activities. It is important to remember that neurodiversity itself is not a mental illness; however, children and young people who are neurodivergent like children and young people with a disability can experience a mental health issue during their childhood and adult lives.

5.2 Policy Context

The Health and Care Act (2022) S21A requires all 'service providers' to have training on autism and learning disability 'relevant to their role'. There is a clear emphasis through all child policy and legislation that we must work in a person-centred way, placing the child (and their family) at the centre of all decision-making. This means more than a tokenistic approach, with a real commitment to involve children and young people at all stages. Using creative ways of working with children and young people is crucial to enabling children with learning disabilities and those who are neurodivergent to have a voice. This will be explored later in this chapter.

It is useful to consider the legal framework that sets out the rights of children with learning disabilities and neurodivergent children. It is important to remember that all children are children first, thus included in all legislation and policy, which is child focused. The reader here is directed towards Chap. 8 (safeguarding) regarding international and UK law that protects children. There are, however, specific acts, policies and statutory guidance, which aim to ensure the rights of children with learning disabilities and autistic children have the same opportunities as all children for education, good health and inclusion in their local communities. The Children Act (1989) is the main legislation in England and Wales, which aims to protect children from harm and provides the statutory basis for most children's services. Within this Act, the welfare of the child is paramount, and the child's needs and wishes must be considered in all decisions made. Whilst the best place for a child to grow up is often within their family, however, if this is considered to place the child at risk of harm, they become a 'child in need'. This status places extra duties on local authorities to provide services for the child(ren) and their families. The Children Act (2004) extends a duty to other agencies including the police and health services, when working with children to consider the need to safeguard and promote the welfare of children (section 11). The statutory guidance Working Together to Safeguard Children (Gov.uk 2023a) advocates a multi-agency approach to safeguarding. This is important because disabled children are more likely to be victims of sexual violence than non-disabled children, particularly those living in residential special schools at some distance from their home (Jay et al. 2022). Some children with learning disabilities may have communication difficulties, which could mean they are unable to communicate this violence or that family members, carers, teaching staff or other professionals may not be able to understand and respond to their disclosures (Gov.uk 2023a, b). Health and social care staff and others encountering children in the course of their work roles must be alert to the possibility that sexual violence may be happening and pay close attention to children who seem to be trying to communicate this to adults.

According to the Human Rights Act (1998), all children and young people with a learning disability or neurodivergence should not be denied the right to education. In addition, the Equality Act (2010) in the UK protects children with a learning disability or neurodivergence from discrimination at school on the grounds of their disability. This means schools must know who is disabled and make reasonable adjustments so they can have the same academic and other school opportunities as all children (Stobbs 2022). Inclusive education for all children is a global priority (UNESCO 1994), legislated for in England and Wales through the Children and Families Act (2014). An important feature of this Act focuses on supporting all children to have access to mainstream education, where they can learn alongside their peers. This also can be achieved by joint working between agencies working for children and young people. There are two levels of support within the Act: Special Educational Needs and Disabilities (SEND) provision for children with special educational needs who may not be disabled (e.g. some autistic children) and a multi-agency Education, Health and Care Plan (EHCP) for children with learning disabilities and additional health needs. The EHCP has clear objectives based on each child's health support and education needs, which should mean each child can attend mainstream school, but in England and Wales, some children attend specialist educational provision where children's complex health and social care needs are met through pooling of resources, facilities and specially trained staff.

For autistic children, whilst the Autism Act (2009) addressed only the need of autistic adults, the 5-year strategy (DHSC 2021b) includes autistic children and young people. The strategy aims to help people to understand autism, thus enabling autistic children and young people at school and making health and care and the criminal justice system more responsive to the needs of autistic children and young people. Children and adults with learning disabilities are more likely to die prematurely (Sleap et al. 2024; Heslop et al. 2022; Mazars 2015). Many of these deaths may be because of life-limiting illness but many are avoidable (Heslop et al. 2022). Following the Mazars report and campaigning by families and disability rights organisations, the Confidential Inquiry into Premature Deaths (Cipold) analysed the deaths of people with learning disabilities aged 4 years and over. This programme identified that 42% of these deaths could have been prevented with better care and support (Heslop et al. 2022). Recent figures indicate that whilst approximately 2.5% of children have learning disabilities, they account for a large proportion of child deaths: 40% of 4–9-year-olds, 34% of 10–14-year-olds and 20% of 15–17-year-olds (Sleap et al. 2024). Additionally, this research identified this figure is much higher in children of Asian/Asian British ethnicity (Sleap et al. 2024).

Following this Inquiry, the Learning (Intellectual) Disabilities Mortality Review (LeDeR) programme was developed in England in 2015 (Heslop et al. 2022). LeDeR reviews aim to disseminate learning and recommendations from avoidable deaths. Adjustments are vital when working with children and young people with learning disabilities and neurodivergence. Heslop et al. (2019) separate these into system-level and individual-level adjustments, both needed for equitable access to health and social care. System-level adjustments aim to make person-centred care possible and include making environments accessible, using easy to read information and hospital passports and interpreters. Individual-level adjustments are specific to the child and are developed with the child and people that know them well. Hospital passports are documents that should travel with the chid or young person to provide key information regarding them and should be referred to whilst in hospital and taken home again upon discharge. The passport tells you important information, which includes what you must know about the child, along with what is important to and for the individual, their likes and dislikes, how to best communicate with the child and how to interpret a child's behaviour. The hospital passport also includes useful contact numbers for the child/young person and possibly their community learning disability nurse (see Reflective Activity 5.1).

Reflective Activity 5.1
Read about hospital passports via https://www.mefirst.org.uk/resource/hospital-passport/ have you seen these or contributed to the development of one of these through the course of your professional role. Reflect whether these passports would be useful for you when working with children and young people with an intellectual disability or who are neurodiverse.

The consequences of not using such personalised information were starkly evidenced in cases of Oliver McGowan and Connor Sparrowhawk who were young autistic people with learning disabilities (both 18) who died whilst being cared for in hospital (see Table 5.1 for case study of Oliver and Connor).

Table 5.1 Case study of Oliver and Connor

Case study 1	
Oliver McGowan (Richie 2020)	Connor Sparrowhawk
Oliver was autistic and had cerebral palsy and mild learning disabilities following meningitis as a baby. Oliver was popular, achieving success at GCSE/BTEC, and went on to college. He had played schoolboy football for England	Connor was admitted to a specialist NHS unit for assessment because of a change in his behaviour but died 107 days later
Oliver had epilepsy, and when he was 17 years old, his seizures became more frequent, and he was admitted several times to hospital. Oliver was scared and anxious about what was happening to him, which exacerbated some of his autistic behaviours. Rather than offering him reassurances, staff medicated Oliver with antipsychotic medication, despite there being no diagnosis of psychosis. The medication did not calm Oliver; instead, it made things much worse, making Oliver feel very unwell and increasing his seizures. This was recorded on Oliver's hospital passport. When he was 18, he was admitted to A&E because of seizures, but no reasonable adjustments were made, and Oliver was prevented from walking around, which helped when he was having seizures. He was restrained and became increasingly anxious. Despite Oliver and his parents trying to ensure that he was not given antipsychotic medication, including emails, warnings on case notes, verbal instructions and Oliver himself telling staff what would happen, he was again given antipsychotic medication, which caused neuroleptic malignant syndrome, and he subsequently died (McGowan n.d.) [see also Richie 2020]	Connor's death was initially recorded as natural causes, but following an independent investigation, it was ruled that his death was preventable, because the staff knew he had epilepsy and could have taken steps to mitigate the risks (Salman 2014). There was no care plan or safe observation strategies, and the staff did not manage his epilepsy (Inquest.org 2014), but also family were excluded, and there was a lack of clinical leadership, and the unit did not give Connor the opportunity to join in activities (Salman 2014)

5.2.1 Causes of Learning Disabilities and Neurodiversity and Common Conditions

As has already been established, a learning disability needs to have 'started before adulthood, with a lasting effect on development' (Department of Health 2001). There are many causes of learning disabilities; some are known and understood, others less so. The term 'learning disability' is a broad term under which those who are affected may be described as having some degree of challenge in terms of intellectual and social functioning (Watson 1997). A learning disability is the result of single or multiple factors that occur before birth (prenatal), during birth (perinatal) or after birth (postnatal). Within these stages, Schalock et al. (2019) identify four categories of risk factors that can potentially occur within each of the three stages: biomedical, social, behavioural and educational (Table 5.2).

For some babies, their learning disability is evident at birth due to physical characteristics—for example, Down syndrome. This is probably one of the most well-known conditions, perhaps because of the distinct physical characteristics that a child might have. Down syndrome is the result of a chromosomal abnormality, where an individual has a full or partial extra copy of chromosome 21. Typical characteristics might include (to varying degrees) an upward slant to the eyes, a single deep crease across the centre of the palm, small stature and low muscle tone (National Down Syndrome Society 2024). Fragile X is a condition that is the result of genetic abnormality that is believed to be the most common cause of learning disability after Down syndrome (Gates 2015). Again, there may be common physical characteristics such as a long narrow face with prominent jaw bones and ears;

Table 5.2 Examples of risk factors that might cause learning disabilities

	Prenatal	Perinatal	Postnatal
Biomedical risks (relating to biological processes)	Chromosomal and genetic disorders	Trauma during birth (e.g. lack of oxygen), prematurity	Traumatic brain injury through disease or accident
Social risks (relating to external risks in the home or local community)	Domestic abuse, poverty	Lack of access to healthcare	Institutionalisation, lack of stimulation
Behavioural risks (relating to behaviours that might cause a baby or child to develop learning disabilities)	Parental drug or alcohol use	Absence of caretaking of the child	Child neglect or abuse
Educational risks (relating to risks around the availability of educational support that promotes good health and wellbeing)	Lack of support during pregnancy	Lack of referrals if interventions are needed at discharge	Lack of early diagnosis and intervention; poor family support

Schalock et al. (2019)

however, these features are hard to see in young children, which is why diagnosis can sometimes be delayed (Mencap n.d.).

Other conditions are less easy to identify, which means that a learning disability may not be picked up until there are clear delays in common developmental milestones. This is also the case with autism, which shall be covered in more depth shortly, but the causes of autism are still being researched. The National Autistic Society (n.d.) states that evidence suggests that autism may be genetic and may be likely to have multiple genes responsible rather than a single gene. Whilst an autistic child may not have learning disabilities, it should also be noted that many conditions that mean that a child has a learning disability do also carry with them a higher prevalence of autism. Foetal alcohol spectrum disorder (FASD) is an umbrella term that describes the effects that alcohol might have on a developing foetus. This is a growing area of research as diagnosis is often late or even completely missed (Morello et al. 2022). Whilst there are no single or unique symptoms of FASD, there can be a pattern of physical and neurological abnormalities that may also include learning disabilities, autism and ADHD (Department of Health and Social Care 2021a). The support that is put in place will of course vary from child to child, but it is vital that people working with children have an awareness of FASD so that support can be appropriately tailored (Moulds 2022).

Some people with learning disabilities and/or who are neurodivergent never receive a diagnosis or may receive a diagnosis much later in life. The consequences of a lack of or late diagnosis for children and young people mean that appropriate interventions are not put in place or are put in place too late, which in turn can affect educational attainment, skill development and the forming of relationships, and the consequences of missing out on these can in turn affect mental health and the opportunity to fulfil one's potential. A literature review carried out by No One Knows (research commissioned by the Prison Reform Trust) noted that between 20% and 30% of adult offenders have learning disabilities or learning difficulties (Talbot 2011). Additionally, she notes that an assessment of children who had offended in England and Wales found that 23% had an IQ of less than 70 and 36% had an IQ of 70–79. This disproportionate number of children and adult offenders who have additional needs is an indication of the possible consequences for individuals if they do not receive a diagnosis and subsequent support when they are young.

Every person who has a learning disability and/or who is neurodivergent is different and must be treated as an individual—what is effective support for one person might not work for another. Recent guidance (Public Health England 2023) defines learning disability as follows:

> as a significantly reduced ability to understand new or complex information, to learn new skills (impaired intelligence), with a reduced ability to cope independently (impaired social functioning), which started before adulthood.

However, despite this, people continue to be labelled, to aid eligibility for support, or arrangement of support. It is acknowledged that classification of learning disability is still commonly used—this relates to how far an individual moves away from the normal distribution of IQ for the general population; therefore, people are categorised as having *mild* learning disabilities (IQ range 50–69), *moderate* learning disabilities (IQ range 35–49), *severe* learning disabilities (IQ range 20–34) and finally *profound and multiple* learning disabilities, which is a term used when people have additional and complex needs that are related to their disability (Gates 2015).

5.3 Neurodiversity

As noted earlier, neurodiversity means recognising the range of ways people's brain works, receiving and processing information and recognising and responding to a range of stimuli. Terminology is important here. The term neurodiversity refers to the heterogeneity of our human brain. Part of this neurodiversity includes conditions such as attention-deficit disorder, attention-deficit/hyperactivity disorder, dyslexia and severe learning difficulties. But individuals are not neurodiverse, because this is a generic term for difference and cannot apply to individuals. Rather they may be described as neurodivergent. Sometimes people use these terms interchangeably, but many autistic people feel this is a disablist attitude to autism and other ways of being. Not all children with learning disabilities are autistic, and not all autistic children have learning disabilities; a recent study suggested high rates of co-existing learning disability, autism and OCD (Martin et al. 2020). There may be symptoms or characteristics of autism such as repetitive movements or communication issues, which may also indicate learning disability (Lord and Bishop 2010). Autistic children, young people and adults (16–96) are 80% more likely to have poor mental health including anxiety, depression, post-traumatic stress disorder, seasonal affective disorder, obsessive-compulsive disorder and sleep problems and are more likely to die by suicide (Weir et al. 2022). The respondents also reported difficulties with describing symptoms within their bodies or the pain they were feeling, along with sensory overload in healthcare settings, which led to feeling overwhelmed and have shutdowns/meltdowns (Weir et al. 2022).

Recognising the symptoms of these conditions in children and young people is improving, and more and more children are being diagnosed. But sadly, there is usually a long delay in getting a diagnosis. Yet a diagnosis can open the door to increased support, and for children with ADD or ADHD, treatments are available including stimulant medication such as Ritalin, which may help a child to focus for longer periods of time. However, there are difficulties for many children with diagnosis, and it remains a postcode lottery; girls are less likely to be diagnosed as autistic or with ADD/ADHD than boys but instead misdiagnosed/diagnosed as having eating disorders, obsessive-compulsive disorder, bipolar disorder or borderline personality disorder (Young et al. 2018). Many people are coming to be diagnosed in adulthood, which means decades of lost opportunities and support through school and beyond. Many children and young people with learning disabilities, autistic children and those with learning difficulties face exclusion from their peers. They are more likely to be bullied and suffer from having fewer peer network supports to protect them or offer support (Humphrey and Hebron 2014). Childhood and even more so adolescence is a time of fitting in. Stigma remains an issue unfortunately, and autistic and neurodivergent children may be bullied in school, on social media and in their local community (Maiano et al. 2016). Differences in communicating, understanding other's needs, relating in so-called neurotypical ways to others and needing quieter spaces or personal spaces are often difficult in a school environment. In a hospital or healthcare environment, there may be added challenges of lack of privacy, anxiety, pain and difficulties with communicating.

There has been criticism of the prevailing deficit model of autism (Pellicano et al. 2014; Dinishak 2016; Kapp 2020) focusing on explanations of autism, which suggest individuals have difficulties with theory of mind, executive functioning and central coherence, rather than meeting individual's real need. This could instead be considered a double empathy problem (Milton et al. 2023), which recognises that non-autistic people appear to have as much difficulty understanding autistic minds as vice versa but also that autistic people develop a greater understanding of society than non-autistic people develop of autism and autistic people have a similar ability to empathise with other autistic people as non-autistic people have with peers (affinity with other autistic people). Thus, neurotypical people fail to understand how and what other individuals are communicating and demand that they adapt to neurotypical ways. There has been some success in using therapy to change (preschool) children's communication and reduce the severity of 'autistic' behaviours, including social communication and repetitive behaviours, in the parent-mediated communication-focused treatment (PACT) (Pickles et al. 2016). However, it is useful to consider alternative approaches to reducing stigma and developing more empathetic ways of understanding and communicating with autistic children. This should be a two-way process. We can learn to communicate with individuals in a way that they find less traumatic, not demanding eye contact, understanding the need for some children to move around, to stim and to vocalise their happiness or anxiety. The implications of this for working with autistic children and young people are that trying to make children adapt to neurotypical ways of communicating can cause damage. Masking is one way that autistic children act non-autistic to fit in, damaging their mental health (Chapman et al. 2022). Instead, we can help autistic children and young people by using intensive interaction (Caldwell 2013) or helpful resources such as the SPELL framework, which offers a way of organising help through moderating both the environment and our interactions with autistic children (Sergeant et al. 2007):

- **S**tructure to help individuals predict what will happen.
- **P**ositive approaches to help the individual develop and grow.
- **E**mpathy by trying to understand the individual's perspective.
- **L**ow arousal keeping stressors to a minimum including noise, lights, smells and demands.
- **L**inks to make sure support is consistent.

5.3.1 Possible Consequences for Children and Young People Who Have Learning Disabilities and/or Are Neurodivergent

Children grow and develop by interacting with the world around them, by observing and copying others and by having the opportunity to develop skills and understanding through play and learning (Vygotsky 1978; Cohen 2018). Children who have learning disabilities or who may be autistic or neurodivergent often experience fewer opportunities to engage in play (Stillianesis et al. 2021). This might be due to anxious parents or caregivers, who feel that to permit their child to engage in play with other children might place them in harm's way; it might be due to a lack of friendships and relationships, therefore decreasing the opportunity for a child to play with others; it might be due to service providers being risk averse and not wanting to place their accountability in jeopardy (Heaslip and Hewitt-Taylor 2014). As children grow up and become adolescents, these same factors may prevent a child from having exposure to experiences that a child who is not learning disabled/neurodivergent/autistic might have exposure to. Niehues et al. (2015, p. 809) state that risk and uncertainty are 'not only valuable, but necessary, contributors to children's healthy development of happiness, well-being and resilience'; therefore, it can be concluded that if a child does not have the opportunity to take risks through play or experience, this could negatively impact their mental health. Reflective Activity 5.2 asks you to consider your role in ensuring children and young people with a learning disability or neurodivergence have the same opportunities as other children.

Reflective Activity 5.2

- Consider how you might work alongside parents, caregivers and others to ensure that learning-disabled and/or neurodivergent children and young people have the same opportunities to play, experience risk and therefore develop as their peers
- Consider how you would sensitively work with a family who are very protective of their child and do not want their child to go on a day trip with the rest of their peers (this could be a school trip or a trip through a sports club or short breaks service). Think about how the parents/caregivers might be feeling and what is prompting their fears. What might be the implications of the child not joining their peers? How would you work constructively with the family?

Another challenge for learning-disabled and/or neurodivergent children and adults is that of 'diagnostic overshadowing', and it is important to also be mindful of this when we are considering the mental health needs of this population. Diagnostic overshadowing is what happens when the symptoms that a person is experiencing are inaccurately attributed to their learning disability or autism, rather than being part of an illness or other specific condition. Woods et al. (2023) note that a blurring of the lines can occur between what is autism and what is not, meaning that diagnostic overshadowing can be a risk for autistic people in areas such as anxiety and personality disorders, where people have motor coordination difficulties or conditions that involve seizure activity. Missing or misdiagnosing the original cause of the symptom(s) means that people do not get the treatment or support they need and the consequences of this can be fatal. Children who do not use words to speak can be particularly vulnerable to this, and it is imperative that practitioners work in partnership with families who know their child best, including the intricate ways that they might communicate. When thinking about the mental health needs of children and young people who have learning disabilities and/or are neurodivergent, practitioners must look and listen very carefully, to truly try and understand what the child is experiencing and be mindful not to attribute their symptoms to the wrong aetiology or cause.

5.4 Communication with Children or Young People with a Learning Disability or Neurodiversity

Communication is a dynamic and cyclical process that involves a message being transmitted, received and understood (McCabe and Timmins 2013). Communication is essential to human interaction, and it makes people feel seen, heard and understood (Money et al. 2016). It is also a vital part of life that is crucial to wellbeing (Daly 2017). Neurodiverse individuals and people with learning disabilities can experience significant challenges with communication—although they will have widely varying communication abilities and needs. Generally, the more severe the learning disability is, the more challenging communication becomes (Lacono et al. 2019). People with learning disabilities may experience issues with expressive communication, which is the ability to express oneself, verbally and/or non-verbally, using facial expressions or body language, and receptive communication, which is the ability to understand other people's verbal language and/or their non-verbal cues (Beukelman and Mirenda 2013; Marrus and Hall 2017).

That said, it is important to take a strength-based approach (Saleebey 1996) that shifts the focus away from the challenges of individuals with neurological differences in favour of finding ways to work with their strengths to enable them to participate. In this approach, the strengths and interests of the person with lived experiences are the starting point for designing effective way of communication, which then results in value-based approach for offering interventions and support (Lerner and Johns 2015). Article 9 of the Convention on the Rights of Persons with Disabilities (United Nations 2006) calls for appropriate measures to ensure that people with disabilities have equal access to information and communications technologies and systems. So, communicating with children who are neurodiverse involves the ability to adopt the strength-based model by people who are involved in their care to ensure effective and supportive interaction and engagement.

By employing some of the strategies below, professionals can create a supportive and effective communication environment for children with learning disabilities and neurodiversity (see Case Study of Donald, Table 5.3).

Donald would benefit from a positive behaviour support plan, which includes his communication preferences. For example, Donald uses some communication aids like pictures, idiosyncratic signs and gestures and some words to communicate, and he also gets more support from specialist services like the Speech and Language Team. It is important that everyone working with Donald is aware of his positive support and communication plan, so there is consistency in the way in which staff communicate with him.

5.4.1 Multi-agency Working

Both case study 1 (Oliver and Connor) and case study 2 (Donald) highlight the importance of multi-agency working in planning and delivering care with people with complex health needs. The importance of working with professionals and to collaborate with speech therapists, special education teachers and other professionals who can provide specialised strategies and support (American Speech-Language Hearing Association (ASHA) 2024) cannot be overemphasised. In the same vein, professionals must encourage family involvement, and there must be active participation of family members in communication practices to ensure consistency and support at home (Centre for Parent Information and Resources (CPIR) 2024). It is also important for everyone who is involved in the care of the young person to engage with ongoing education and training about the specific needs and preferences of the child to improve communication efforts (National Centre for Learning Disability (NCLD 2024)).

Table 5.3 Case study of Donald

Donald is a 12-year-old boy who was diagnosed with ADHD and ASD at age 2, and he also has a learning disability. Donald is generally healthy although he has recently been diagnosed with asthma, he is prescribed an inhaler, and his asthma is well managed by his GP. He has difficulty with small spaces where many people are congregated. Donald attends a special education at a local elementary school
Donald finds communication challenging, and he is impulsive and displaying behaviours, which include having tantrums, being aggressive, throwing things and being impulsive when he is in public places and property destruction. These challenges have made it difficult for Donald to participate in activities with peers, and his parents and teachers are increasingly finding it difficult to engage with him and to calm him down whenever he is agitated
If you were working with Donald, what information do you need to be able to communicate and work with him to help him to express verbally how he feels?

5.4.2 Communication Techniques

When working with children or young people who are neurodivergent, it is important to be person centred. This includes flexibility and willingness to adjust communication style based on the child's responses and needs (ASHA 2024). To achieve this, it is important you observe and learn the child or young persons' communication cues and preferences and be open to adapting communication approaches accordingly. Patience is also important as the child or young person may require extra time to process information and to respond (CPIR 2024). Time is also needed to establish a trusting relationship, and this is facilitated by being consistent, reliable and understanding (Wehmeyer and Webb 2014). It is important in all interactions with the child or young person to show empathy and respect for the child's feelings and perspectives (Autism Speaks 2024).

Below are some strategies and techniques that can be used to promote effective communication with children and young people with a learning disability or who are neurodivergent:

- Use clear and simple language: Use straightforward, concrete language. Avoid idioms, metaphors and abstract concepts unless you are going to explain them (Autism Speaks 2024).
- Use visual supports, such as pictures, symbols and written words to support verbal communication. Tools like visual schedules can help children understand and anticipate routines (Wehmeyer and Webb 2014).
- Consider gestures and body language: Complement words with gestures and facial expressions to convey meaning (ASHA 2024).
- Know the importance of repetition and rephrasing where appropriate: Repeat information and rephrase it if the child does not understand initially (Autism Speaks 2024).
- Use encouragement and praise: Provide positive reinforcement to build the child's confidence and encourage further communication (NCLD 2024).
- Minimise distractions: Create a quiet and distraction-free environment to help the child focus on communication (Wehmeyer and Webb 2014).
- Use of technology: Employ assistive technology and communication devices if needed, such as speech-generating devices or apps designed for communication support (Leaf and McEachin 2018).
- Active listening technique: Pay close attention to the child's attempts to communicate, whether through words, gestures or behaviours (CPIR 2024).
- Use of interactive activities: Engage in activities that the child enjoys and can participate in actively, such as games, storytelling or role-playing (Leaf and McEachin 2018).

Lastly, Rees (2023) provides ten helpful tips when assessing the mental health of neurodivergent children and young people, which we argue would also be useful for children and young people with a learning disability (Table 5.4).

Table 5.4 Helpful tips in assessing mental health of children who are neurodivergent

Hint	Key question
Continuum of mental health and wellbeing	Which factors (e.g. environment, peers, activities) contribute to the child moving up (or down) the mental health continuum?
Consider the child and then their diagnosis	How does a child's diagnosis help you to understand their strengths and contribute to a positive sense of who they are?
Take time to get to know the child or young person	What regular and motivating activities can you do with the child?
Liaise with those who know them best	Are there other multi-agency professionals who have been working with the child who can contribute to a holistic assessment of how they are coping?
Don't underestimate the impact of the environment	How do smaller transitions such as a change from one activity to another or a change in teacher for the day influence a child's wellbeing?
Think about what has happened to them (not what is wrong with them)	Have there been any recent events (e.g. a difficult change or loss) which have impacted on the child's presentation or which have triggered previous feelings of grief, anger or anxiety?
Work out their sensory profile	How can your knowledge of a child's sensory preferences support them to stay regulated? (E.g. do they need more movement activities or time outside, or do they need time away from noise and in a small and quiet space?)
Match your communication with theirs	How do you adapt the strategies you use to support the communication of a child or young person (e.g. the words you use objects, visuals, gestures, movement, etc.)?
Emphasise exceptions, motivators and strengths	How can you tell when a child is motivated or engaged in an activity? (e.g., what is their expression like, how do they communicate, move etc.)?
Assessment is intervention	What approaches and strategies have you used as part of the assessment process which have helped to enhance a child's mental health and wellbeing?

Rees (2023)

5.5 Conclusion

Despite a variety of international and UK laws and policies, this chapter has highlighted that often the needs of children or young people with a learning disability or neurodivergence are often not met. This may be because of the intricate interplay between a lack of knowledge and skills of the practitioner and a lack of flexibility within service provision to meet the complex needs of these children and their families. Yet the number of children with a disability globally is large, and indeed the number of children and young people with a neurodivergence is growing. Communicating with children and young people with a learning disability or neurodivergence can be more challenging, which often results in their voices not being heard. We assert it is vitally important that all practitioners working with children and young people feel confident in communicating with them irrespective of their communication needs. Due to the complex needs of such children and young people, multidisciplinary working is key, and failure to do so can result in tragic consequences.

References

American Speech-Language-Hearing Association (ASHA). 2024. Available from: https://www.asha.org. Accessed 24 July 2024.

Autism Act 2009. c.15. Available from: Autism Act 2009. legislation.gov.uk. Accessed 24 July 2024.

Autism Speaks. 2024. Available from: https://www.autismspeaks.org. Accessed 24 July 2024.

Beukelman DR, Mirenda P. Augmentative and alternative communication: supporting children and adults with complex communication needs. 4th ed. Baltimore: Paul H Brookes; 2013.

British Psychological Society. Guidance on the assessment and diagnosis of intellectual disabilities in adulthood. 2015. Available from: https://www.rcpsych.ac.uk/docs/default-source/members/faculties/intellectual-disability/id-assessment-guidance.pdf?sfvrsn=fd3c2aea_2. Accessed 24 July 2024.

Caldwell P. Intensive interaction: using body language to communicate. J Dev Disabil. 2013;19(1):33–9.

Centre for Parent Information and Resources. 2024. Available from: https://www.parentcenterhub.org/. Accessed 26 July 2024.

Chapman L, Rose K, Hull L, Mandy W. "I want to fit in… but I don't want to change myself fundamentally": a qualitative exploration of the relationship between masking and mental health for autistic teenagers. Res Autism Spectr Disord. 2022;99:102069. https://doi.org/10.1016/j.rasd.2022.102069. ISSN 1750-9467.

Children Act 1989. c.41. Available from: https://www.legislation.gov.uk/ukpga/1989/41/contents. Accessed 26 July 2024.

Children Act 2004. c.41. Available from: https://www.legislation.gov.uk/ukpga/2004/31/contents. Accessed 24 July 2024.

Children and Families Act. 2014. Available from: https://www.legislation.gov.uk/ukpga/2014/6/contents. Accessed 26 July 2024.

Cohen D. The development of play. New York: Routledge; 2018.

Daly L. Effective communication with older adults. Nurs Stand. 2017;31(41):55–63. https://doi.org/10.7748/ns.2017.e10832.

Department of Health. Valuing people: a new strategy for learning disability for the 21st century. London: HMSO; 2001.

Department of Health & Social Care. Fetal alcohol spectrum disorder: health needs assessment. 2021a. Available from: https://www.gov.uk/government/publications/fetal-alcohol-spectrum-disorder-health-needs-assessment. Accessed 26 July 2024.

Department of Health & Social Care. National strategy for autistic children, young people and adults: 2021 to 2026. 2021b. Available from: GOV.UK. www.gov.uk. Accessed 26 July 2024.

Dinishak J. The deficit view and its critics. Disabil Stud Q. 2016;36. https://doi.org/10.18061/dsq.v36i4.5236. Accessed 26 July 2024.

Equality Act 2010. c.15, Available from: .legislation.gov.uk. Accessed 26 July 2024.

Gates B. The nature of learning disabilities and their relationship to learning disability nursing. In: Gates B, Mafuba K, editors. Learning disability nursing: modern day practice. London: CRC Press; 2015. p. 1–26.

Gov.uk. Working together to safeguard children. 2023a. Available from: GOV.UK. www.gov.uk. Accessed 26 July 2024.

Gov.uk. IICSA: report of the Independent Inquiry into Child Sexual Abuse, part K and annexes. 2023b. Available from: https://www.gov.uk/government/publications/iicsa-report-of-the-independent-inquiry-into-child-sexual-abuse/the-report-of-the-independent-inquiry-into-child-sexual-abuse-part-k-and-annexes-accessible#contents. Accessed 9 June 2024.

Health and Social Care Act 2022. Available from: https://www.legislation.gov.uk/ukpga/2022/31/section/181. Accessed 26 July 2024.

Heaslip V. Health and disability in adults. In: Parker J, Ashencaen Crabtree S, editors. Critical perspectives on human growth and development in adults. Bristol: Bristol University Press; 2020.

Heaslip V, Hewitt-Taylor J. Vulnerability and risk in children living with a physical disability. J Child Young People's Nurs. 2014;26(10):24–9.

Heslop P, Turner S, Read S, Tucker J, Seaton S, Evans B. Implementing reasonable adjustments for disabled people in healthcare services. Nurs Stand. 2019;34(8):29–34.

Heslop P, Byrne VM, Calkin RA, Gielnik KT, Huxor AP. Establishing a national mortality review programme for people with intellectual disabilities: the experience in England. J Intellect Disabil. 2022;26(1):264–80. https://doi.org/10.1177/1744629520970365.

Human Rights Act 1998. c.42. Available from: legislation.gov.uk. Accessed 26 July 2024.

Humphrey N, Hebron J. Bullying of children and adolescents with autism spectrum conditions: a 'state of the field' review. Int J Incl Educ. 2014;19(8):845–62. https://doi.org/10.1080/13603116.2014.981602.

Inquest.org. Independent investigation finds death of 18-year old Connor Sparrowhawk at a learning disability in-patient unit in Oxford was preventable. 2014. Available from: https://www.inquest.org.uk/connor-sparrowhawk-independent-investigation-conclusions. Accessed 25 July 2024.

Jay A, Evans M, Frank I, Sharpling D. The residential schools investigation. Phase 1: music schools, residential schools. Phase 2: Safeguarding: day and boarding schools. Investigation report. 2022 March. https://www.iicsa.org.uk/key-documents/28486/view/residential-schools-investigation-report-march-2022.pdf. Accessed 26 July 2024.

Kapp SK. Conclusion. In: Kapp S, editor. Autistic community and the neurodiversity movement. Singapore: Palgrave Macmillan; 2020. https://doi.org/10.1007/978-981-13-8437-0_22.

Lacono T, Bould E, Beadle-Brown J, Bigby C. An exploration of communication within active support for adults with high and low support needs. J Appl Res Intellect Disabil. 2019;32(1):61–70. https://doi.org/10.1111/jar.12502.

Leaf JB, McEachin J. Applied behaviour analysis: implementing strategies for success. New York: Springer; 2018.

Lerner J, Johns BH. Learning disabilities and related disabilities: strategies for success. Stamford: Cengage Learning; 2015.

Lord C, Bishop S. Autistic spectrum disorders. Diagnosis, prevalence, and services for children and families. Sharing child and youth development knowledge. Soc Policy Rep. 2010;24(2). ISSN 1075-7031. www.srcd.org/spr.html

Maiano C, Normand CL, Salvas MC, Moullec G, Aime A. Prevalence of school bullying among youth with autism spectrum disorders: a systematic review and meta-analysis. Autism Res. 2016;9(6):601–15.

Marrus N, Hall L. Intellectual disability and language disorder. Child Adolesc Psychiatr Clin. 2017;26(3):539–54. https://doi.org/10.1016/j.chc.2017.03.001.

Martin AF, Jassi A, Cullen AE, et al. Co-occurring obsessive–compulsive disorder and autism spectrum disorder in young people: prevalence, clinical characteristics and outcomes. Eur Child Adolesc Psychiatry. 2020;29:1603–11. https://doi.org/10.1007/s00787-020-01478-8.

Mazars. 2015. Independent review of deaths of people with a Learning Disability or Mental Health problem in contact with Southern Health NHS Foundation Trust April 2011 to March 2015. Available from: FINAL REPORT of the Review of MH and LD deaths at Southern Health NHSFT- 16.12.15. Accessed 10 April 2025.

McCabe C, Timmins F. Communication skills for nursing practice. 2nd ed. Basingstoke: Palgrave Macmillan; 2013.

McGowan T. "An avoidable death" by Oliver's father. Blogpost (n.d.). https://www.olivermcgowan.org/post/an-avoidable-death-by-oliver-s-father-s. Accessed 26 July 2024.

Mencap. Fragile X syndrome (online). (n.d.). Available from: https://www.mencap.org.uk/learning-disability-explained/learning-disability-and-conditions/fragile-x-syndrome?gad_source=1&gclid=EAIaIQobChMItoKejNOkhwMVYJRQBh0Qlg4BEAAYAiAAEgKGmfD_BwE. Accessed 25 July 2024.

Milton DE, Waldock KE, Keates N. Autism and the 'double empathy problem'. In: Conversations on empathy: interdisciplinary perspectives on empathy, imagination and othering. London: Routledge; 2023. p. 78–97.

Money D, Hartley K, McAnespie L, et al. Inclusive communication and the role of speech and language therapy. Royal College of speech and language therapists position paper. 2016. Available from: http://www.rcslt.org/wp-content/uploads/2021/02/20162209_InclusiveComms_final.pdf. Accessed 26 July 2024.

Morello R, Cook P, Coffey M. *"Now, with a bit more knowledge, I understand why I'm asking those questions."* midwives' perspectives on their role in the Greater Manchester health and social care partnership's programme to reduce alcohol exposed pregnancies. Midwifery (online). 2022 July;110.

Moulds C. Understanding FASD. Commu Pract (online). 2022;95(5):26–9.

National Autistic Society. The causes of autism (n.d.). Available from: https://www.autism.org.uk/advice-and-guidance/what-is-autism/the-causes-of-autism. Accessed 13 July 2024.

National Centre for Learning Disabilities. 2024. Available from: https://www.ncld.org. Accessed 25 July 2024.

National Down Syndrome Society. About Down Syndrome (online). 2024. Available from: https://ndss.org/about. Accessed 13 July 2024.

NHS England. Neurodiversity (undated). Available from: https://www.hee.nhs.uk/our-work/pharmacy/transforming/initial/foundation/resources/edi/neurodiversity#:~:text=Neurodiversity%20describes%20the%20population%20as,as%20the%20societal%20%E2%80%9Cnorm%E2%80%9D. Accessed 25 July 2024.

Niehues AN, Bundy A, Broom A, Tranter P. Parents' perceptions of risk and the influence on children's everyday activities. J Child Fam Stud. 2015;24(3):809–20. https://doi.org/10.1007/s10826-013-9891-2.

Olusanya BO, Kancherla V, Shaheen A, Ogbo FA, Davis AC. Global and regional prevalence of disabilities among children and adolescents: analysis of findings from global health databases. Front Public Health. 2022;23(10):977453. https://doi.org/10.3389/fpubh.2022.977453. PMID: 36249226; PMCID: PMC9554924

Pellicano E, Dinsmore A, Charman T. What should autism research focus upon? Community views and priorities from the United Kingdom. Autism. 2014;18(7):756–70. https://doi.org/10.1177/1362361314529627.

Pickles A, Le Couteur A, Leadbitter K, Salomone E, Cole-Fletcher R, Tobin H, et al. Parent-mediated social communication therapy for young children with autism (PACT): long-term follow-up of a randomised controlled trial. Lancet. 2016;388(10059):2501–9.

Public Health England. Learning disability – applying all our health. 2023. Available from: https://www.gov.uk/government/publications/learning-disability-applying-all-our-health/learning-disabilities-applying-all-our-health. Accessed 24 July 2024.

Rees K. Assessing the mental health of neurodivergent children and young people at school. 2023. Available from: https://www.bps.org.uk/psychologist/assessing-mental-health-neurodivergent-children-and-young-people-school. Accessed 25 July 2024.

Richie F. Independent review into Thomas Oliver McGowan's LeDeR process phase two. Final Report. 2020. Available at: Independent-Review-into-Thomas-Oliver-McGowans-LeDeR-Process-phase-two-_20-October-2020.pdf. england.nhs.uk. Accessed 26 July 2024.

Saleebey D. The strengths perspective in social work practice: extensions and cautions. Soc Work. 1996;41(3):296–305.

Salman S. Why did Connor Sparrowhawk die in a specialist NHS unit? Sara Ryan on her fight for justice for her son. 2014. Available from: https://www.theguardian.com/society/2014/mar/19/connor-sparrowhawk-death-nhs-care-unit-slade-house-learning-disabilities?CMP=share_btn_url. Accessed 25 July 2024.

Schalock RL, Luckasson R, Tassé M. The contemporary view of intellectual and developmental disabilities: implications for psychologists. Psicothema. 2019;31(3):223–8. https://doi.org/10.7334/psicothema2019.119.

Sergeant L, Dewsbury G, Johnstone S. Supporting people with complex behavioural difficulties and autistic spectrum disorder in a community setting: an inclusive approach. Hous Care Support. 2007;10(1):23–30. https://doi.org/10.1108/14608790200700005.

Sleap V, Williams T, Odd D, Stoianova S, Garstang J, Kendall B, White A, Geoghegan L, Tranter S, Nettleton-Burrows J, Luyt K. 2024. Learning from deaths: Children with a learning disability and autistic children aged 4 - 17 years. National Child Mortality Database. Available from: NCMD-Learning-disability-and-autism-report_FINAL.pdf. [Accessed 10 April 2025].

Stillianesis S, Spencer G, Villeneuve M, Sterman J, Bundy A, Wyver S, Beetham KS. Parents' perspectives on managing risk in play for children with developmental disabilities. Disabil Soc. 2021;37(8):1272–92. https://doi-org.ezproxy.bolton.ac.uk/10.1080/09687599.2021.1874298

Stobbs P. Disabled Children and the Equality Act 2010: What teachers need to know and what schools need to do. Council for Disabled Children; 2022. March. https://councilfordisabledchildren.org.uk/sites/default/files/uploads/attachments/SchoolsEqAWordformatFINAL.pdf. Accessed 25 July 2024

Talbot J.. Prisoners with learning disabilities and learning difficulties Prison Reform Trust (Blog) 2 June 2011. Available from: https://prisonreformtrust.org.uk/prisoners-with-learning-disabilities-and-learning-difficulties/#:~:text=A%20literature%20review%20undertaken%20by,within%20the%20criminal%20justice%20system

UNESCO. The Salamanca statement and framework for action on special needs education. Paris: UNESCO; 1994. Available from: https://unesdoc.unesco.org/ark:/48223/pf0000098427.locale=en. Accessed 24 July 2024.

UNICEF. Seen, counted, included: using data to shed light on the well-being of children with disabilities. 2022. Available from: https://data.unicef.org/resources/children-with-disabilities-report-2021/. Accessed 24 July 2024.

United Nations. Convention on the rights of persons with disabilities. 2006. Available from: https://www.ohchr.org/en/instruments-mechanisms/instruments/convention-rights-persons-disabilities. Accessed 26 July 2024.

United Nations. Disability and employment (undated). Available from: https://www.un.org/development/desa/disabilities/resources/factsheet-on-persons-with-disabilities/disability-and-employment.html. Accessed 24 July 2024.

Vygotsky LS. The role of play in development. In: Early years education: histories and traditions. New York: Routledge; 1978. p. 199–211.

Watson D. Causes and manifestations. In: Gates B, editor. Learning disabilities. 3rd ed. London: Churchill Livingstone; 1997. p. 21–32.

Wehmeyer ML, Webb KW. Understanding and supporting neurodiversity in education. Baltimore: Brookes Publishing; 2014.

Weir E, Allison C, Baron-Cohen S. Autistic adults have poorer quality healthcare and worse health based on self-report data. Mol Autism. 2022;13(1):23. https://doi.org/10.1186/s13229-022-00501-w.

Woods R, Williams K, Watts C. "Profound autism": the dire consequences of diagnostic overshadowing. Autism Res. 2023;16:1656–7. https://doi-org.ezproxy.bolton.ac.uk/10.1002/aur.2985

Young H, Oreve MJ, Speranza M. Clinical characteristics and problems diagnosing autism spectrum disorder in girls. Arch Pediatr. 2018;25(6):399–403. https://doi.org/10.1016/j.arcped.2018.06.008.

6 Transgender and Gender Variance in Young People

Gemma Trainor and Corey Hartley

G. Trainor (✉)
Mental Health Nursing, Directorate of Nursing and Midwifery, University of Salford, Salford, UK
e-mail: gemma.trainor@outlook.com

C. Hartley
Expert by Experience, Burnley, UK

G. Trainor, V. Heaslip (eds.), *Needs of Children and Young People Living with Complex Mental Health Difficulties*,
https://doi.org/10.1007/978-3-031-84532-1_6

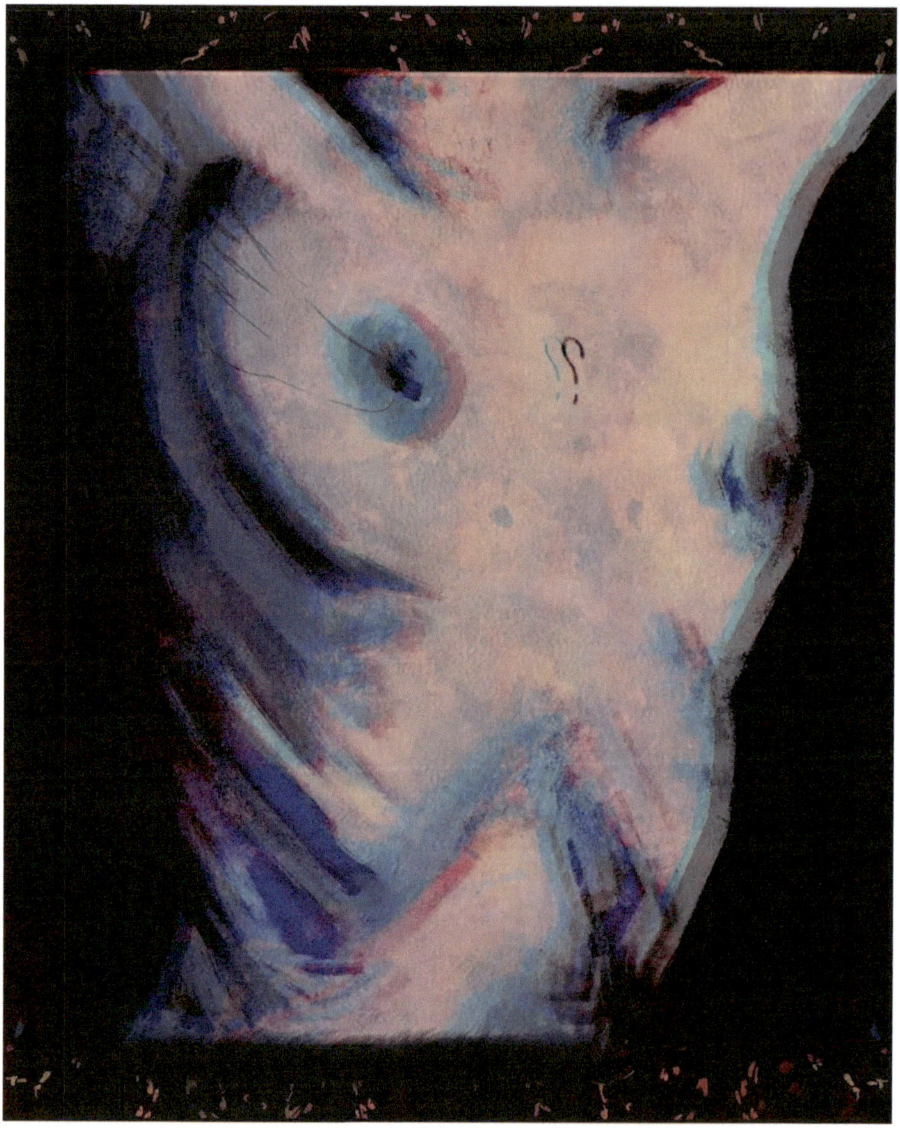

6.1 Key Terminology

Trans* is an inclusive umbrella term that is used to describe people who identify with a different gender than their assigned gender at birth. The term trans* is inclusive of all gender identities and gender variations that transgress binary gender narratives (Fiani and Han 2018). In this chapter, the term trans star (trans*) has been used, as this captures a wide range of individuals who identify with a gender that is different from their assigned sex, including people who are non-binary or gender diverse.

To understand the differing terms used by young people who identify as trans*, it is essential to emphasise the key differences between assigned sex at birth, gender identity, and gender expression, which are often conflated, but for trans* young people, it is an essential point to separate these key elements of gender. Another key element that is often coalesced is trans* gender identity and sexual orientation; again, it is vital to underline how separate these are:

> Despite being out as gay since the age of 12 a lingering sense of unease persisted. While my sexual orientation felt authentic my adherence to traditional masculine issues did not. I embarked on a journey of self-exploration experimenting with my outward presentation by growing my hair longer, wearing nail varnish and selecting more feminine attire. (CH chapter co-author)

A detailed discussion on terminology would be beyond the scope of this chapter; therefore, Table 6.1 describes the more commonly encountered terms. Additionally,

Table 6.1 Key terms and definitions

Term	Definition
Trans	Is an umbrella term used to describe those whose gender identity differs from their assignment at birth
Trans*	Trans star (*) is a term used to describe individuals whose gender identity differs from their assigned sex, including those who transgress gender norms and do not identify as cisgender, but not necessarily as male or female
Gender identity	This refers to a person's knowledge of their own gender and everyone has an identity. For some young people, this may match their assigned gender at birth; however, for others, their identity does not fit into two binary genders
Gender expression	This is when a person has an external manifestation of their gender through use of names, pronouns, clothing, speech, and behaviour/mannerisms
Cisgender	Used to describe people who identify with their assigned sex at birth
Sexual orientation	Used to describe a person's physical, romantic, and/or emotional attraction to another person
Transfeminine male to female (MTF)	Used to describe an individual who was assigned male at birth (AMAB) and whose gender/expression is feminine
Transmasculine female to male (FTM)	Used to describe an individual who was assigned female at birth (AFAB) and whose gender/expression is male

(continued)

Table 6.1 (continued)

Term	Definition
Genderqueer/gender diverse/gender creative	Used to describe individuals whose gender identity/expression falls outside the binary characteristics of male and female. They may describe feeling somewhere in between categories of male and female or have a different term for themselves
Gender affirming	Used to refer to behaviours or treatments that affirm a transgender person's gender identity, e.g. use of cross-sex hormones
Sex	At birth, infants are assigned a sex based on their external anatomy, which is a combination of hormones, chromosomes, internal and external reproductive organs, and secondary sex characteristics
Non-binary	Used to describe people who experience their gender identity/expression as falling outside the binary gender category of man or woman. It encompasses various ways of understanding one's gender. It is also an umbrella term for individuals who do not prescribe to traditional gender roles and identify as having both male and female or a fluctuation of their identity
Gender fluid	An individual whose gender identity fluctuates along the gender spectrum. This can occur more than once a day up to every few years
Gender dysphoria	Psychological and emotional distress which a person feels regarding their assigned gender and their identification with a gender other than that associated with assigned sex at birth
Gender euphoria	An experience an individual faces when their intrinsic/subconscious gender is affirmed physically, i.e. *affirmed by others and affirmed in physical expression (dress, make-up,* etc.*)*
Sex assigned at birth	The sex label given to a baby that is assigned based on physical sex characteristics
Differences in sex development (DSD)/intersex	Umbrella terms that cover over 40 biological conditions that affect a young person's sexual development. Intersex individuals are born with ambiguous sexual characteristics, which often are unable to be used to assign a definitive sex at birth

the language around this subject area is constantly evolving, and Table 6.1 provides some examples of the key terminologies.

6.2 Historical and Social Context

Understanding gender identity and its impact on mental health in young people under 16 is important for recognising their unique challenges and needs. Historically, terms like 'transvestite', 'transsexual', 'transgender', and 'trans*' have evolved, reflecting societal attitudes and cultural perspectives. While older terms such as 'transvestite' and 'transsexual' were often used as slurs, 'transgender' is now preferred for its inclusivity within the trans* community.

While some authors have suggested that transgender and diversity of gender identity are a relatively new phenomenon, there are historical accounts of children within Western society expressing their gender identity (Gill-Peterson 2018). Gill-Peterson argues that historical documents evidence that trans* children have always existed, with social transitions occurring long before medical interventions, despite prevailing cisnormativity cultural and sociopolitical factors. Non-Western cultural perspectives from India, Polynesia, and the Americas also offer valuable insights into how trans* identities have existed throughout time. For instance, the Hijra community in South Asia has long been recognised as a third gender, challenging Western-centric views (Nanda 2014). Other examples of non-Western gender variance come from Indigenous communities in the Americas, such as the two-spirit identity. This identity represents a reclamation of traditional suprabinary gender roles with cultural roots deeply tied to the land. It challenges colonial gender binaries while preserving and reaffirming Indigenous values and identities (Robinson 2019).

Although the concept of transgenderism has historical roots, over the past two decades, there has been an increased visibility of gender-variant youths seeking treatment, which traditional Western cisnormative services have been underprepared for. Rates in the UK of individuals identifying as transgender have increased since 2002 in all age groups with individuals aged 16–17 years showing the greatest proportionate increase from 0.19 per 10,000 in 2002 to 16.23 per 10,000 in 2018, with a sharp increase from 2015 onwards (McKechnie et al. 2023). More research is needed to understand this phenomenon and the transgender, gender-variant, and gender nonconforming identity development in children and young people, as identity development occurs during adolescence (Aitken et al. 2015).

> My journey as a trans* woman has been marked by moments of introspection, resilience and self-discovery. Struggling with gender dysphoria and its accompanying emotional turmoil I found solace in coping mechanisms such as writing, music and self-care rituals. (CH chapter co-author)

6.3 Gender Dysphoria Among Children and Adolescents

Understanding the prevalence of gender dysphoria (GD) among children and adolescents is needed for all those supporting these young people. The landscape of gender identity in younger populations is evolving, and some people may find they are confused by terms new to them. Healthcare professionals may find themselves in an environment where there are strong differences of opinion, which challenge clinicians to navigate an evolving understanding of gender identity in the younger populations. This is heightened by the ever-changing recognition and acceptance of not only transgender identities but also non-binary and other gender-diverse identities among youths.

6.3.1 Diagnostic Criteria

The updated versions of the two main mental disorder classifications, the World Health Organization's *International Classification of Diseases—11th Edition* (ICD-11) (WHO 2024) and the American Psychiatric Association's *Diagnostic and Statistical Manual Mental Disorders 5th Edition* (DSM-5) (APA 2023), differ substantially in relation to transgender identity.

- DSM-5 uses the term gender dysphoria (GD).
- ICD-11 uses the term gender incongruence (GI).

GD in DSM-5 is considered to be a mental health condition and implies discomfort and distress a person may experience because of the accompanying conflict regarding their assigned gender and their identification with a different gender. The term gender identity disorder was used in a previous edition of DSM (i.e. DSM-4) but is no longer used. Likewise, terms such as gender identity and transexual have been removed from ICD-11 and renamed gender incongruence (GI) and also moved from the chapter on mental and neurodevelopmental disorders to a separate chapter entitled "Conditions related to sexual health". Under this definition, trans* people are no longer classified as having a mental illness, which moves away from pathologising identities and reducing stigma. Additionally, there are differences in diagnostic criteria in the duration/persistence of the condition. ICD-11 provides more flexibility, e.g. a condition persisting for several months, *whereas* in DSM-5, it requires *a* minimum of 6 months. Both definitions have, however, identified four main features for the diagnoses of gender incongruence or gender dysphoria:

- A strong aversion to or discomfort with one's primary and/or secondary sex characteristics.
- A strong desire to be rid of some of or all of one's sex characteristics.
- A strong desire to be treated, accepted, and affirmed as the gender the young person identifies as.
- A strong desire to have the primary/secondary sex characteristics or appearance of their experienced gender.

All those involved in supporting young people need to understand and familiarise themselves with the criteria laid out in DSM-5 and ICD-11 regarding children and adolescents. Gender can be viewed as being a continuum with youngsters expressing themselves in different ways at different times of their lives. A lot of trans* young people may or may not transition and may not experience comorbid health issues. In fact, being trans* in itself is not a mental illness. However, there are many people who are very sceptical about using this type of diagnostic criteria as it can be potentially pathologising (Tordoff et al. 2022). The medicalisation of transgender identities and gender related to distress has been a controversial topic for decades, and there are concerns about further stigmatisation of an already marginalised population.

6.4 Gender Expression and Early Manifestation of Dissatisfaction with Gender Identity

Gender exploration, argued to be a key aspect of understanding gender dysphoria and gender nonconformity, can appear quite early in childhood. Butler (1990) suggests that gender exploration and nonconforming gender expression may manifest in children as young as 2–4 years. This may be due to gender schemas and cognitive frameworks that help individuals understand and process information about gender, which begins to form at a very young age. These schemas are influenced by a myriad of factors including family, culture, media, and peer interactions. Children internalise gender schemas, which then shape understanding of gender roles and influence gender expression. Gender play in childhood is a natural and common part of development. It involves children experimenting with roles, behaviours, and activities that are traditionally associated with different genders. It is important for healthcare professionals to recognise that gender play is a normal, healthy part of childhood and not inherently indicative of a child's gender identity. While gender play is about exploration and does not necessarily reflect deep-seated feelings about one's gender identity, early signs of gender dysphoria are different. Gender dysphoria (GD) involves a persistent discomfort with the gender assigned at birth and a strong identification with a different gender. This is more than just a preference for the toys or clothes traditionally associated with the other gender. Children who experience gender dysphoria may consistently express that they are, or want to be, another gender. They might also show distress about their physical sex characteristics or social roles that are associated with their assigned gender.

Current discourse around GD and transgender identities in youth is heavily influenced by social, political, and cultural factors. The polarised nature of this discourse can impact the mental health and well-being of gender-diverse youth. People supporting young people must, therefore, navigate these discussions carefully, ensuring that their practice is informed by the most current research and is sensitive to the individual experiences of their young clients (Rafferty et al. 2018; Telfer et al. 2018). It is important for people working with young people to be aware of how sociopolitical narratives shape how we approach working with this client group, shape the services for them, and affect young people and their families/carers and siblings.

6.4.1 Prevalence of Gender Dysphoria

The DSM-5 (2024) gives a gender dysphoria prevalence of 0.005% to 0.014% of people assigned male at birth (5–14 per 100,000) and 0.002% to 0.003% of people assigned female at birth (2–3 per 100,000). While these figures might seem low, it is significant, pointing towards a growing recognition and diagnosis of GD. In the UK, there was a sharp rise in the past decade in referrals to the Tavistock and Portman NHS Mental Health Trust (the home of the UK Gender Identity Development Service—see later in this chapter) from 250 referrals in 2011–2012 to

5000 in 2021–2022. This change has been observed not just in the UK but also in Canada, the USA, and Finland with a preponderance of those assigned female at birth (Graham 2023).

This increase in reported cases can be partly attributed to a broader societal awareness and acceptance of gender diversity. However, it is important to note that these statistics only account for formally diagnosed cases, potentially omitting a wider range of gender nonconformity experiences among young people. The variability in GD prevalence, as indicated by Steensma and Cohen-Kettenis (2011) and Zucker (2017), underscores the diverse and fluid nature of gender experiences in youth.

There's an observable trend in the increasing number of young people reaching out for support related to GD. de Graaf et al. (2018) and Kaltiala et al. (2020) have both noted a rise in referrals to specialist gender clinics. This uptrend can be linked to several societal shifts. For one, there's a change in attitudes towards seeking help, with less stigma attached to gender diversity. The increased visibility of diverse gender identities in the media and public discourse also plays a crucial role, as does heightened public awareness. These factors collectively contribute to a more supportive environment where individuals feel more comfortable seeking help and expressing their gender identities.

6.4.2 Longitudinal and Epidemiological Data

One of the challenges in understanding GD among children and adolescents is the scarcity of comprehensive epidemiological studies to understand the prevalence, experiences, and health outcomes of these diverse gender identities in youth populations. There is a gap in the research landscape: the absence of extensive, formal studies specifically targeting youth with nonconforming gender identities (Zucker 2017). Recent efforts have aimed to address this gap, with emerging studies attempting to gather more inclusive and detailed data. For instance, studies are now being designed to capture a broader range of gender experiences, including those of non-binary and genderqueer youth, which were often overlooked in earlier research. However, as new studies are being developed and piloted, concerns around design and methodology are being raised. Future studies need to be mindful on the importance of using language that respects and reflects the self-identified gender of participants.

6.4.3 Comorbid Mental Health Issues

Gender incongruence and gender dysphoria can pose significant challenges to the mental health and well-being of young people, particularly those under the age of 16. As they navigate their gender identity and expression, they may encounter various psychosocial stressors and experiences that can exacerbate mental health difficulties. Understanding the complex interplay between gender identity and mental health is crucial for developing supportive interventions and promoting positive outcomes for young individuals.

There are social consequences of expressing gender identity deemed transgressive within Western society, for example, Cooper et al. (2020) identified through qualitative enquiry that trans* people can experience social ostracisation due to lack of societal acceptance for nonconformity to traditional gender norms. This can lead to feelings of loneliness, invisibility, invalidation, and a reduced sense of belonging. Trans* young people may experience body dissatisfaction, which can contribute towards an eating disorder (Avila et al. 2019). Furthermore, transgender youths can experience concurrent attention deficit disorders and be neurodiverse. There is a consistent observation about the prevalence in gender-diverse young people, which is identified as being three to six times higher than their cis counterparts (Warrier et al. 2020). Research suggests that young people grappling with gender incongruence and dysphoria often experience psychiatric comorbidity and coexisting problems (Olson et al. 2016). These challenges can manifest in various forms, including depression, anxiety, self-harm, and suicidal ideation. Stigma, prejudice, and discrimination contribute to the heightened vulnerability of these individuals, exacerbating their mental health struggles.

> From a personal experience of self-harm and trauma I can attest to the transformative power of compassionate and inclusive care in fostering healing and resilience. (CH chapter co-author)

6.4.4 Coexisting Problems

Supportive environments, both within the family and broader community, can play a crucial role in mitigating the adverse effects of gender incongruence and dysphoria on mental health (Spencer et al. 2021). Unfortunately, many trans* young people experience rejection and marginalisation, particularly within their families (McCann and Brown 2019). This rejection can lead to social isolation and exacerbate mental health issues. Conversely, parental support has been identified as a protective factor against the development of depression in trans* adolescents (Simons et al. 2013).

Trans* youths are disproportionately exposed to bullying, harassment, and discrimination in school settings, which can have profound implications for their mental health and educational outcomes (Javda et al. 2023; McCann and Brown 2019). Feeling unsafe at school can contribute to a negative educational experience and exacerbate mental health difficulties. Addressing homophobic, biphobic, and transphobic bullying requires concerted efforts from school leadership, staff, and community stakeholders to create anti-bullying strategies as identified in other chapters in this book.

> I felt like I couldn't be myself or express my true gender identity without facing discrimination, bullying and rejection from those around me. This caused me to feel isolated and alone which only exacerbated any feelings of depression and anxiety. (CH chapter co-author)

6.4.5 Healthcare Access and Risks

Accessing healthcare services can be particularly challenging for trans* young people due to several factors, including discrimination, a lack of understanding among healthcare providers, and the limited availability of gender dysphoria clinics (Wright et al. 2021). These barriers often result in inadequate and inappropriate care, exacerbating the mental and physical health issues that trans* youth may face. In this context, online forums have emerged as a valuable resource, offering much-needed emotional support and community. However, these platforms also present risks such as exposure to misinformation and online bullying (Pardoe and Trainor 2017), which can further complicate the mental health landscape for trans* young people.

The discourse surrounding medical interventions for trans* youth is complex and has sparked considerable debate. Critics argue that medical interventions may not always be the best approach for supporting young people who are questioning their gender identity (Edwards-Leeper et al. 2016). Despite this, there is growing evidence to suggest that social affirmation can be an effective and supportive strategy (Spivey and Edwards-Leeper 2019).

Social affirmation involves recognising and validating a young person's gender identity, which can significantly reduce distress and improve mental health outcomes. Studies have shown that children who have socially transitioned demonstrate no elevations in depression compared to their peers, highlighting the potential protective effects of social affirmation (Olson et al. 2016). However, other studies on "gender-affirming care" criticise this approach and suggest a more conservative approach that addresses psychiatric comorbidities and psychotherapeutically exploring the developmental aetiology of the trans* identity (Levine and Abbruzzese 2023). It is important to recognise that this is a topic over which there are conflicting views. Gender-affirming care including social affirmation is currently one of the most debated conversations, particularly whether this is appropriate for minors.

Research by Bhatt et al. (2022) highlights that even if a young person ultimately decides not to transition medically, the experience of having their gender identity affirmed by others can be crucial. This affirmation, whether temporary or permanent, provides essential support during a critical period of identity exploration and development. It can help build a sense of belonging and self-worth, which are vital for the overall well-being of trans* youth.

In addition to the challenges faced by trans* individuals, there are other factors that can significantly impact their experiences in health and social care settings. One such factor is the intersectionality of gender identity and neurodiversity. For instance, in an exploration of autistic trans* people's experiences of healthcare, Adams et al. (2024) found that autistic transgender and non-binary (TNB) individuals were misgendered more frequently by mental healthcare providers compared to their allistic (non-autistic) TNB counterparts. This misgendering can lead to increased distress and negatively affect their mental health and overall well-being.

Further research is essential to identify and address the specific barriers that lead to misgendering in healthcare settings for autistic TNB individuals. Understanding these factors will help develop targeted interventions and training programmes for healthcare providers, ensuring that they can offer more respectful, affirming, and effective care.

An essential component of care is the education of parents, peers, and community members about trans issues, creating an environment that fosters support for the well-being of trans* youth.

6.5 Gender Identity Services in the UK and the Cass Review

In the UK, a national Gender Identity Development Service (GIDS) was established in 1989 at the Tavistock Clinic in London, and at that time, it saw fewer than ten children a year, taking referrals from Child and Adolescent Mental Health Services (CAMHS) or general practitioners (GPs). Originally GIDS main focus was therapeutic, with only a small proportion referred for hormone treatment by around age 16. The approach to treatment changed with the emergence of the so-called the Dutch Protocol, which involved the use of puberty blockers from early puberty. In 2014, and without published evidence of positive outcomes, puberty blockers moved from a research-only protocol to being available in routine clinical practice, which included those under 18.

A series of key events in 2020 prompted an evaluation of GIDS in a review headed by Dr. Hilary Cass (2024); these included:

- Publication of the results of the 2011 research studies, which showed there was a lack of positive measurable outcomes from the use of puberty blockers.
- A significant increase in the number of referrals to the GIDS year on year, reaching to nearly 3000 in 2020 with waiting times stretching to almost 3 years (Cass 2024).
- A High Court ruling that those under the age of 16 did not have the competence to make their own decisions about receiving medical interventions, particularly in light of a lack of evidence of the long-term impacts of these treatments.

The interim review in 2022 (Cass 2022) found 'gaps in the evidence' over the use of puberty blockers and supported the National Institute for Clinical and Social Care Excellence's (NICE) opinion that there was 'not enough evidence to support the safety or clinical effectiveness of puberty suppressing hormones to make the treatment routinely available at this time' (NICE 2020). The ban was originally a short-term solution; however, at the time of writing this chapter, it is being extended for an indefinite period of time. As a result, NHS England stopped prescribing them to children. However, concerns remain that this emphasis has disregarded the necessity for prescription of puberty blockers, to delay onset of puberty as a highly distressing experience for trans* youths that can worsen gender dysphoria. This is especially pertinent as recent research from Australia suggests that as little as 1% of young people who seek gender identity services reidentify with their birth-registered sex (Blake et al. 2024). However, allowing for more time to understand the reason and mitigate gender dysphoria that is harmful to trans* young people, children experiencing significant gender dysphoria may seek intervention outside of NHS services, resulting in young people going to private clinics abroad or purchasing medication online. Concerns also centre around children who may be able to demonstrate capacity to give consent to medical treatment without parents' knowledge or consent (also known as "Gillick competence") but who may now be excluded from such conversations with health professionals. However, these topics are under serious discussion at present, and recommendations may change in the future.

In July 2022, the NHS announced the closure of the Gender Identity Development Service (GIDS) and the establishment of new regional healthcare services aimed at providing holistic care by linking into local mental health services. These new services opened in 2024 at Alder Hey Hospital, Liverpool, in the north and Great Ormond Street Hospital, London, in the south of England. More recently, a clinic has opened in Bristol, and there are plans to open a fourth clinic in the East of England in Spring 2025. The Tavistock centre is now closed.

The Cass Review has led to significant disappointment and concern within the trans* community, largely due to unresolved questions about potential bias in the report's development. Community members are calling for greater transparency regarding the criteria used for inclusion and exclusion in the review, underscoring a need for further clarification to address their concerns effectively. The Mermaids charity has published their concerns; however, there is consensus that the review recognises the plight of young people in accessing services and the failures of services to provide adequate care (Mermaids 2024). Ahead of the Cass Review, NHS England announced in 2024 a pause on the prescription of puberty blockers for children, citing a need for more evidence to support their safe usage and clinical effectiveness. During the summer of 2024, an emergency ban prohibited UK private prescribers from the European Economic Area (EEA) or Switzerland from prescribing these medicines for puberty suppression in new patients under 16 experiencing gender dysphoria (RPS 2024). The Cass Review has faced significant critiques from multiple academic and professional sources regarding its methodology, evidence base, and implications for the transgender and gender-variant community. Yale Law School has criticised the review for its methodological flaws and selective use of evidence, noting that its conclusions are unsupported by broader scientific literature and have been misrepresented to justify restrictive measures on gender-affirming care (McNamara et al. 2024). Similarly, the Society of Gender Based Medicine in Germany has responded, highlighting the review's lack of rigorous scientific methodology and inadequate evidence base due to its failure to systemically appraise the literature. Concern around gender conservative recommendations is that the findings are not aligned with international standards and may harm transgender youth by restricting access to necessary treatments (Society of Gender Based Medicine 2024). Furthermore, the exclusion of trans* healthcare experts and individuals with lived experience from the review process has been highlighted as a significant limitation, arguing that its flawed evidence and recommendations could lead to adverse outcomes by limiting access to essential medical interventions (Horton 2024).

While recent actions do not proscribe puberty blockers on the grounds of risks to patient safety, puberty blockers have positive effects. Rew et al. (2021) identify risks associated with the use of puberty blockers but also highlight these medications can significantly reduce suicidality and improve psychological functioning and social life, potentially alleviating aspects of gender dysphoria by providing more time for gender identity exploration without the stress of ongoing pubertal development. Additionally, puberty blockers can prevent the need for extensive and often traumatic bodily surgeries in the future. By delaying the development of unwanted secondary sexual characteristics, such as breast tissue in transmasculine individuals, the necessity for procedures like top surgery (breast removal) can be reconsidered or potentially avoided.

Some young people and their families themselves feel that there are now 'limits' imposed on their gender expression.

> It is important to note that trans* identity does not in itself cause gender dysphoria and comorbid mental health issues, but instead it is the reaction of socialisation affects to that identity that causes problems to an individual's mental health. (CH chapter co-author)

This section has provided an overview of some of the current debates and anomalies of treating young people with gender dysphoria in the UK. The authors have tried to provide a balanced narrative, which suggests that GD youths should have access to both gender services and psychiatric treatment, and which are individualised to each person's unique circumstances. However, the picture is dynamic and ever-evolving, and the reader should also access current guidance and opinions of authoritative bodies on this topic.

6.6 Supporting Trans* Young People in Schools

The recent guidance from the Department for Education (2023) in England stresses the necessity of caution and parental involvement in supporting gender-questioning children within educational settings. Crucially, the guidance asserts that decisions about social transitions should be influenced by parental views, and teachers are advised against initiating such transitions. Additionally, it mandates that single-sex spaces must remain so, with alternative facilities to be considered for gender-questioning children. The guidance also addresses sports participation, suggesting that physical differences be considered for safety and fairness. Name and pronoun changes are to be rare, with legal names and assigned sexes recorded, and schools may allow flexibility in uniform policies, especially with gender-neutral options (Department for Education 2023).

This has led to concerns by the trans* community about inclusivity and support. Some advocates argue that the guidance may not go far enough in creating an environment where gender-diverse students feel fully respected and understood. Evidence from Durwood et al. (2017) and Ehrensaft et al. (2018) indicates that socially transitioning children, when supported by adults, generally experience good well-being and positive mental health opposed to those individuals who are denied affirmation having adverse effects on their health and well-being (Cawley et al. 2019). Furthermore, the guidance's parent-first approach is contentious, as parental consent may not always align with the child's best interests. Research by Klein and Golub (2016) has shown that family rejection significantly increases the risks of suicide attempts and substance misuse among trans* individuals, highlighting the need for safeguarding measures for trans* young people, should circumstances require it.

> Reflecting on my school years, I realise how profoundly challenging they were, primarily due to the inability to express my true self. Physical Education (P.E.) was particularly harrowing. Despite the school's attempt to accommodate me by allowing me to change in the disabled toilet, I was still placed in the boys' group for lessons. This experience was agonising, as I already had a strong aversion to sports, and being among boys who bullied me compounded the distress. Meanwhile, my friends were in the girls' P.E. group, which intensified my feelings of isolation and discomfort. The segregation of groups in P.E., and other school activities, can be particularly traumatic for trans* individuals. Such rigid structures often leave those in distress without adequate support or recourse. It is imperative for educational institutions to provide alternative arrangements and support mechanisms for students experiencing similar challenges. The lack of such provisions contributes to feelings of marginalisation and alienation.
>
> The necessity of having supportive and affirming environments in schools cannot be overstated. Reducing or eliminating the already minimal support available can have devastating consequences for young people. My own experience is a testament to this: avoiding P.E. due to fear and discomfort led to significant educational setbacks and severely impacted my already poor mental health. (CH chapter co-author).

People supporting trans* youths in schools should be aware of the shifting landscape in this area and act in accordance with legislation, guidance, and the best interest of the young person.

6.7 Principles of Working with Those Supporting Gender Dysphoric Young People

As frontline staff become more involved in supporting these youngsters, this chapter concludes with some 'do's' and 'don'ts' and some principles of care from one of the authors (Table 6.2).

2024 was a year in which trans healthcare in young people has been under scrutiny and where there is a lack of consensus, and the void can be filled with anxiety and emotion; therefore, it is important to adopt some principles of care when supporting these young people and their families.

Principles

- Validate the young person's emotions and help them with techniques to alleviate the accompanying distress they may feel.
- Actively treat the comorbid mental health conditions using the best available evidence.
- Be inclusive, non-judgemental, compassionate, and respectful.
- Take a watchful waiting approach to see how things develop.
- Each young person should be treated individually and with the involvement of parents and carers and educational and community networks.
- Adopt an accepting approach without trying to influence decisions.
- Allow exploration of the reasons for the presence of gender dysphoria.
- Decisions about change of name, pronoun, use of toilets, etc. need to be negotiated, and adults need to be open-minded and sympathetic to what are the young person's wishes.
- The increasing visibility and inclusion of trans* young people mean that those supporting young people need to understand the needs of these youngsters and their families and develop supporting pathways and onward referral to appropriate support.
- As sibling relationships are often the longest and most influential relationships in a young person's life, siblings of transgender youth may also need support in the same way as parents.

Table 6.2 DO's and DON'Ts for interacting with gender dysphoric young people (CH chapter co-author)

DO's for interacting with gender dysphoric young people
Be positive and genuine and above all be patient
Create a safe space for a young person to explore their feelings
Listen carefully to what the family and young people are saying and try to worth out where everyone is up to on the journey
Explore the concept of gender within the family considering role models
Ask the young person and family what support they may require helping them including involving the wider family and community
Introduce yourself with your name and pronoun
Do not rush to offer solutions and allow the young person and the family to come up with issues they are facing
Be flexible as family members may experience different reactions at different time points
Check if it is OK to ask intrusive or personal things:
Give up-to-date and relevant advice
Let the young person to self-identify

(continued)

Table 6.2 (continued)

DON'Ts for interacting with gender dysphoric young people
Don't pretend that you know what they are going through when you don't
Don't ever say it's just a phase that they are going through and they will grow out of it
Don't say they have to dress in a particular way unless the young people feel strongly about it is up to them to take the lead
Don't refuse to use the individuals' preferred name or preferred pronouns; if you make a mistake, correct yourself or allow someone to correct you and move on
Avoid disclosing any individual's gender-diverse identity unless you have permission from the young person as many trans and gender-diverse young people are not open to everybody*
Don't talk over the young person to family members or other adults
Don't pretend that you are the expert

6.8 Reflective Task

Reflective practice is an essential component in developing a deeper understanding and enhancing the quality of care and support provided to young people. This reflective task aims to guide you through a process of introspection, helping to identify personal knowledge gaps and biases, while fostering an empathetic and informed approach to supporting trans* people. By engaging in this activity, you will be able to assess your current understanding of trans* identities, the psychosocial stressors faced by these young people, and the specific challenges related to coexisting mental health issues. The task encourages honest self-reflection and proactive learning, providing a framework to develop practical action plans. These plans will not only enhance your knowledge, skills, and confidence when working with trans* young people but also promote a more inclusive and supportive environment. As you undertake this activity, take the time to thoroughly contemplate each question, jotting down your thoughts and feelings honestly. This exercise is designed to be a transformative step towards becoming a more effective and compassionate advocate for young people.

Reflective Task: Enhancing Support for Trans* Youths

This reflective activity aims to help you identify and overcome barriers related to understanding and supporting trans* youths, particularly those experiencing gender dysphoria and coexisting mental health issues. Reflect on the provided questions to develop an action plan that enhances your knowledge and confidence in supporting trans* youths effectively.

Reflect on Your Current Understanding

- What do you currently know about trans identities, including gender identity, gender expression, sexual orientation, gender dysphoria, and gender incongruence?

(continued)

- How familiar are you with the psychosocial stressors faced by trans youths, such as societal rejection and bullying?
- How confident do you feel in your ability to distinguish between gender dysphoria and coexisting mental health issues and to support trans* youths effectively?

Action

Take a few minutes to jot down your initial thoughts. Be honest about any knowledge gaps or areas of less confidence. Note definitions and examples you are familiar with and any uncertainties you have.

Identify Personal Concerns and Challenges

- What specific concerns or challenges do you have regarding understanding and supporting trans* youths, especially those with coexisting mental health issues?
- Consider obstacles that might hinder your support, such as personal biases, lack of knowledge, or institutional limitations. Reflect on how sociopolitical narratives and cultural factors might influence your approach.

Action

Reflect on potential barriers, exploring their origins—whether from past experiences, societal norms, or gaps in understanding. Consider the impact of sociopolitical and cultural factors on your approach.

Develop an Action Plan

- What specific actions can you take to improve your understanding and support of trans* youths?
- What resources (books, articles, online courses, local support groups) are available to help you enhance your knowledge and skills?

Action

List practical steps to increase your knowledge and confidence. Consider resources such as:

- *Books written by trans people on trans identities and gender diversity.*
- *Articles and research papers on gender dysphoria and trans issues.*
- *Online courses or webinars on supporting trans* youths.*
- *Engaging with your local LGBTQ+ community for firsthand insights.*
- *Be aware of the current landscape for those youngsters under 18.*

6.9 Resources and Services for Supporting and Signposting Non-binary Youth

For people working with children and young prolific who are trans*, there is a need for greater awareness of services and advice tailored to these individuals. As detailed earlier in this chapter, trans* youth often face unique challenges that can impact their mental health and well-being. These challenges include, but are not limited to, societal stigma, discrimination, lack of family support, and internal conflicts regarding their gender identity. Mental health professionals play a vital role in providing the emotional support and guidance necessary to help these young individuals thrive. Understanding their needs and knowing where to direct them for additional support can make a significant difference in their lives. For all health and social care professionals, it is important to be informed about the resources available to support transgender and non-binary youths and their families.

Some useful resources are listed below.

- *Mermaids* (https://mermaidsuk.org.uk/): The organisation offers a variety of services that are essential for trans youth and their families.
- *Childline* (https://www.childline.org.uk/): A service for young people in need of support. It provides a free confidential service where young people can talk about anything.
- *NSPCC* (https://www.nspcc.org.uk/): The NSPCC offers general support for children and young people and provides guidance for parents with gender-diverse children.
- *YoungMinds* (https://www.youngminds.org.uk/) are a mental health charity for children, young people, and their parents, making sure all young people can get the mental health support they need.

For all adults supporting transgender, non-binary, and gender-diverse youth, understanding and signposting the appropriate resources and services is important to supplement their day-to-day practices. By leveraging appropriate resources, professionals can ensure that transgender, non-binary, and gender-variant youth are able to obtain resources and support they need to navigate their journeys with confidence and resilience.

6.10 Final Words

The objective of this chapter is to present the various viewpoints, debates, and controversies surrounding this uniquely challenging topic. In this ever-shifting environment, the reader should also be aware of the developing legislation, up-to-date guidance from authoritative bodies, opinions of relevant charities, and evidence from peer-reviewed publications.

The final words are from the personal perspective of one of the authors who has shared their personal insights throughout this chapter to help those supporting young people.

> Building in strength, courage and resilience to continue my journey forward, hoping that my story can help not just trans* people but those around them in understanding, accepting and supporting them to being able to live their own life in the way they are supposed to, as themselves. (CH chapter author)

References

Adams N, Jacobsen K, Li L, Francino M, Rutherford L, Tei C, Bauer G. Health and health care access of autistic transgender and nonbinary people in Canada: a cross-sectional study. Autism in Adulthood; 2024. https://doi.org/10.1089/aut.2023.0024.

Aitken M, Steensma TD, Blanchard R, VanderLaan DP, Wood H, Fuentes A, Spegg C, Wasserman L, Ames M, Fitzsimmons CL, Leef JH, Lishak V, Reim E, Takagi A, Vinik J, Wreford J, Cohen-Kettenis PT, de Vries AL, Kreukels BP, Zucker KJ. Evidence for an altered sex ratio in clinic-referred adolescents with gender dysphoria. J Sex Med. 2015;12(3):756–63. https://doi.org/10.1111/jsm.12817. Epub 2015 Jan 22.

American Psychiatric Association. DSM-5 diagnostic and statistical manual of mental disorders. Updates to the Fifth edition DSM-5™. 2023. Available from: https://www.psychiatry.org/psychiatrists/practice/dsm/updates-to-dsm/updates-to-dsm-5-tr-criteria-text. Accessed 7 Oct 2024.

Avila JT, Golden NH, Aye T. Eating disorder screening in transgender youth. J Adolesc Health. 2019;65(6):815–7. https://doi.org/10.1016/j.jadohealth.2019.06.011.

Bhatt N, Cannella J, Gentile JP. Gender-affirming care for transgender patients. Innov Clin Neurosci. 2022;19(4–6):23.

Blake S, Cavve BS, Bickendorf X, Ball J, et al. Reidentification with birth-registered sex in a Western Australian pediatric gender clinic cohort. JAMA Pediatr. 2024;178(5):446–53. https://doi.org/10.1001/jamapediatrics.2024.0077.

Butler J. Gender trouble: feminism and the subversion of identity. New York: Routledge; 1990. ISBN 0415900425.

Cass H. The independent review of gender identity services for children and young people. Interim report. 2022. Available from: https://cass.independent-review.uk/home/publications/interim-report/. Accessed 7 Oct 2024.

Cass H. The independent review of gender identity services for children and young people. Final report. 2024. Available from: https://cass.independent-review.uk/home/publications/final-report/. Accessed 7 Oct 2024.

Cawley R, Pontin EE, Touhey J, Sheehy K, Taylor PJ. What is the relationship between rejection and self-harm or suicidality in adulthood. J Affect Disord. 2019;242:123–34.

Cooper K, Russell A, Mandy W, Butler C. The phenomenology of gender dysphoria in adults: a systematic review and meta-synthesis. Clin Psychol Rev. 2020;80:101875.

de Graaf NM, Cohen-Kettenis PT, Carmichael P, de Vries AL, Dhondt K, Laridaen J, Steensma TD. Psychological functioning in adolescents referred to specialist gender identity clinics across Europe: a clinical comparison study between four clinics. Eur Child Adolesc Psychiatry. 2018;27:909–19.

Department of Education. Gender questioning children: everything you need to know about new draft guidance for schools. London: Department of Education; 2023.

Durwood L, McLaughlin KA, Olson KR. Mental health and self-worth in socially transitioned transgender youth. J Am Acad Child Adolesc Psychiatry. 2017;56(2):116–23.e2.

Edwards-Leeper L, Leibowitz S, Sangganjanavanich VF. Affirmative practice with transgender and gender nonconforming youth: expanding the model. Psychol Sex Orientat Gend Divers. 2016;3(2):165.
Ehrensaft D, Giammattei SV, Storck K, Tishelman AC, Keo-Meier C. Prepubertal social gender transitions: what we know; what we can learn—a view from a gender affirmative lens. Int J Transgend. 2018;19(2):251–68.
Fiani CN, Han HJ. Navigating identity: experiences of binary and non-binary transgender and gender non-conforming (TGNC) adults. Int J Transgend. 2018;20(2–3):181–94. https://doi.org/10.1080/15532739.2018.1426074.
Gill-Peterson J. Histories of the transgender child. University of Minnesota Press; 2018. https://www.upress.umn.edu/book-division/books/histories-of-the-transgender-child
Graham P. Transgender children and young people: how the evidence can point the way forward. BJPsych Bull. 2023;47(2):98–104. https://doi.org/10.1192/bjb.2022.3.
Horton C. The Cass review: cis-supremacy in the UK's approach to healthcare for trans children. Int J Transgender Health. 2024:1–25. https://doi.org/10.1080/26895269.2024.2328249.
Jadva V, Guasp A, Bradlow JH, Bower-Brown S, Foley S. Predictors of self-harm and suicide in LGBT youth: The role of gender, socio-economic status, bullying and school experience. J Public Health (Oxf). 2023;45(1):102–108. https://doi.org/10.1093/pubmed/fdab383. PMID: 34850220; PMCID: PMC10017085.
Kaltiala R, Bergman H, Carmichael P, de Graaf NM, Egebjerg Rischel K, Frisén L, Waehre A. Time trends in referrals to child and adolescent gender identity services: a study in four Nordic countries and in the UK. Nord J Psychiatry. 2020;74(1):40–4.
Klein A, Golub SA. Family rejection as a predictor of suicide attempts and substance misuse among transgender and gender nonconforming adults. LGBT Health. 2016;3(3):193–9. https://doi.org/10.1089/lgbt.2015.0111.
Levine SB, Abbruzzese E. Current concerns about gender-affirming therapy in adolescents. Curr Sex Health Rep. 2023;15:113–23. https://doi.org/10.1007/s11930-023-00358-x.
McCann E, Brown M. Homelessness among youth who identify as LGBTQ+: a systematic review. J Clin Nurs. 2019;28(11–12):2061–72.
McKechnie DGJ, O'Nions E, Bailey J, Hobbs L, Gillespie F, Petersen I. Transgender identity in young people and adults recorded in UK primary care electronic patient records: retrospective, dynamic, cohort study. BMJ Med. 2023;28;2(1):e000499. https://doi.org/10.1136/bmjmed-2023-000499. PMID: 38034075; PMCID: PMC10685922.
McNamara M, Baker K, Connelly K, Janssen A, Olson-Kennedy J, Pang K, Scheim AJ, Turban J, Alstott A. An evidence-based critique of "the Cass review" on gender-affirming care for adolescent gender dysphoria. Yale: Yale University; 2024. Available at: https://law.yale.edu/sites/default/files/documents/integrity-project_cass-response.pdf
Mermaids. Mermaid's response to the Cass review. 2024. Available from: https://mermaidsuk.org.uk/news/mermaids-response-to-the-cass-review-in-depth/. Accessed 7 Oct 2024].
Nanda S. Gender diversity: crosscultural variations. Long Grove: Waveland Press; 2014.
National Institute for Health and Social Care Excellence. Evidence review: gender affirming hormones for children and adolescents with gender dysphoria. 2020. Available from: https://cass.independent-review.uk/nice-evidence-reviews/. Accessed 7 Oct 2024.
Olson KR, Durwood L, DeMeules M, McLaughlin KA. Mental health of transgender children who are supported in their identities. Pediatrics. 2016;137(3):e20153223.
Pardoe J, Trainor G. Transgender youths who self-harm: perspectives from those seeking support. Mental Health Today. 2017 Jan 27. Available from: https://www.mentalhealthtodaycouk/transgender-youths-who-self-harm-perspectives-from-those-seeking-support
Rafferty J, Committee on Psychosocial Aspects of Child and Family Health; Committee on Adolescence; Section on Lesbian, Gay, Bisexual, and Transgender Health and Wellness. Ensuring comprehensive care and support for transgender and gender-diverse children and adolescents. Pediatrics. 2018;142(4):e20182162. https://doi.org/10.1542/peds.2018-2162.

Rew L, Young CC, Monge M, Bogucka R. Puberty blockers for transgender and gender diverse youth—a critical review of the literature. Child Adolesc Mental Health. 2021;26(1):3–14.
Robinson M. Two-Spirit identity in a time of gender fluidity. J Homosex. 2019;67(12):1675–90. https://doi.org/10.1080/00918369.2019.1613853.
Royal Pharmaceutical Society. New restrictions on the prescription and supply of puberty blockers. 2024. Available from: https://www.rpharms.com/about-us/news/details/New-restrictions-on-the-prescription-and-supply-of-puberty-blockers#:~:text=Why%20has%20the%20ban%20been,Cass%20Review)%20earlier%20this%20year. Accessed 3 July 2024.
Simons L, Schrager SM, Clark LF, Belzer M, Olson J. Parental support and mental health among transgender adolescents. J Adolesc Health. 2013;53(6):791–3.
Society of Gender Based Medicine. Response to the Cass review. 2024. Available at https://segm.org/German-draft-guidelines-gender-dysphoria-children-adolescents-2024. Accessed 7 Oct 2024.
Spencer KG, Berg DR, Bradford NJ, Vencill JA, Tellawi G, Rider G. The gender-affirmative life span approach: a developmental model for clinical work with transgender and gender-diverse children, adolescents, and adults. Psychotherapy. 2021;58(1):37.
Spivey LA, Edwards-Leeper L. Future directions in affirmative psychological interventions with transgender children and adolescents. J Clin Child Adolesc Psychol. 2019;48(2):343–56.
Steensma TD, Cohen-Kettenis PT. Gender transitioning before puberty. Arch Sex Behav. 2011;40:649–50.
Telfer M, Tollit M, Pace C, Pang KC. Australian standards of care and treatment guidelines for transgender and gender diverse children and adolescents. Med J Aust. 2018;209(3):132–6. https://doi.org/10.5694/mja17.01044.
Tordoff D, Wanta J, Colin A, et al. Mental health outcomes in transgender and nonbinary youths receiving gender-affirming care. JAMA Netw Open. 2022;5(2):e220978. https://doi.org/10.1001/jamanetworkopen.2022.0978.
Warrier V, Greenberg DM, Weir E, et al. Elevated rates of autism, other neurodevelopmental and psychiatric diagnoses, and autistic traits in transgender and gender-diverse individuals. Nat Commun. 2020;11:3959. https://doi.org/10.1038/s41467-020-17794-1.
World Health Organization. International statistical classification of diseases and related health problems. 11th ed. WHO; 2024. Available from: https://icd.who.int/. Accessed 7 Oct 24
Wright T, Nicholls EJ, Rodger AJ, Burns FM, Weatherburn P, Pebody R, McCabe L, Wolton A, Gafos M, Witzel TC. Accessing and utilising gender-affirming healthcare in England and Wales: trans and non-binary people's accounts of navigating gender identity clinics. BMC Health Serv Res. 2021;21:1–1.
Zucker KJ. Epidemiology of gender dysphoria and transgender identity. Sex Health. 2017;14(5):404–11.

7 Impact of Social Exclusion, Intersectionality, and Discrimination on Children and Young People's Mental Health

Patience Udonsi, Miriam Collett, and Vanessa Heaslip

P. Udonsi (✉)
Directorate of Social Sciences, University of Salford, Salford, UK
e-mail: p.udonsi@salford.ac.uk

M. Collett · V. Heaslip
Directorate of Nursing and Midwifery, University of Salford, Salford, UK
e-mail: m.collett1@salford.ac.uk; V.A.Heaslip@salford.ac.uk

G. Trainor, V. Heaslip (eds.), *Needs of Children and Young People Living with Complex Mental Health Difficulties*,
https://doi.org/10.1007/978-3-031-84532-1_7

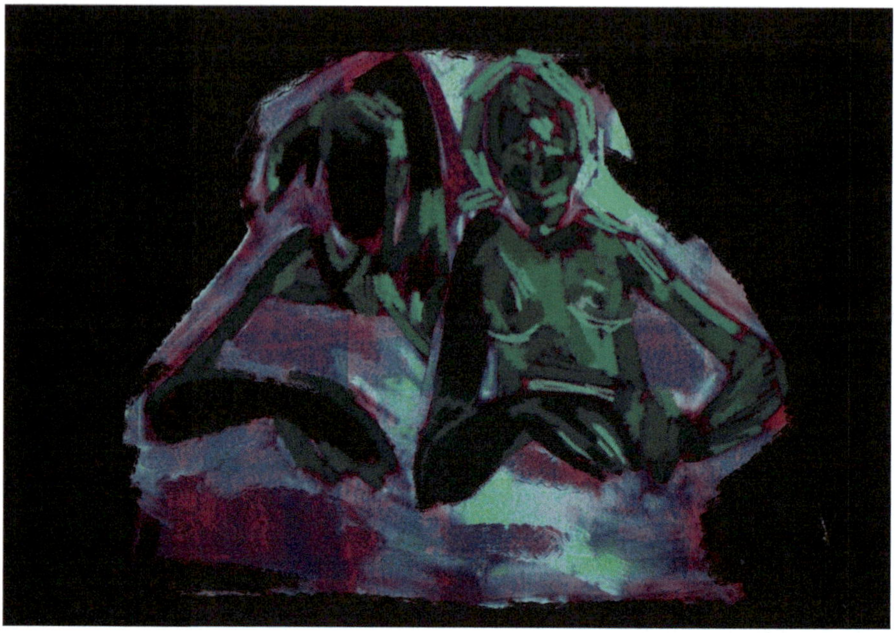

7.1 Health Inequalities and Mental Health

In 2010, Michael Marmot published a groundbreaking report that identified a social gradient in health; this social gradient identified that the lower the individual's position in society, the worse their health and, conversely, the higher the social position, the better their health (Marmot 2010). To understand this further, there is a need to understand the wider social determinants of health. The World Health Organization (WHO) defines social determinants as 'non-medical factors that influence health outcomes. They are the conditions in which people are born, grow, work, live, and age, and the wider set of forces and systems shaping the conditions of daily life' (WHO 2024). The social determinants of health are widely used within public health as accepted factors that impact upon health and well-being (see Fig. 7.1).

As it can be seen in Fig. 7.1, social determinants of health can affect every aspect of an individual's life; furthermore, it affects young people's social, psychological, cognitive, and emotional development (Atashbahar et al. 2022). The WHO recognises that the wider social determinants of health also have a significant impact upon mental health (WHO 2014) as the risk factors for many common mental disorders are linked to social inequalities that can exist before birth, during early childhood, through adolescence, and into adult life. Indeed, Marmot (2015) argues that social disadvantage has profound effects on developing brains limiting children's intellectual and social development (Marmot 2015). Ten years on from this initial

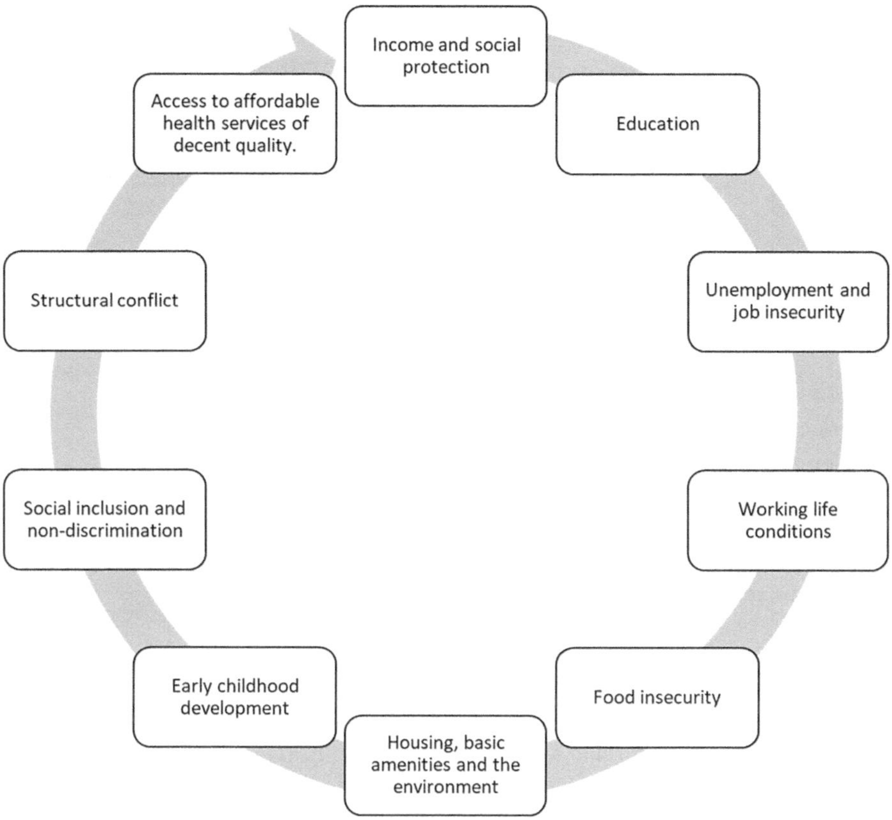

Fig. 7.1 Social determinants of health. (Adapted from World Health Organization 2024. https://www.who.int/health-topics/social-determinants-of-health#tab=tab_1)

review, Marmot published another report that identified a widening of health inequalities in England, most notably for women (Marmot et al. 2020). Furthermore, the gradient in healthy life expectancy is steeper than the life expectancy gradient meaning that not only do people living in deprived areas die younger but also they spend more of their shorter lives in ill-health (Marmot et al. 2020).

Due to this recognition of health inequities within the UK, NHS England has developed the Core20PLUS5 framework (NHS England 2021) to reduce health inequalities for adults, children, and young people at both national and system levels within England (see Fig. 7.2).

The Core20PLUS5 for children and young people's framework focuses attention in three areas: firstly, it focuses on the most deprived 20% of the population (see section on poverty later in this chapter for rationale); secondly, it focuses on the PLUS population groups (see Fig. 7.2) who are well known to experience social exclusion (NHS England 2020); and lastly, it focuses on five clinical areas (asthma, diabetes, epilepsy, oral health, and mental health) in recognition of the health

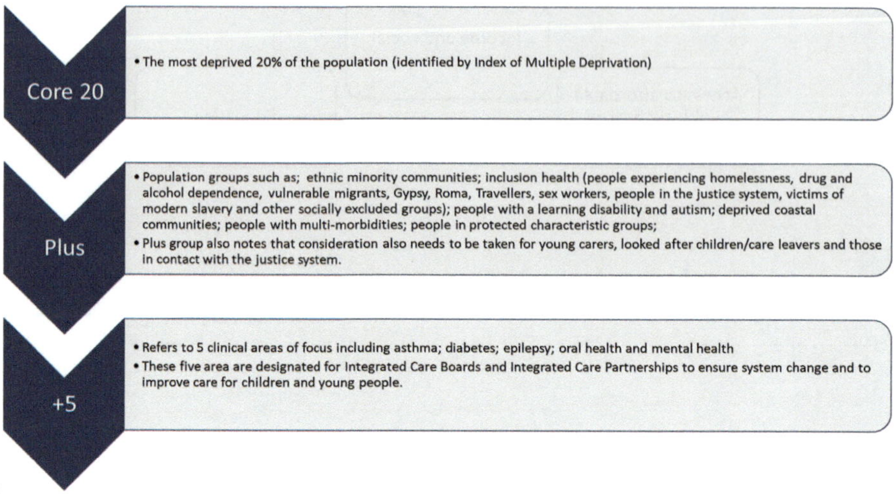

Fig. 7.2 Core20PLUS5 for children and young people. (Adapted from NHS England 2021. https://www.england.nhs.uk/about/equality/equality-hub/national-healthcare-inequalities-improvement-programme/core20plus5/core20plus5-cyp/)

challenges faced by children and young people (NHS England 2020). Social exclusion is an important concept here, and it is defined as 'a state in which individuals are unable to participate fully in economic, social, political and cultural life, as well as the process leading to and sustaining such a state' (United Nations 2016a: 8). Factors that influence an individual's experience of social exclusion include a lack of access to material resources (such as income, housing, or employment) or access to services (such as education or healthcare), a lack of agency over choices (such as a lack of capacity or ability to articulate choices), and/or a lack of feeling of being valued in the society (such as experiences of discrimination and alienation) (United Nations 2016a).

7.2 Discrimination and Stigma

In the UK, discrimination is defined within the Equality Act (2010) as 'treating someone less favourably than someone else because of a protected characteristic'. There are nine protected characteristics covered by the Equality Act (see Table 7.1) and which seek to protect those (with these protected characteristics) from discrimination through a legal framework, which covers many aspects of life such as employment, healthcare, and education (Equality Act 2010).

However, there are many people that experience discrimination who are not covered by the Equality Act (2010), for example, people with a lower socioeconomic status, people living in poverty, people with bigger bodies, and people with regional

Table 7.1 Protected characteristics (Equality Act 2010)

The Equality Act (2010) identifies the following protected characteristics:
Age
Disability
Gender reassignment
Marriage and civil partnership
Pregnancy and maternity
Race
Religion and belief
Sex
Sexual orientation

accents (Marmot 2020; Sanchez 2020; Wood and Elliott 2020; Brown et al. 2022; Thornicroft et al. 2022; Levon et al. 2021). This broader reflection on discrimination can be defined as 'Any distinctions, exclusion or preference made on the basis of race, [skin] colour, sex, religion, political opinion, national extraction or social origin, which has the effect of nullifying equality of opportunity or treatment in employment or occupation' (UNICEF 2022: 8).

The term 'stigma' means 'mark' and originated in ancient Greece, where a tattoo or mark was put on the bodies of slaves or criminals to signify to all their status (Thornicroft et al. 2022). Those with the mark had a low status and were treated poorly, with judgements being made about them based on their 'mark'. Modern concepts of stigma reflect this experience, where people who display 'socially undesirable' characteristics are treated poorly by others (Economou et al. 2020). Stigma occurs where there is a combination of 'labelling, stereotyping, separation, status loss and discrimination' (Link and Phelan 2001: 377). This always happens within the context of power imbalance, with those that are in positions of power deciding what characteristics are (or are not) socially acceptable, dictating who will experience stigma (Link and Phelan 2001; Thornicroft et al. 2022).

Discrimination and stigma are a major concern for children and young people, both nationally and globally. The United Nation (UN) Convention on the Rights of the Child (UN 1990) asserts that all children have the right to grow up without discrimination and asserts that member states take appropriate measures to ensure that children are protected against all forms of discrimination. Discrimination and stigma can have catastrophic effects on the mental health and well-being of children, their long-term outcomes, and, more broadly, the success of a sustainable future for all (Atashbahar et al. 2022; WHO 2014). Due to the links between poverty, social determinants, and social exclusion (identified earlier), addressing poverty and discrimination is at the core of many of the UN Sustainable Development Goals (SDGs) (UN 2016b); see Reflective Activity 7.1.

Reflective Activity 7.1: United Nations Sustainable Development Goals
Watch the video by the UN on the SDGs—https://www.youtube.com/watch?v=0XTBYMfZyrM—and following this, read:

- UN SDGs—https://sdgs.un.org/goals
- The Sustainable Development Goals Report 2022—accessed from https://unstats.un.org/sdgs/report/2022/

Choose from the following SDGs and look at the specific subtargets for that goal:

1—No poverty
3—Good health and well-being
5—Gender equality
7—Reduced inequalities

What progress do you think is being made towards the goals?

Consider what contribution you can make in your role or organisation towards achieving these within your role.

In 2022, the United Nations Children's Fund (UNICEF) published a report exploring the impact of discrimination on children. This report reported on a study with 407,000 young people and identified that 63% of respondents said discrimination was common in their environments (school, community, or workplace). Of these, 44% identified that the discrimination had a 'significant' impact on their lives or the lives of someone they know, whereas only 17% said that the discrimination had a 'little' effect on their life (UNICEF 2022). In terms of stigma and mental illness, a report by the YMCA (2016) with 2072 young people aged between 11 and 24 years across England and Wales (of which 1098 had experienced mental health difficulties) identified that:

- Seventy-five per cent of the sample believed that people experiencing difficulties with their mental health are treated negatively due to stigma.
- Thirty-eight per cent of those with mental health difficulties had experienced the negative effects of stigma.
- Thirty-seven per cent who experienced the stigma experienced it at least once a week.
- Fifty-nine per cent experienced this stigma whilst at school.
- Fifty-four per cent who experience this stigma said it came from their friends.

Not only does stigma worsen an individual's mental health but it also reduces the likelihood they will access professional support. Research by the YMCA (2016) noted that 85% of young people who experienced stigma said it affected their confidence, whilst 56% identified it made them less likely to seek professional help. The negative impact of stigma in mental health affecting young people's willingness to access professional services has also been reported by Villatoro et al. (2022), whose research with adolescents identified that they were more willing to seek help for peers who were struggling than they would for themselves.

7.3 Intersectionality

Initially conceptualised by Kimberlé Crenshaw in 1989, the theory of intersectionality has become instrumental in recognising the compounded effects of marginalisation and discrimination faced by individuals belonging to multiple marginalised groups, such as racial minorities or those experiencing economic hardship, particularly among young people (Nayak 2015). Intersectionality refers to the complex interplay of various aspects of identity, such as race, class, and gender, and how they intersect to shape individuals' experiences (Cho et al. 2013). It underscores the understanding that individuals can face challenges stemming from multiple sources of discrimination and disadvantage, rather than solely one factor (Bernard 2022).

In the context of mental health, intersectionality highlights that the difficulties encountered by children and young people stem from a combination of social determinants and identities. For instance, a young person experiencing homelessness who also belongs to a marginalised racial group may face distinct mental health challenges compared to someone who is homeless but does not share the same racial identity. Understanding intersectionality can enhance the effectiveness of interventions aimed at supporting children and young people. By acknowledging the various dimensions of their identity, practitioners can tailor their approaches to address specific needs. Additionally, this perspective informs strategies to combat discrimination, ensuring interventions consider the diverse aspects of an individual's identity.

To understand the experiences of belonging to a socially excluded group and the associated implications on children and young people's mental health and wellbeing, three groups of children and young people have been identified: living in poverty, living in a racialised community, and living with a bigger body.

7.4 Children and Young People Living in Poverty

During 2021 and 2022, 4.2 million children were identified as living in poverty (Child Poverty Action Group 2023); this equates to around 9 children in every class of 30 children (Child Poverty Action Group 2024). The recent cost of living crisis has led to many more families experiencing economic disadvantage; indeed, 75% of children living in poverty have at least one parent working in at least one job. In addition, other groups that are more likely to be living in poverty are children from Black and minority ethnic families (47% living in poverty) and children in lone families (44% living in poverty) (Child Poverty Action Group 2024).

Childhood poverty invokes significant human and economic costs. In terms of economics, recent analysis has identified that childhood poverty equates to £39.5 billion a year (Child poverty Action Group 2023). In terms of human costs, the Royal College of Paediatrics and Child Health (2018) argues that the links between poverty and ill-health are unequivocal in that children living in poverty have higher infant mortality rates and are more likely to experience acute infections and mental illness. A longitudinal cohort study of 10,500 children by (Adjei et al. 2024) identified that children living in poverty with a caregiver with poor mental health were at an increased risk long term of socioemotional behavioural problems, poor mental health, and cognitive disability. The study concluded that 40% of socioemotional behavioural problems experienced by young people by the age of 17 were attributable to persistent parental caregivers' mental health problems and poverty (Adjei et al. 2024).

A rapid review of children and young people's views and experiences of poverty (Bidmead et al. 2023) identified that young people were aware of their parent's difficult financial situation and in response to this chose to hide their emotional feelings in order not to add to their parent's sense of shame and stress. Furthermore, many of the young people in the review actively tried to support their parents by not asking for things that they wanted but knew their parents could not afford (such as not asking for money for clothes or activities) as well as using their own money for household items to reduce their parent's burden. The review also identified that many children and young people experienced feeling torn between their individual wants and desires and their responsibility to their family by constraining these desires (Bidmead et al. 2023). To understand the emotional impact on the young people, the findings from the review are presented in Table 7.2.

Table 7.2 Rapid review of young people's experiences of poverty

Theme	Evidence presented in the review. Poverty impacted upon
Education	Inability to have correct uniform and learning resources (such as books, pencil cases, etc.) Inability to attend extracurricular activities Increased experiences of bullying and harassment in school due to the issues raised above. Not only did young people experience this from their peers but also children identified that poverty was often linked to behavioural issues such as detentions, exclusions for incorrect uniform wearing, and not having correct equipment
Housing and neighbourhood	Homes were identified as cold, damp, and having mould There was a lack of space at home, and this negatively impacted upon their ability to study Young people reported feeling embarrassed about their living conditions resulting in them not inviting friends to come over to socialise Homes were in areas of deprivation meaning that young people felt unsafe in their communities, which had increased criminal activity, drugs, rubbish, and mess
Food insecurity	Missing meals (especially at weekends) and associated hunger Parent struggling to afford nutritionally balanced diets, often not having access to food at home, parents not eating so they could feed their children
Social exclusion	Feeling excluded as not able to join in activities with friends; this led to feelings of jealously and embarrassment for young people

Bidmead et al. (2023)

Having developed a better understanding of the impact of poverty on health and well-being as well as the experiences of young people living in poverty, Reflective Activity 7.2 requires you to critically assess your knowledge and practice in terms of addressing poverty in families.

Reflective Activity 7.2: Self-Assessment of Knowledge and Skills in Supporting Families Living in Poverty

- Critically reflect regarding your knowledge of local support services (such as food banks, charities, and statutory services).
- Critically examine the degree to which your assessment focuses upon financial assessment of families.
- What more could you do in your service to address poverty experienced by children and young people?

7.5 Children and Young People Living in Racialised Community

Welsing (1991) characterises racism as a power system that operates on both local and global scales, maintained by those who consider themselves White, whether they do so intentionally or not. This system includes established ways of thinking, reasoning, creating symbols, understanding, speaking, and responding emotionally. These ingrained patterns perpetuate the marginalisation of non-White individuals, leading to environments that exacerbate health inequity and oppression. Assuming that the needs of young racialised individuals with mental health difficulties mirror those of dominant societal groups overlooks the reality of inequality. Whilst it is recognised that race is a social construct devoid of biological grounding, the impact of racism on marginalised racialised groups can be profound (Ellis 2021; Wesp et al. 2018). Consider the hypothetical case study of Aisha (see Table 7.3) detailed below, which illustrates how intersectional identities can exacerbate mental health difficulties for racialised young people.

The case study of Aisha demonstrates how intersectional identities of race, class, and poverty can create a complex web of challenges that can worsen mental health outcomes. This case study underscores the importance of understanding and addressing the unique challenges faced by children and young people at the intersection of multiple marginalised identities. Young people's generic mental health services need to recognise and respond to microaggressions, racism, and poverty. Ellis (2021) alludes to the transgenerational traumatising impact of racism; as such, a trauma-informed care (TIC) approach is recommended. A trauma-informed care (covered more extensively in Chap. 10) essentially involves understanding, recognising, and responding to the effects of all types of trauma by creating physical, psychological, and emotional safety for young people enabling them to regain their power (Levenson 2017).

Table 7.3 Case study of Aisha

Case Study: Aisha's Story
Aisha is a 16-year-old young person of East African heritage, living in an area with high levels of poverty. Her family is of low socioeconomic status, and they reside in a poorly maintained housing complex that is often neglected by the local authority. Aisha faces regular microaggressions and systemic racism at her school and in her neighbourhood. She often feels misunderstood and stereotyped by her peers and teachers, which leads to a sense of isolation and a lack of belonging. Coming from a low-income family, Aisha struggles with the stigma associated with poverty. She cannot afford the same opportunities as her classmates, such as extracurricular activities or tutoring, which impacts her self-esteem and academic performance. The condition of Aisha's home, with issues such as mould and inadequate heating, contributes to chronic health problems, adding another layer of stress. The stigma of living in substandard housing also affects her social interactions and self-image
The intersection of these identities means that Aisha experiences compounded stressors that significantly impact her mental health and well-being. She develops symptoms of anxiety and depression, feeling overwhelmed by the weight of her circumstances. When Aisha seeks help, she encounters barriers. Mental health services are not easily accessible in her community, and when she does reach out, she feels that her concerns are not fully understood or taken seriously by healthcare providers who do not share her lived experiences
Having read the case study, what marginalised identities intersect in Aisha's life?
Now read the University of Bristol (n.d.) Microaggressions Guide on the following link https://www.bristol.ac.uk/media-library/sites/equality/documents/microaggressions-guide.pdf and consider the questions below:
What is the modern definition of microaggressions?
How do microaggressions affect the mental and emotional Well-being of young people from minority ethnic groups?
What steps would you take to respond to Aisha's complex needs?

7.6 Children and Young People with Bigger Bodies

The language practitioners use to describe adults, children, and young people with bigger bodies can have a significant impact on individuals (Brown et al. 2022). The language around body size was somewhat standardised when the World Health Organization (WHO) endorsed the body mass index (BMI) as a recognised measurement in 1997, formalising the definition of 'overweight' and 'obese' (WHO 2000). Despite their frequency of use, these words can be loaded with judgement, and many people in bigger bodies would reject them, citing them as offensive and stigmatising (Brown et al. 2022). It is essential that practitioners are mindful of this and take the lead from the individuals they work with around choice of language.

Since 2006, the National Child Measurement Programme (NCMP) has gathered the heights and weights of children across England and Wales in reception and year 6 class (Office for Health Improvements and Disparities [OHID] 2023; NHS Digital 2023). In 2023, 9.2% of children in reception and 22.7% of children in year 6 class were obese (OHID 2023). Furthermore, children living in areas of high deprivation are twice as likely to be obese as those living in areas of affluence, and the proportion of children living with obesity was highest for Black children (NHS Digital 2023).

Obesity, inequalities, and deprivation are intrinsically linked, and these connections are consistently demonstrated year after year in NCMP results (OHID 2023). It has long been acknowledged that there are many factors that contribute to a person's body fat percentage, including access to safe green space, quality of housing, access to affordable fresh food, advertising, isolation, mental health, food production, climate change, ethnicity, and education level (Government Office for Science 2007). Research evidences the significant impact of social and health inequalities, poverty, and deprivation on a person's obesity, things which are largely outside of an individual's control (Government Office for Science 2007; Mauldin et al. 2022). As such, professionals need to shift the direction of responsibility and accountability towards the provision of good public health provision, rather than focus solely on individual. Individualised messages around the need to lose weight or conform to thin ideals can be harmful for children and young people, particularly for those who experience deprivation or social exclusion as they have very little agency to change the structural inequalities they face (Mauldin et al. 2022; Noonan 2018).

Whilst there is evidence that some children with bigger bodies have an increased incidence of poor long-term health outcomes, the causal factors of the poor health outcomes are complex and not solely due to increased body fat percentage (Tylka et al. 2014). One of the evidenced contributing factors to poorer health outcomes for people with bigger bodies is 'weight stigma' or 'weight bias' (Mauldin et al. 2022; Mold and Forbes 2013). Weight stigma can be defined as the 'inclination to form unreasonable judgements based on a person's weight' (Washington 2011: 1) or where people experience prejudice or discrimination because of their weight (Brown et al. 2022). Many health and care professionals hold stigmatising and negative views of people in bigger bodies, expressing that people with bigger bodies are lazy, unmotivated, unintelligent, and non-compliant with treatment (Darling and Atav 2019; Sabin et al. 2012; Vartanian 2010). This can lead to increased risks such as delayed presentation accessing healthcare due to fear of stigma and delayed or inappropriate treatment (Brown et al. 2022; Phelan et al. 2015; Rand et al. 2017).

Children and young people with bigger bodies are at increased vulnerability of bullying, stigmatising comments, or verbal abuse, not only from peers but also from adults and professionals (Pudney et al. 2019; Puhl et al. 2016). Furthermore, experiences of weight stigma and anti-fat attitudes are well evidenced to contribute to poor body image, low body satisfaction, and increased incidence of disordered eating behaviours (Brown et al. 2022; Neves et al. 2017). This is particularly true for overweight children, more so for overweight girls, as they are the most at risk of low body satisfaction, with overweight children as young as 6 presenting a strong desire for a body that conforms to the thin ideal (Truby and Paxton 2002; Vander Wal and Thelen 2000; Jongenelis et al. 2014) (more information on eating disorders is presented in Chap. 3). Social media is increasingly having a negative impact on body image, with content feeds being flooded with weight loss and diet industry messages such as #thinspiration and #fitspo (Rodgers et al. 2023; Be Real 2017). Research from social media platform 'BeReal' found that over 50% of adolescents surveyed had considered going on a diet to change their appearance and 10% had considered cosmetic surgery (Be Real 2017). The links between poor body satisfaction and increased incidence of depression or anxiety are well established, with a much higher incidence of both for children and young people with bigger bodies (Goldfield et al. 2010; Quek et al. 2017). Additionally, the incidence of depression and anxiety symptoms is highest in obese female teens from 'non-Western' backgrounds; this included Iran, Turkey, China, India, and South Korea, highlighting the potential impact of intersecting inequalities on mental health (Quek et al. 2017).

An alternative approach of 'weight-neutral healthcare' has been gathering momentum and would be a way for practitioners to reduce weight stigma and the associated impact on mental health for children and young people with bigger bodies. Weight-neutral or weight-inclusive approaches to care focus on encouraging evidence-based health behaviours that are independent of a person's weight (Tylka et al. 2014). The premise of this approach is that the advice given would be the same for a person with a bigger body as it is with a smaller body, thus reducing weight stigma (Willer et al. 2019). Encouraging children and young people to engage with movement or sports and mindfulness activities, increasing the amount of fruit and vegetables they eat, and improving sleep quality are all evidenced health- and well-being-promoting behaviours (Matheson et al. 2012). Many people with bigger bodies feel self-conscious when doing exercise or moving their bodies and have experienced weight stigma in exercise contexts (Thedinga et al. 2021; Be Real 2017). This can result in the avoidance of PE lessons, sport, or group exercise, even more so for those living in deprivation due to issues around appropriate clothing or funds to pay for activities (Thedinga et al. 2021, Be Real 2017). Children and young people that do engage in activities where they can enjoy moving their bodies have a higher sense of positive regard for their body than those that do not (Foley Davelaar 2021; Tylka and Homan 2015). For children and young people in bigger bodies to have those opportunities to engage in health- and well-being-promoting activities, practitioners must ensure they are providing welcoming and inclusive services (Thedinga et al. 2021; Foley Davelaar 2021). Reflective Activity 7.3 provides further opportunities to reflect on your professional practice.

Reflective Activity 7.3: Review of Weight Stigma and Opportunities to Reduce Discrimination

- Consider your personal views about body weight, obesity, and people with bigger bodies.
- Critically examine the potential ways in which these views could influence your professional practice.
- Consider the environments that you work in with children and young people. What messages do they receive in that environment? Consider posters, online information, size of furniture, equipment suitable for bigger bodies, and information available in advance for bigger bodies.
- How might the words you use, or messages you give to the children or young people you work with, negatively impact on their mental health and well-being?
- Look at implementing opportunities to embed a more weight-neutral approach in your service.
- Identify three actions that could be taken in your practice to reduce the weight stigma experienced by the children and young people you work with.

The three examples presented above (poverty, racialised community, and children with bigger bodies) have resulted in three groups of children and young people who experience stigma and discrimination. However, it must be remembered there are many other children who will experience discrimination and stigma due to the nature of the group they belong to (e.g. disability, mental illness, care-experienced children, parents in prison, etc.). Therefore, there is a need to consider how practitioners can address this ensuring that children grow up free from discrimination as espoused in the UN Convention on the Rights of the Child (UN 1990).

7.7 Challenging Discrimination

Children and young people learn discriminatory attitudes from observing the behaviours of those around them such as family or wider social institutions (such as the media) (Child Rights International Network 2018); as such, any approach to challenging discrimination needs to be multifactorial. There needs to be an understanding of the social construction of categories such as race, disability, gender, and religion and how these constructions create systemic discrimination (Thompson 2017). As such, practitioners working with children and young people need to be aware of their own privilege and power, being insightful of how these impact on the diverse communities that they are working with. The Personal, Cultural, and Structural (PCS) model suggested by Thompson (2020) is a helpful theoretical framework for identifying and responding to discrimination at all levels. This PCS model posits that power and discrimination operate on three distinct but interconnected levels:

1. Personal Level: Individual beliefs and prejudices that are shaped by personal experiences.
2. Cultural Level: Shared societal norms and values that dictate behaviour and reinforce stereotypes.
3. Structural Level: Institutionalised discrimination within policies and societal structures, influenced by media and laws.

The PCS model underscores that these levels interact to perpetuate oppression and that recognising this is vital for addressing and challenging discrimination in society (Thompson 2020).

Despite a wealth of research highlighting discrimination and stigma experienced by children and young people living in socially marginalised and excluded groups, as presented to date in this chapter, there appears to have been little movement in practice to support young people. Research by UNICEF (2022) with 407,000 young people noted that only 18% were confident to confront the other person and a further 12% reached out to someone else for support. In contrast, 33% internalised the feelings of the discrimination and responded by working harder to prove the person wrong and 27% took no action. This research highlights that much more needs to be done to support young people who are experiencing discrimination. The Equality

Table 7.4 Online resources

Online resources to support children, young people, families, and professionals in addressing stigma and bullying:
Equality and Human Rights Commission—https://www.equalityhumanrights.com/sites/default/files/tips_for_tackling_discriminatory_bullying.pdf
NSPCC—https://www.nspcc.org.uk/keeping-children-safe/support-for-parents/children-race-racism-racial-bullying/
Anti-Bullying Alliance—https://anti-bullyingalliance.org.uk/anti-bullying-week-2023-make-noise-about-bullying/odd-socks-day
Body Happy Org—https://www.bodyhappyorg.com/
Challenging Weight Stigma—Public Health Scotland E-Learning Hub https://learning.publichealthscotland.scot/course/view.php?id=622

and Human Rights Commission (undated) identifies that schools are key places in which children and young people can be supported to develop the confidence to challenge discrimination. They argue it requires a whole school approach in which there is a culture of an inclusive and supportive community, where differences are celebrated and where staff and student feel empowered to make changes for the inclusion of all. Furthermore, research conducted by Wallrich et al. (2020) with 639 adolescents identified that a 30-min group discussion on discrimination experiences that focuses upon perspectives and action planning can prompt higher self-efficacy in individuals to address discriminatory language.

It is evident that more work needs to be done to support practitioners to feel confident to implement strategies to address the experiences of stigma and discrimination of children and young people from socially excluded groups. Table 7.4 identifies a variety of resources and organisations, which provide support to children, young people, and their families.

7.8 Conclusion

This chapter has offered a comprehensive exploration of the intricate interplay between social determinants of health and discrimination, in shaping the mental well-being of children and young people. It navigates through the complex landscape of factors such as poverty, racialisation, and weight stigma, shedding light on their profound adverse impact on mental health outcomes. Frameworks have been suggested to understand and respond to health inequities, promoting holistic health for all, at the individual, cultural, and systemic levels. An intersectional lens is recommended to mitigate against the compounded effects of multiple marginalisations on mental health outcomes, emphasising the need for tailored interventions and trauma-informed care. There is a call for further education, community engagement, and empowerment in challenging discriminatory attitudes and fostering inclusive environments. Indeed, for an effective paradigm shift towards equity and inclusion in mental health services for children and young people, commissioners and providers of mental health services must recognise the multifaceted nature of health inequalities and the imperative of collective action to dismantle systemic barriers, thereby promoting holistic well-being for all children and young people. Finally, you are invited to draw up a personal action plan (Reflective Activity 7.4: Personal Action Plan).

Reflective Activity 7.4: Personal Action Plan

Review the activities presented in this chapter and develop an action plan which you shall work on over the next 6 months to help you further develop your knowledge and skills to work more inclusively with children, young people, and their families. In developing your plan, identify immediate-, medium-, and long-term learning and development needs. Once you have identified your needs, consider what actions and resources you need to achieve your action plan. Check this over the next 6 months and add and adjust as necessary.

References

Adjei N, Schlüter DK, Melis G, Straatmann VS, Fleming KM, Wickham S, Munford L, McGovern R, Howard LM, Kaner E, Wolfe I, Taylor-Robinson DC. Impact of parental mental health and poverty on the health of the next generation: a multi-trajectory analysis using the UK millennium cohort study. J Adolesc Health. 2024;74(2024):60e70.

Atashbahar O, Sari AA, Takian A, Olyaeemanesh A, Mohamadi E, Barakati SH. The impact of social determinants of health on early childhood development: a qualitative context analysis in Iran. BMC Public Health. 2022;2022(22):1149. https://doi.org/10.1186/s12889-022-13571-5.

Be Real. Somebody like me: a report investigating the impact of body image anxiety on young people in the UK. [Internet]. 2017. Available from: https://www.berealcampaign.co.uk/research/somebody-like-me. Accessed 15 May 2024.

Bernard C. Intersectionality for social workers: a practical introduction to theory and practice. Abingdon: Routledge; 2022.

Bidmead E, El Zerbi C, Cheetham M, Frost S. A rapid review of children and young people's views of poverty and welfare in the context of Universal Credit. Child Soc. 2023;2023(37):1–19. https://doi.org/10.1111/chso.12728.

Brown A, Flint SW, Batterham RL. Pervasiveness, impact, and implications of weight stigma. EClinicalMedicine. 2022;47:101408. https://doi.org/10.1016/j.eclinm.2022.101408.

Child Poverty Action Group., 2023. Official child poverty statistics: 350,000 more children in poverty and numbers will rise. Available from: https://cpag.org.uk/news/official-child-poverty-statistics-350000-more-children-poverty-and-numbers-willrise#:~:text=350%2C000%20more%20children%20were%20pulled%20into%20relative%20poverty%20(after%20housing,youngest%20child%20aged%20under%20five. Accessed 17 Apr 2024.

Child Poverty Action Group. Poverty: facts and figures. CPAG; 2024. Available from: Poverty: facts and figures. Accessed 17 Apr 2024.

Child Rights International Network. Challenging discrimination. CRIN; 2018. Available from: Accessed 18 Apr 2024.

Cho S, Crenshaw KW, McCall L. Toward a field of intersectionality studies: theory, applications, and praxis. J Women Cult Soc. 2013;38(4):785–810. https://doi.org/10.1086/669608.

Darling R, Atav AS. Attitudes toward obese people: a comparative study of nursing, education, and social work students. J Prof Nurs. 2019;35(2):138–46. https://doi.org/10.1016/j.profnurs.2018.07.009.

Economou M, Bechraki A, Charitsi M. Psychiatrike = Psychiatriki. 2020;31(1):36–46. https://doi.org/10.22365/jpsych.2020.311.36.
Ellis E. The race conversation—an essential guide to creating life-changing dialogue. London: Confer Books; 2021.
Equality Act. 2010. Available from: https://www.legislation.gov.uk/ukpga/2010/15/contents. Accessed 7 May 2024.
Equality and Human Rights Commission. Tips for tackling discriminatory bullying. undated. Available from: tips_for_tackling_discriminatory_bullying.pdf. equalityhumanrights.com. Accessed 18 Apr 2024.
Foley Davelaar CM. Body image and its role in physical activity: a systematic review. Cureus. 2021;13(2):e13379. https://doi.org/10.7759/cureus.13379.
Goldfield GS, Moore C, Henderson K, Buchholz A, Obeid N, Flament MF. Body dissatisfaction, dietary restraint, depression, and weight status in adolescents. J Sch Health. 2010;80(4):186–92. https://doi.org/10.1111/j.1746-1561.2009.00485.x.
Government Office for Science. Foresight: tacking obesities: future choices—project report. 2nd ed.; 2007. https://assets.publishing.service.gov.uk/media/5a759da7e5274a4368298a4f/07-1184x-tackling-obesities-future-choices-report.pdf
Jongenelis MI, Byrne SM, Pettigrew S. Self-objectification, body image disturbance, and eating disorder symptoms in young Australian children. Body Image. 2014;11(3):290–302.
Levenson J. Trauma-informed social work practice. Soc Work. 2017;62(2):105–13. https://doi.org/10.1093/sw/swx001.
Levon E, Sharma D, Watt DJ, Cardoso A, Ye Y. Accent bias and perceptions of professional competence in England. J Engl Ling. 2021;49(4):355–88.
Link BG, Phelan JC. Conceptualizing stigma. Annu Rev Sociol. 2001;27(1):363–85. https://doi.org/10.1146/annurev.soc.27.1.363.
Marmot M. Fair society, healthy lives; the Marmot Review. 2010. Available from: instituteofhealthequity.org/resources-reports/fair-society-healthy-lives-the-marmot-review/fair-society-healthy-lives-full-report-pdf.pdf. Accessed 17 Apr 2024.
Marmot M. The health gap: the challenge of an unequal world. Lancet. 2015;386(10011):2442–4. https://doi.org/10.1016/S0140-6736(15)00150-6.
Marmot M, Allen J, Boyce T, Goldblatt P, Morrison J. 2020. Health Equity in England: The Marmot Review 10 years on. Available from: Health Equity in England: The Marmot Review 10 Years On - The Health Foundation [accessed 28.7.23].
Matheson EM, King DE, Everett CJ. Healthy lifestyle habits and mortality in overweight and obese individuals. J Am Board Fam Med. 2012;25(1):9–15. https://doi.org/10.3122/jabfm.2012.01.110164.
Mauldin K, May M, Clifford D. The consequences of a weight-centric approach to healthcare: a case for a paradigm shift in how clinicians address body weight. Nutr Clin Pract. 2022;37(6):1291–306. https://doi.org/10.1002/ncp.10885.
Mold F, Forbes A. Patients' and professionals' experiences and perspectives of obesity in healthcare settings: a synthesis of current research. Health Expect. 2013;16(2):119–42. https://doi.org/10.1111/j.1369-7625.2011.00699.x.
Nayak S. The activism of black feminist theory: race, gender, and social change. Abingdon: Routledge; 2015.
Neves CM, Cipriani FM, Meireles JFF, Morgado FFDR, Ferreira MEC. Body image in childhood: an integrative literature review. Rev Paul Pediatr. 2017;35:331–9. https://doi.org/10.1590/1984-0462/;2017;35;3;00002.
NHS Digital. The national child measurement programme, England 2022/2023 school year. 2023. Available from: https://digital.nhs.uk/data-and-information/publications/statistical/national-child-measurement-programme#summary
NHS England., 2021. Core20PLUS5 – An approach to reducing health inequalities for children and young people. Available from: https://www.england.nhs.uk/about/equality/equality-hub/national-healthcare-inequalities-improvement-programme/core20plus5/core20plus5-cyp/ Accessed 17 Apr 2024.

Noonan RJ. Poverty, weight status, and dietary intake among UK adolescents. Int J Environ Res Public Health. 2018;15(6):1224.

Office for Health Improvements & Disparities. National child measurement programme: operational guidance 2023. 2023. https://www.gov.uk/government/publications/national-child-measurement-programme-operational-guidance/national-child-measurement-programme-operational-guidance-2022. Accessed 17 Apr 2024.

Phelan SM, Burgess DJ, Yeazel MW, Hellerstedt WL, Griffin JM, Ryn M. Impact of weight bias and stigma on quality of care and outcomes for patients with obesity. Obes Rev. 2015;16(4):319–26. https://doi.org/10.1111/obr.12266.

Pudney EV, Himmelstein MS, Puhl RM. The role of weight stigma in parental weight talk. Pediatr Obes. 2019;14(10):e12534. https://doi.org/10.1111/ijpo.12534.

Puhl RM, Latner JD, O'Brien K, Luedicke J, Forhan M, Danielsdottir S. Weight-based bullying in youth. Pediatr Obes. 2016;11(4):241–50. https://doi.org/10.1111/ijpo.12051.

Quek YH, Tam WWS, Zhang MWB, Ho RCM. Exploring the association between childhood and adolescent obesity and depression: a meta-analysis. Obes Rev. 2017;18(7):742–54. https://doi.org/10.1111/obr.12535.

Rand K, Vallis M, Aston M, Price S, Piccinini-Vallis H, Rehman L, Kirk SFL. It is not the diet; it is the mental part we need help with. A multilevel analysis of psychological, emotional, and social well-being in obesity. Int J Qual Stud Health Well Being. 2017;12(1):1306421. https://doi.org/10.1080/17482631.2017.1306421.

Rodgers RF, Laveway K, Zalvino J, Cardone W, Wang L. #BodyPositive: a qualitative exploration of young people's responses to body positive social media content. Body Image. 2023;47:101613. https://doi.org/10.1016/j.bodyim.2023.08.005.

Royal College of Paediatrics and Child Health. 2018. The impact of poverty on child health. Available from: https://www.rcpch.ac.uk/news-events/news/impact-povertychild-health Accessed 17 Apr 2024.

Sabin JA, Marini M, Nosek BA. Implicit and explicit anti-fat bias among a large sample of medical doctors by BMI, race/ethnicity and gender. PLoS ONE. 2012;7(11):e48448. https://doi.org/10.1371/journal.pone.0048448.

Sanchez N. Women with polycystic ovary syndrome: a marginalized population in the United States. Health Soc Work. 2020;45(1):40–6.

Thedinga HK, Zehl R, Thiel A. Weight stigma experiences and self-exclusion from sport and exercise settings among people with obesity. BMC Public Health. 2021;21(1):565. https://doi.org/10.1186/s12889-021-10565-7.

Thompson N. Promoting equality: working with diversity and difference. 4th ed. London: Bloomsbury Publishing Plc; 2017.

Thompson N. Anti-discriminatory practice: equality, diversity and social justice. London: Bloomsbury Publishing Plc; 2020.

Thornicroft G, Sunkel C, Aliev AA, Baker S, Brohan E, Chammay R, Davies K, Demissie M, Duncan J, Fekadu W, Gronholm PC, Guerrero Z, Gurung D, Habtamu K, Hanlon C, Heim E, Henderson C, Hijazi Z, Hoffman C, et al. The lancet commission on ending stigma and discrimination in mental health. Lancet. 2022;400(10361):1438–80. https://doi.org/10.1016/s0140-6736(22)01470-2.

Truby H, Paxton SJ. Development of the children's body image scale. Br J Clin Psychol. 2002;41(2):185–203.

Tylka TL, Homan KJ. Exercise motives and positive body image in physically active college women and men: exploring an expanded acceptance model of intuitive eating. Body Image. 2015;15:90–7. https://doi.org/10.1016/j.bodyim.2015.07.003.

Tylka TL, Annunziato RA, Burgard D, Daníelsdóttir S, Shuman E, Davis C, Calogero RM. The weight-inclusive versus weight-normative approach to health: evaluating the evidence for prioritizing Well-being over weight loss. J Obes. 2014;2014:1–18. https://doi.org/10.1155/2014/983495.

United Nations. The United Nations Convention on the Rights of the Child. 1990. Available from: Layout 1. unicef.org.uk. Accessed 7 May 2024.

United Nations. Identifying social inclusion and exclusion. 2016a. Available from: chapter1.pdf. un.org. Accessed 17 Apr 2024.
United Nations. Leaving no one behind: equality and non-discrimination at the heart of sustainable development. 2016b. Available from: https://www.un.org/esa/socdev/rwss/2016/chapter1.pdf. Accessed 31 July 2023.
United Nations Children's Fund. Rights denied: the impact of discrimination on children. 2022. Available from: rights-denied-discrimination-children-EN.pdf. unicef.org. Accessed 18 Apr 2024.
University of Bristol. Microaggressions guide. n.d.. Available from: https://www.bristol.ac.uk/media-library/sites/equality/documents/microaggressions-guide.pdf. Accessed 7 May 2024.
Vander Wal JS, Thelen MH. Eating and body image concerns among obese and average-weight children. Addict Behav. 2000;25(5):775–8.
Vartanian LR. Disgust and perceived control in attitudes toward obese people. Int J Obes. 2010;34(8):1302–7. https://doi.org/10.1038/ijo.2010.45.
Villatoro A, DuPont-Reyes MJ, Phelan JC, Link BG. 'Me' vs. 'them': how mental illness stigma influences adolescent help-seeking behaviors for oneself and recommendations for peers. Stigma Health. 2022;7(3):300–10. https://doi.org/10.1037/sah0000392.
Wallrich L, Palmer SB, Rutland A. Adolescents challenging discrimination: the benefits of a perspective-taking and action-planning intervention on self-efficacy. J Community Appl Soc Psychol. 2020;2021:1–7. https://doi.org/10.1002/casp.2530.
Washington RL. Childhood obesity: issues of weight bias. Prev Chronic Dis. 2011;8(5):A94.
Welsing FC. The Isis papers: the keys to the colours. Chicago: Third World Press; 1991.
Wesp SV, Ruiz A, Walker K, Weitzel J, Shaw L, Kako PM, Mkandawire-Valhmu L. An emancipatory approach to cultural competency: the application of critical race, postcolonial, and intersectionality theories. Adv Nurs Sci. 2018;41(4):316–26. https://doi.org/10.1097/ANS.0000000000000230.
Willer F, Hannan-Jones M, Strodl E. Australian dietitians' beliefs and attitudes towards weight loss counselling and health at every size counselling for larger-bodied clients. Nutr Diet. 2019;76(4):407–13. https://doi.org/10.1111/1747-0080.12519.
Wood E, Elliott M. Opioid addiction stigma: the intersection of race, social class, and gender. Subst Use Misuse. 2020;55(5):818–27.
World Health Organisation. Obesity: preventing and managing the global epidemic: report of a WHO consultation. Geneva: WHO; 2000.
World Health Organisation. Social determinants of mental health. 2014. Available from: https://iris.who.int/bitstream/handle/10665/112828/9789241506809_eng.pdf?sequence=1. Accessed 17 Apr 2024.
World Health Organisation. Social determinants of health. 2024. Available from: https://www.who.int/health-topics/social-determinants-of-health#tab=tab_1. Accessed 17 Apr 2024.
YMCA. I am whole. 2016. Available from: https://www.ymca.org.uk/wp-content/uploads/2016/10/IAMWHOLE-v1.1.pdf. Accessed 7 May 2024.

Child Protection and Safeguarding 8

Samita Wilson, Trudy Cowan, Jasmin Flynn,
and Vanessa Heaslip

S. Wilson (✉)
Department of Social Work, Norwegian University of Science & Technology,
Trondheim, Norway
e-mail: samita.wilson@ntnu.no

T. Cowan · V. Heaslip
Directorate of Nursing and Midwifery, University of Salford, Salford, UK
e-mail: t.cowan1@salford.ac.uk; V.A.Heaslip@salford.ac.uk

J. Flynn
Directorate of Allied Public Health, University of Salford, Salford, UK
e-mail: j.j.flynn@salford.ac.uk

G. Trainor, V. Heaslip (eds.), *Needs of Children and Young People Living with Complex Mental Health Difficulties*,
https://doi.org/10.1007/978-3-031-84532-1_8

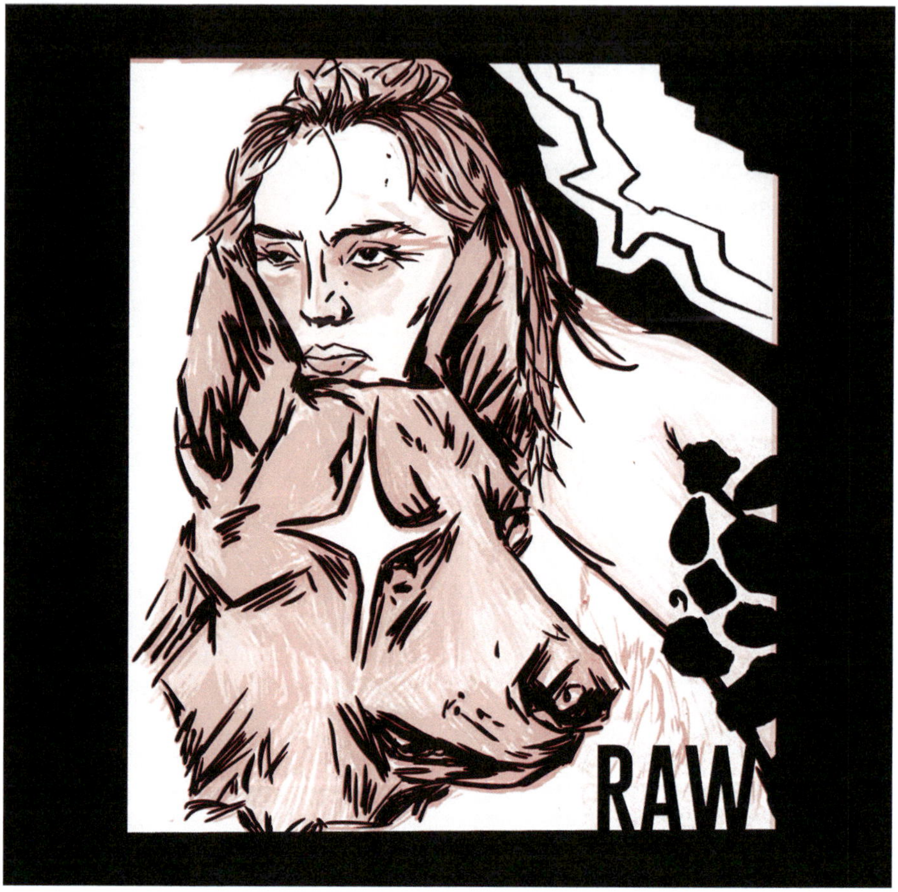

© Robyn Heaslip

8.1 Global Picture and Vulnerabilities

There are currently estimated to be over 2 billion children and young people under the age of 18 (World Population Review 2024). While global birth rates have dropped, these vary between countries, for example, they are higher in low-income countries and lower in high-income countries which impacts the number of children. For example, in Niger, 48.85% of its population is aged 0–14 years compared to the UK, which has 17.47% (World Population Review 2024). In the 2021 census, 12,392,240 (20.7%) of the UK population were aged 0–17 (UK Gov 2023a), representing a significant part of the UK population.

Children and young people are often identified as vulnerable, due in part to their physical size and strength which makes them less able to defend themselves, but also because they are still developing their social, cognitive, and emotional skills, which impacts on their decision-making (Hewitt-Taylor and Heaslip 2012). In addition to this, children and young people are often reliant upon others to meet many of their basic needs, such as food, shelter and other essentials, and have little autonomy in choices affecting their daily lives (Bagattini 2019). While many children have supportive and happy childhoods, this is not true for all children. In 2023 in the UK, there were 403,090 children identified as a child in need, defined as needing help and protection because of risks to their development or health and includes the following (UK Gov 2023b):

- Those with a child in need plan
- Those with child protection plans
- Those looked after by local authorities
- Care leavers
- Disabled children

Many of the children identified as a child in need will have experienced an adverse childhood experience (ACE). This term refers to some of the most difficult and stressful experiences that children and young people may face, which can include abuse, neglect, violence, and/or living in households with drug or alcohol abuse (Anda et al. 2010; Berens et al. 2017); see Chap. 1 for full list and long-term health impact of ACEs. In terms of prevalence, a systematic review across 22 countries with 546,458 participants by Madigan et al. (2023) identified:

- 39.9% of the sample had experienced five ACEs.
- 16.1% of the sample had experienced five ACEs.
- 8.7% of the sample three ACEs.
- 13% of the sample one ACE.

The review also identified that the prevalence of four or more ACEs was higher in contexts involving mental illness, substance abuse/addiction, low income, homelessness, or minoritised ethnic communities. Reflective Activity 8.1 explores this further, supporting your knowledge and understanding of ACEs.

Reflective Activity 8.1

Consider how much you know about adverse childhood experiences (ACEs) and the impact these have on young people's health and well-being.

- Read the section about ACEs in Chap. 1
- Watch the YouTube video developed by NHS Health Scotland available from https://www.youtube.com/watch?v=VMpIi-4CZK0&feature=youtube
- Critically reflect on the degree to which you consider the possibilities of ACEs among the young people you work with. If you do not currently consider ACEs, reflect on ways to integrate this into your professional practice.

8.2 Global Policies

Advocacy for children's right to protection through state intervention dates back to the nineteenth century, with policies designed to govern childhood towards achieving social goals sanctioned by the state (Mason and Fattore 2021). Child protection and welfare policies in the UK are significantly influenced by the United Nations Convention on the Rights of the Child (UNCRC; UNICEF 1990), which promotes a comprehensive approach to children's safeguarding and protecting them from maltreatment (United Nations 1989). This approach recognises children's rights to protection as well as broader rights to survival, access to resources, development, and participation. The UNCRC also gives precedence to the child's best interests in all decision-making in cases that involve them (Article 3, UNCRC), making it pertinent to child protection policies and practice. The convention is viewed as a 'suggested' contract between the child and adults, where the adults are responsible for ensuring the child's access to provisions, protection, and participation in all matters concerning them (Bardy 2000). While all articles of the UNCRC are indivisible and must be considered holistically, Article 19 is of particular importance as it obliges state parties to establish systems for safeguarding and protecting children (see Box 8.1).

Box 8.1: Article 19 UN Convention on the Rights of the Child (United Nations 1989 from https://www.ohchr.org/en/instruments-mechanisms/instruments/convention-rights-child)

1. States parties shall take all appropriate legislative, administrative, social, and educational measures to protect the child from all forms of physical or mental violence, injury or abuse, neglect or negligent treatment, maltreatment, or exploitation, including sexual abuse, while in the care of parent(s), legal guardian(s), or any other person who has the care of the child.
2. Such protective measures should, as appropriate, include effective procedures for the establishment of social programmes to provide necessary support for the child and for those who have the care of the child, as well as for other forms of prevention and for identification, reporting, referral, investigation, treatment, and follow-up of instances of child maltreatment described heretofore and, as appropriate, for judicial involvement.

This highlights the obligation of state parties to actively protect children from 'all' forms of violence, neglect, sexual abuse, and exploitation, emphasising a multifaceted approach that includes legal, administrative, educational, and social strategies and services, as well as a supportive infrastructure. This ensures mechanisms are in place for reporting and responding to instances of maltreatment, with the aim of comprehensively safeguarding children's well-being and rights.

The family is an integral unit of society, with the primary responsibility for upbringing of children in a safe and nurturing environment so they can reach their full potential. While families may require assistance to fulfil this purpose, there is a risk that some families and homes are not the safe places for children they are supposed to be (Wilson et al. 2020). Thus, state intervention that can involve separating children from their families, may be necessary for the child's best interest (Article 3, UNCRC). While not specifically a children's rights instrument, the European Convention on Human Rights, to which the UK adheres, has provisions that indirectly protect children's rights, such as the right to life, the prohibition of torture, the right to private life, and the right to a fair trial (Council of Europe 1950). These provisions have implications for child protection policies and practices. For instance, under the convention, the UK is obliged to implement measures that prevent ill-treatment, investigate any allegations thoroughly, and ensure effective remedies for violations, thereby creating a comprehensive legal framework and minimum standards for the protection of children's rights against both public and private actors (O'Mahony 2019).

8.3 UK Child Protection Policies

The terms 'safeguarding children' and 'child protection' are often mistakenly used interchangeably (Chambers et al. 2021). Section 17 of the Children Act (1989) notes that safeguarding is keeping children safe from harm and promoting their welfare, whereas child protection is defined as 'the set of multi-agency activities and processes that follow a concern that a child is suffering or likely to suffer significant harm'. Safeguarding children is noted to be everyone's business (Department for Education 2023b, c; Criminal Justice Inspectorates 2015), and a preventative multi-agency approach is advocated. Such approaches embrace the notion of 'making every contact count' (Public Health England (PHE) 2016), ensuring that any interaction with babies, children, young people, and their families and caregivers is conducted in a supportive format (PHE 2018).

Child protection is a supportive part of the safeguarding process and is highlighted as everyone's responsibility (DfE 2015; Children and Social Work Act 2017; NICE 2019; Foster 2023). Under section 47 of the Children Act 1989, 'the local authority has a duty to make enquiries when there are safeguarding concerns, and where necessary, take decisive action to protect a child from abuse, neglect, and exploitation' (DfE 2023a, p. 79). Brandon et al. (2020) and MacAlister (2022) assert that such assessments must be multimodal in nature to ensure that the needs of babies, children, and young people are being effectively supported. The use of the assessment framework (DfE 2023b, p. 57) enables a systematic approach to investigation.

Not only are there different assessment tools, but their application and implementation also vary depending upon where you live in the UK (Clements 2018). This makes it difficult for practitioners attempting to navigate their local processes (Taylor et al. 2024). Furthermore, Casey and Hackett (2021) also note that referral for support depends on the practitioner's subjective view of whether the threshold is met. Yet early support improves outcomes for children, which can include referral to children's centres, parenting programmes, and behaviour change schemes (Asmussen et al. 2022). Despite the evidence of effective interventions (Ofsted 2022), in times of austerity and political change, the rationing of finite resources is common that has consequences for practitioners, who often must navigate these limitations while trying to provide appropriate support to families (Devaney 2018).

8.3.1 Threshold Criteria and Escalation

Determining safeguarding need is often misjudged and misinterpreted (Clements 2018), and to assist with this, local authorities, police, and health commissioners are required to jointly publish threshold documents (DfE 2023b). These documents serve as a resource for professionals working across children and young people's services and for those making referrals to assess whether a child protection inquiry should be carried out. Each area's threshold criteria have common principles to aid assessment, which include:

- The safeguarding and referrals processes in the local area
- Legal definitions of children in need and the forms of abuse
- Differing levels of intervention and support

The national framework (DfE 2023c) identifies principles for practice to ensure that children thrive. This guidance offers a standardisation of what is expected for children to ensure they receive care that enables them not only to reach adulthood, but also supports them in achieving their potential. Lines et al. (2020) assert that although escalation policies exist, and practitioners may have awareness of them, the process is often difficult to navigate, and as a result concerns are often dealt retrospectively. Reflective Activity 8.2 asks you to explore your national and local safeguarding processes and threshold criteria.

Reflective Activity 8.2: National and Local Processes

- Please visit the NSPCC Child Protection site https://learning.nspcc.org.uk/child-protection-system and look at the processes relevant to where you live (England, Northern Ireland, Scotland, or Wales).
- Access and read your local safeguarding threshold criteria.
- Read your employer's safeguarding procedures to make sure you are aware of to whom you should report concerns.

8.4 The Impact of Child Protection Services on Children's Mental Health and Well-Being

It is important to remember that children should be considered as service-users, who have the right to be heard in matters concerning them, as well as the right to appropriate and effective social services (Wilson et al. 2020). Within this context, children as 'citizens and service users share the same fundamental rights to participate as others', in decisions regarding their welfare and well-being (Sinclair and Franklin

2000, p. 1). This highlights the importance of incorporating children's participation in protection and welfare policies and practices, which improves the decision-making processes and outcomes for children and their families by ensuring that decisions are more inclusive and responsive and meet the specific needs and lived realities of children (Toros 2021). Conversely, a lack of participation in child protection processes risks children feeling vulnerable, stressed, helpless, and angry (Wilson et al. 2020). These feelings combined with the long-term physical, psychological, emotional, and social consequences of child maltreatment, can have adverse implications across the lifespan (Afifi et al. 2018). Therefore, it is important for practitioners to understand children's experiences with and perspective of Child Protection Services (CPS).

8.4.1 Children's Experiences of Disclosures in CPS Settings

Disclosure is an important step in helping children in abusive situations. However, considering how children disclose, as well as the processes involved in recognising and understanding the different forms of maltreatment and accessing help, is an important aspect of the broader context (Cossar et al. 2019). Research with children shows that for them, the experience of recognising and disclosing maltreatment is deeply personal and can be fraught with confusion and fear (Wilson et al. 2020). Often, children may not even recognise their experiences as abusive, or they may acknowledge them but fear the consequences of disclosure. Disclosure is hindered by numerous elements, including developmental factors such as age and cognitive and linguistic development; emotional barriers such as self-blame for abuse, conflicted loyalties, love for parents, and fear of consequences; and cultural dynamics such as family honour and shame (Wilson et al. 2020, 2023; Cossar et al. 2019).

Furthermore, disclosure is a process and not a one-time event for children. The role of professionals is crucial in this respect, as children often talk to a safe and trusted adult first about their maltreatment (Wilson et al. 2020). However, a study by Cossar et al. (2019) also noted that children may express distress (intentionally or unintentionally) through their behaviour and overall demeanour. Although such signs are not conclusive evidence of maltreatment, they warrant careful consideration and investigation into their underlying causes. A trusting, professional relationship with children is a prerequisite for encouraging them to talk, and this entails spending time with children to build rapport and actively listening to them (Finn 2011).

8.4.2 Identifying and Addressing Emotional Responses of Being in CPS

Children in CPS experience a spectrum of emotions that can impact their mental health, regardless of whether they initially entered the system with pre-existing mental health issues. Research with children in CPS has identified that they frequently experience feelings of guilt, regret, and anger, arising not only from their family dynamics but also from their interactions with CPS (Wilson et al. 2020). Thus, it is important for professionals to explore and understand children's emotional experiences, enabling them to adopt a sensitive and informed approach that addresses these complex experiences and provides better support for the overall well-being of the children they are in contact with.

Children's emotions and emotional experiences within CPS are influenced by their social, cultural, and political contexts (Wilson et al. 2023; Drake et al. 2019). In CPS, children's emotions shape their relationships and sense of self, and vice versa. These emotions are generated through their interpersonal (e.g. how CPS made their parents feel) and intrapersonal (e.g. how CPS fulfilled their expectations) relations (Wilson et al. 2023). Many children express the importance of emotional connections with family, friends, and even places for their feelings of safety and well-being (Drake et al. 2019). Thus, being in CPS sometimes creates moral and emotional dilemmas for children, as they feel compelled to navigate irreconcilable options, such as choosing between saving the family honour and seeking help from CPS for their own safety (Wilson et al. 2023).

Child protection services have the potential to provide essential safety and protection for children. However, children have expressed that while CPS usually provides protection from physical violence, it could not help children escape the emotional violence such as manipulation and stress that resulted from contacting CPS (Wilson et al. 2020, 2023). This highlights that meeting children's 'being needs' such as love, belonging, self-esteem, and recognition, is as important as basic necessities such as food, shelter, and safety. Moreover, children in CPS often experience hopelessness, which can be attributed to several factors, including a lack of appropriate responses from CPS that may lead children to believe that nothing will change and a feeling that neither CPS nor their parents can restore their lost childhood or reverse the trauma they have suffered (Font et al. 2023; Wilson et al. 2023).

8.4.3 Agency and Safety: Empowering Children and Promoting Child Participation

Children often associate safety with having agency, that is, control over their environment and decisions affecting their lives (Drake et al. 2019). Children's participation, which entails listening to their voices and involving them in the decision-making process, is generally considered beneficial (Toros 2021). Participation is useful for children as it improves their emotional well-being and feeling of safety, while also benefitting CPS and other professionals, as it helps them provide better quality services and support to children (Wilson et al. 2020). However, Wilson et al. (2023) emphasise the need to consider the complex emotional consequences participation may have for them. For instance, children who report maltreatment at home may subsequently struggle with feelings of guilt and regret for upsetting their parents or bringing shame to the family. The distribution of complex emotions is shaped by social hierarchies and inequalities; hence, some groups of children, particularly those in marginalised positions or those burdened by societal expectations, may be more susceptible to experiencing these emotions (Ahmed 2014). Therefore, it is critical that professionals understand the emotional impact on children receiving support from CPS. In addition, professionals should provide children with information and counselling to identify and report maltreatment, as well as create an emotionally and psychologically safe environment that encourages children to disclose experiences of abuse. Reflective Activity 8.3 asks you to reflect on how you feel about having conversations with children about any concerns they may have.

Reflective Activity 8.3

- How confident do you feel about having conversations with children and young people when you are concerned they may be at risk of abuse?
- Are you aware of your roles and responsibilities with regard to this?
- If you are unsure, do you know where can you access training and support to help you develop your professional practice?

Continual professional development in safeguarding and child protection is supported by the Royal College of Nursing (RCN 2019) and the Royal College of Paediatrics and Child Health (RCPCH 2019). Practitioners who work with children often report feeling underprepared to support certain children (Bierman et al. 2024), particularly those with mental health difficulties or those who are gender-questioning (Becerra-Culqui et al. 2018) (see Chap. 6).

8.5 Multi-agency Working in Safeguarding

As previously noted, multi-agency working is essential in safeguarding children and young people (Children Act 1989). Understanding and respecting each other's roles and responsibilities is important to comprehending the landscape of the safeguarding process. No single practitioner can have a full picture of a child's needs and circumstances, but it may feel this way if individual practitioners are not connected or specialised roles are misunderstood (Forrester 2024). Differences in opinion do not necessarily mean the collaborative approach is breaking down; rather, the varied perspectives from different professionals help support a fuller understanding of the child's situation and enables informed decision-making. Throughout the safeguarding process, staff should be empowered to utilise professional curiosity and raise concerns (Mansoor and Mansoor 2019). It is expected that practitioners comment, challenge, and jointly deliberate, before making a final decision about the likelihood of significant harm and considering further actions (Department for Education 2023a, b, c). To understand this process and the role of different professionals, please read the Alex's case study (Box 8.2).

Box 8.2: Case Study of Alex

Alex is 12 years old and has a diagnosis of autism spectrum disorder (ASD). Alex is known to the special educational needs coordinator (SENCO) who recognises that Alex has struggled with the transition from primary school to secondary school. The school nurse has referred Alex to the following:

- A dietician, as Alex has a low appetite and is underweight
- A physiotherapist, as Alex reports pain in their legs after P.E. class
- An occupational therapist (OT) to explore potential sensory processing difficulties

During the occupational therapy assessment, the schoolteacher, SENCO, and parents engage well and are supportive. They report that Alex is doing well academically but is often isolated from peers, preferring to be alone. This represents a change, as Alex had a few close friends in primary school. The teacher reports that Alex does not like to sit for long periods and is often moving or fidgeting, and covers their ears if the environment becomes noisy. The teacher also notes there have been occasions when Alex has become angry with their peers, and has been asked to leave the classroom to calm down. The parents reported that Alex always seems exhausted after school and needs to go to their room for a period of time before joining the family downstairs. Furthermore, they reflected that Alex has recently been spending increased time in their room and engaging less frequently with the family. Alex is assessed separately and observed in the school environment by the OT. Alex shows signs of sensory processing difficulties and is provided with advice and strategies to support self-regulation. The SENCO and parents are advised on how to support Alex in carrying out these strategies in the home and school environment. An initial assessment report is written including advice and is sent out within 2 weeks to parents and the school.

Three months later, the OT meets Alex (for a review) at school. During this review, Alex discloses that they do not like school because it makes them sad, and they feel they do not want to be there anymore. When asked for clarification, Alex states they do not want to be alive, and while they have considered ways to end their life, they do not have a plan to carry this out at the moment. Alex asks the occupational therapist not to tell anyone because it will make their parents angry. As issues regarding the necessity of breaking confidentiality have been explained at the outset, the OT reiterates this to Alex.

The OT feels anxious about saying the wrong thing and potentially making this situation worse for Alex. They thank Alex for letting them know how they are feeling and acknowledge that these are difficult emotions to experience. The OT expresses that they are pleased Alex does not have a plan to harm themselves at this time. When asked what Alex thinks would make them feel differently, Alex reports they do not know. They reluctantly agree that the OT

(continued)

can inform the school and parents, after receiving assurance that Alex will not be in trouble or made to feel embarrassed.

The OT discusses this with the SENCO before leaving the premises and then calls Alex's parents to share the information. All parties agree to immediate considerations to reduce the short-term risk of harm. The OT then documents this incident and follows the safeguarding policy of the organisation, which includes information sharing with other agencies on a need-to-know basis. This includes Alex's GP, so a mental health assessment can be undertaken. Both the parents and SENCO are updated to inform them of progress and next steps.

Questions

- What other questions could be asked to find out more from Alex?
- Are there any signs that the OT might have missed about what Alex is experiencing?
- How could the OT support their own well-being during this time?

Considering the case study, it is important to gather as much information as possible to inform any potential interventions. Due to Alex living with autism, they may think very literally. This means that clinicians must consider the meaning of what is being asked and ensure questions are direct and clear (Chen et al. 2020). For example, asking 'Do you want to hurt yourself?' and 'Are you planning to hurt yourself?' may elicit different responses. It is important to avoid leading questions such as 'You feel really sad, don't you?'; instead, consider asking 'How does that make you feel?'. It is also important to identify any coping strategies Alex may have by asking, 'Is there anything you have found that makes you feel better?'. Due to Alex's reported suicidal ideation, they are at risk of self-harm and therefore, require a safeguarding intervention. Asking, 'Is there anyone else you feel safe talking to about this?' could provide clarity around Alex's support system. Allowing Alex to consider, 'If I had a magic wand, and you still had to go to school, but we could change something to make it better, what would that be?' could allow Alex to reflect on an outcome that would improve the situation and give the practitioner insight into the situation itself and whether there is a desired outcome (Brennan and McElvaney 2020). It is important that practitioners feel confident in having these conversations with Alex, remembering the importance of children's agency and voice as discussed earlier.

The case study indicates that Alex's parents and the teacher have identified changes in Alex's behaviour, including increased withdrawal, uncharacteristic anger with peers, and loss of appetite. Although it could be considered that these behavioural changes are part of Alex's diagnosis of autism, they could also indicate a change in Alex's emotional well-being or mental health. It may have been beneficial for the occupational therapist to ask more questions about Alex's emotional well-being at the initial assessment stage. For example, questions such as: 'You have reported that Alex has struggled with the transition from primary school to secondary school. What makes you think this specifically? Has Alex told you they are struggling or said how they feel about the change?'. Or, 'You have said Alex has become angry with peers in the school. Are you aware of Alex expressing anger in any other contexts?'. These questions could have provided answers that indicate whether more exploration was required when the OT met Alex for the first time. Consequently, safeguarding concerns might have been identified sooner (Bagattini 2019).

Lastly, it is important to acknowledge that health and social care workers are likely to be impacted emotionally when working with safeguarding cases. For example, the OT in the case study identifies feeling anxious when Alex discloses suicidal ideation. Protection of well-being can be pre-emptive; for example, staying up to date with safeguarding training and having knowledge and an understanding of local safeguarding processes and procedures (see Reflective Activity 8.2). To maintain well-being, it is important to utilise formal and informal supervision and peer support from colleagues, as this can reduce emotional burden and feelings of isolation (Lewis et al. 2022). Furthermore, engaging in reflective practice help practitioners learn from safeguarding events in a way that supports and informs future practice positively (Rolfe et al. 2011).

8.6 Implications for Practice

8.6.1 Working with Children and Young People

As noted in the UK Children Act (1989), professionals must consider a child's welfare to be of the utmost importance and must always act in the best interest of the child (Mansoor and Mansoor 2019). This includes following safeguarding pathways but also listening to the child in a way that supports autonomy, respects privacy and integrity, and maintains dignity and respect (Feldthusen et al. 2022). Building a therapeutic relationship based on this foundation supports children and young people in expressing themselves and helps the practitioner to understand the child's lived experience (Driscoll et al. 2022). The Equality Act (2010) states that specialist provision must be put in place to support dialogue with children who may struggle to convey their experiences. This could include children with communication difficulties, children who do not speak the same language as the practitioner, or victims of modern slavery and/or trafficking (Department for Education 2024).

Research by Kogan (2004) highlighted that children's disclosure of harmful events was facilitated by being asked direct questions from professionals or parents, rather than by organic initiation from the child themselves. A qualitative study focusing on the disclosure process for children by McElvaney (2013) found that parents' questioning of children was prompted by their concern about the young person's emotional distress, which was a manifestation of an unsafe event that the child found difficult to process. It is important to note that proactively creating a supportive and safe therapeutic environment that facilitates engagement for all children is imperative in the safeguarding process, as it may quicken disclosure and enhance the efficiency of safeguarding intervention.

8.6.2 Working with Parents

It must be recognised that the terms 'safeguarding' and 'child protection' can cause significant anxiety for families (Working Together with Parents Network 2021); therefore, clear and honest communication with families is key. Palmer and Jenkins (2014) identified that parents valued key aspects of input from professionals when involved in child safeguarding (see Box 8.3).

Box 8.3: Communication with Parents (Palmer and Jenkins 2014)

- *Feeling involved and up to date:* Regular updates and involvement in decision-making, where appropriate, contribute to parents' sense of inclusion. This also recognises that the child at the centre of safeguarding is part of a family and acknowledges that the family will also be impacted by the intervention.
- *Reliable and consistent contact:* Knowing who to contact, receiving timely responses, and being able to rely on professionals to do what they say they will do is crucial for maintaining trust between the MDT and parents.
- *Feeling that the professionals genuinely care about the welfare of the family:* Professionals who demonstrate empathy and concern for the family's well-being reinforce the intention of safeguarding intervention and support a 'team around the child' approach, preventing parents from feeling isolated during the safeguarding process.

Additionally, parents reflected that they appreciated being contacted with what was perceived as kindness, as they were used to being contacted only when professionals had concerns for their child (Driscoll et al. 2022).

It is important to acknowledge that practitioners may find engaging with parents and building a therapeutic relationship challenging, due to stressors of their role, additional responsibilities outside of an individual case, or the complexities of circumstances that may negatively impact the practitioner's view of the child's support system. Despite personal feelings that may arise for practitioners regarding parents' treatment of their child, it is important that unconditional positive regard is upheld and a genuine professional relationship is built and maintained, where possible (Forrester 2024). This is because the parents may be key to the implementation of positive change for the child, reducing risk and increasing safety.

8.6.2.1 Information Sharing

Practitioners often worry about what information they can share and with whom, as confidentiality is often a source of anxiety for professionals (Baltag and Sawyer 2016). Yet information-sharing guidance sets clear parameters of when to share information, guided by the principles of necessity and proportionality (DfE 2024). Furthermore, the Data Protection Act (2018) does not prohibit practitioners from sharing information to uphold section 11 of the Children Act (2004). Regarding children and young people, while they are entitled to privacy and their preferences, needs, and values, and experiences should be respected, if they are at risk, then early intervention prevents more serious difficulties from developing later (Bell and Pollard 2022). It is important to include the voice of the child or young person and report what they have said in detail, including their wishes, if these have been obtained (Driscoll et al. 2022). Because of the importance of acting quickly in safeguarding situations, consent is not required before raising safeguarding concerns if there is a risk of harm to the child and/or others (DfE 2023a, b, c). However, it is important that the child is made aware that the information will be shared and the reason why, and this must be conveyed with sensitivity and in a way that supports the maintenance of a therapeutic relationship. If safeguarding concerns are reported, then practitioners should share these with others involved in the child's care and escalate them through local safeguarding channels (Department for Education 2024). Closing the communication loop is imperative when providing or receiving information related to safeguarding. Concerns must be escalated in a timely way, but this cannot be at the expense of accuracy (Tufford et al. 2021). It is imperative that safeguarding conversations are followed up with written documentation. When sharing concerns verbally or in writing, it is important to be clear about what you are sharing and why, describing the risk in detail, and only sharing information related specifically to the concern and risk specifically (Nouman et al. 2020). Reflective Activity 8.4 asks you to consider some of the barriers to reporting concerns as well as guidance for practitioners.

Reflective Activity 8.4

- Please read and reflect upon the following: "Barriers for professionals to reporting abuse and neglect" (nspcc.org.uk)
- Please also read and reflect upon the following: "Information sharing: advice for practitioners" (publishing.service.gov.uk)

8.7 Conclusion

Adverse experiences in childhood can profoundly impact not only physical and psychological health but also general well-being later in life. This chapter has explored the multifaceted challenges and critical strategies of child protection and safeguarding within the UK context, highlighting the impact of global policies such as the UNCRC on domestic practices. These discussions contribute to understanding how practitioners must navigate their responsibilities with an awareness of the vulnerabilities of children. By exploring the concepts of 'child protection' and 'safeguarding', we have uncovered significant tensions between the intentions of policies and their practical outcomes. The discussion illuminate how legislative frameworks interact with the lived experiences of children, revealing a critical need for practitioners to balance professional authority with the vulnerabilities of children, who often have limited power. Furthermore, it is important for professionals to gain knowledge about their local policies and reporting procedures. This chapter also emphasises the importance of multi-agency working in safeguarding practices, where children and their adult advocates, such as professionals and parents work together towards the goal of child protection. This partnership, supported by official frameworks and policies in the UK, is vital for ensuring that children's rights and welfare are prioritised in all decisions. Through various modes of engagement and reflective exercises, we encourage practitioners working with children to continuously re-evaluate and refine their approach to safeguarding and child protection, ensuring that it is both child centred and conducive to fostering an environment where children feel safe, respected, and heard.

References

Afifi TO, McTavish J, Turner S, MacMillan HL, Wathen CN. The relationship between child protection contact and mental health outcomes among Canadian adults with a child abuse history. Child Abuse Negl. 2018;79:22–30.

Ahmed S. The cultural politics of emotion. New York: Routledge; 2014.

Anda RF, Butchart A, Felitti VJ, Brown DW. Building a framework for global surveillance of the public health implications of adverse childhood experiences. Am J Prev Med. 2010;39(1):93–8. https://doi.org/10.1016/j.amepre.2010.03.015.

Asmussen K, Waddell S, Molloy D, Moore I. What works to improve the lives of England's most vulnerable children: a review of interventions for a local family help offer. Early Intervention Foundation; 2022. Available at: eif.org.uk. Accessed 9 Apr 2024

Bagattini A. Children's well-being and vulnerability. Ethics Soc Welfare. 2019;13(3):211–5. https://doi.org/10.1080/17496535.2019.1647973.

Baltag V, Sawyer SM. Quality health care for adolescents. In: International handbook on adolescent health and development; 2016. p. 309–24. https://doi.org/10.1007/978-3-319-40743-2_15.

Bardy M. The three P's of children's rights: provision, protection and participation. Cyc-Online. 2000;16. Retrieved from http://www.cyc-net.org/cyc-online/cycol-0500-threepees.html

Becerra-Culqui T, Yuan L, Nash R, Cromwell L, Flanders D, Getahun D, Giammattei S, Hunkeler E, Lash T, Millman A, Quinn V, Robinson B, Roblin D, Sandberg D, Silverberg M, Tangpricha V, Goodman M. Mental health of transgender and gender nonconforming youth compared with their peers. Pediatrics. 2018;141(5):e20173845.

Bell A, Pollard A. No wrong door. NHS Confederation; 2022. Available at: https://www.nhsconfed.org/publications/no-wrong-door. Accessed: 27 Apr 2024

Berens A, Jensen SKG, Nelson CA. Biological embedding of childhood adversity: from physiological mechanisms to clinical implications. 2017;15:135. https://doi.org/10.1186/s12916-017-0895-4.

Bierman R, Ashworth K, Cereso I, Choudhary A, Ott E, Hall A. A randomised controlled trial of a therapeutic intervention for unaccompanied asylum-seeking children. London: Foundations, What Works Centre for Children & Families; 2024.

Brandon M, Sidebotham P, Belderson P, Cleaver H, Dickens J, Garstang J, et al. Complexity and challenge: a triennial analysis of SCRs 2014–2017. London: Department for Education; 2020.

Brennan E, McElvaney R. What helps children tell? A qualitative meta-analysis of Child sexual abuse disclosure. Child Abuse Rev. 2020;29(2):97–113. https://doi.org/10.1002/car.2617.

Casey B, Hackett S. Deconstructing discourses in assessments of child neglect. Br J Soc Work. 2021;51(6):2097–115. Available from: OP-SOCI210044 2097.2115. silverchair.com. Accessed 9 Apr 2024

Chambers D, Cantrell A, Booth A. Recognition of risk and prevention in safeguarding of children and young people: a mapping review and component analysis of service development interventions aimed at health and social care professionals. BMC Health Serv Res. 2021;21:1241. https://doi.org/10.1186/s12913-021-07257-8.

Chen N, Miller S, Milbourn B, Black MH, Fordyce K, Van Der Watt G, Alach T, Masi A, Frost G, Tucker M, Eapen V, Girdler S. The big wide world of school: supporting children on the autism spectrum to successfully transition to primary school: perspectives from parents and early intervention professionals. Scand J Child Adolesc Psychiatry Psychol. 2020;8(1):91–100. https://doi.org/10.21307/sjcapp-2020-009.

Children Act. 1989. Available from: Children Act 1989. legislation.gov.uk. Accessed 20 Feb 2024.

Children Act. 2004. Available from: Children Act 2004. legislation.gov.uk. Accessed 20 Feb 2024.

Children and Social Work Act. 2017. Available from: Children and Social Work Act 2017. legislation.gov.uk. Accessed 20 Feb 2024.

Clements K. An analysis of Local Safeguarding Children Boards' threshold documents. Summary of research carried out on behalf of the All-Party Parliamentary Group for Children. National Childrens Bureau; 2018. Available at: Full threshold documents analysis report.pdf. ncb.org.uk. Accessed 9 Apr 2024

Cossar J, Belderson P, Brandon M. Recognition, telling and getting help with abuse and neglect: Young people's perspectives. Child Youth Serv Rev. 2019;106:104469.

Council of Europe. European Convention on Human Rights (ECHR). Strasbourg Cedex: Council of Europe; 1950.

Criminal Justice Inspectorates. In harm's way. The role of the police in keeping children safe. 2015. Available at: in-harms-way.pdf. justiceinspectorates.gov.uk. Accessed 9 Apr 2024.

Data Protection Act. 2018. Available from: Data Protection Act 2018. legislation.gov.uk. Accessed 9 Apr 2024.

Department for Education. What to do if you're worried a child is being abused advice for practitioners. 2015. Available at: Child abuse concerns: guide for practitioners – GOV.UK. www.gov.uk. Accessed 9 Apr 2024.

Department for Education. Children's social care: stable homes, built on love. 2023a. Available at: Children's social care: stable homes, built on love consultation response. publishing.service.gov.uk. Accessed on 20 Feb 2024.

Department for Education. Working together to safeguard children 2023: a guide to multi-agency working to help, protect and promote the welfare of children. 2023b. Available at: Working together to safeguard children 2023: statutory guidance. publishing.service.gov.uk. Accessed 4 Apr 2024.

Department for Education. Safeguarding and child protection in schools. A guide for schools. 2023c. Available at: Safeguarding & child protection in schools (September 2023)_0. PDF. education-ni.gov.uk. Accessed 9 Apr 2024.

Department of Education. Information sharing: advice for practitioners providing safeguarding services. 2024. Available from: https://www.gov.uk/government/publications/safeguarding-practitioners-information-sharing-advice. Accessed: 27 Apr 1991.

Devaney J. The trouble with thresholds: Rationing as a rational choice in child and family social work. Child Fam Soc Work. 2018;24:458–66.

Drake G, Edenborough M, Falloon J, Fattore T, Felton R, Mason J, Mogensen L. Is there a place for children as emotional beings in child protection policy and practice? Int J Emot Educ. 2019;11(1):115–34.

Driscoll J, Hutchinson A, Lorek A, Stride C, Kisset K. Multiagency safeguarding arrangements during and beyond the COVID-19 pandemic: identifying shared learning. Child Abuse Rev. 2022;31(5) https://doi.org/10.1002/car.2774.

Equality Act. 2010. Available from: Equality Act 2010. Retrieved from: https://www.legislation.gov.uk/ukpga/2010/15/contents.

Feldthusen C, Forsgren E, Wallström S, Andersson V, Löfqvist N, Sawatzky R, Öhlén J, Ung EJ. Centredness in health care: a systematic overview of reviews. Health Expect. 2022;25(3):885–901. https://doi.org/10.1111/hex.13461.

Finn C. Forensic nurses' experiences of receiving child abuse disclosures. J Spec Pediatr Nurs. 2011;16(4):252–62.

Font SA, Kennedy R, Littleton T. Child protective services involvement and exclusionary school discipline. Child Dev. 2023;94(6):1625–41.

Forrester D. Humanist social work. In: The enlightened social worker. Bristol: Policy Press; 2024. Available from: https://doi.org/10.51952/9781447367680.ch007. Accessed 29 Apr 2024.

Foster D. An overview of child protection legislation in England. Research briefing. House of Commons Library. 2023. Available at: SN06787.pdf. parliament.uk. Accessed 8 Apr 2024.

Hewitt-Taylor J, Heaslip V. Protecting children or creating vulnerability? Community Pract. 2012;85(12):31–3.

Kogan SM. Disclosing unwanted sexual experiences: Results from a national sample of adolescent women. Child Abuse Negl. 2004;28(2):147–65.

Lewis S, Willis K, Bismark M, Smallwood N. A time for self-care? Frontline health workers strategies for managing mental health during the COVID-19 pandemic. SSM Mental Health. 2022;2:100053. https://doi.org/10.1016/j.ssmmh.2021.100053.

Lines, E., Grant, J., and Hutton, A., 2020. Nurses' perceptions of systems and hierarchies shaping their responses to child abuse and neglect. Nurs Inq. Available at: Wiley Online Library. Accessed 29 May 2024.

MacAlister J. The independent review of children's social care—final report research report. 2022. Available at: . publishing.service.gov.uk. Accessed 9 Apr 2024.

Madigan S, Deneault AA, Racine N, Park J, Thiemann R, Zhu J, Dimitropoulos G, Williamson T, Fearon P, Cénat JM, McDonald S, Devereux C, Neville RD. Adverse childhood experiences: a meta-analysis of prevalence and moderators among half a million adults in 206 studies. World Psychiatry. 2023;22(3):463–71. https://doi.org/10.1002/wps.21122.

Mansoor T, Mansoor N. Safeguarding children and young people-everyone's responsibility. J Dow Univ Health Sci. 2019;13(3):165–70. https://doi.org/10.36570/jduhs.2019.3.703.

Mason J, Fattore T. Child protection and child participation. In: Fernandez E, Delfabbro P, editors. Child protection and the care continuum. Abingdon: Routledge Taylor and Francis Group; 2021. p. 271–88.

McElvaney R. Disclosure of child sexual abuse: delays, non-disclosure and partial disclosure. What the research tells us and implications for practice. Child Abuse Rev. 2013;24(3):159–69. https://doi.org/10.1002/car.2280.

National Institute for Health and Care Excellence. Child abuse and Neglect QS179. National Institute for Health and Care Excellence; 2019. Available at: Overview | Child abuse and neglect | Quality standards | NICE. Accessed 9 Apr 2024

Nouman H, Alfandari R, Enosh G, Dolev L, Daskal-Weichhendler H. Mandatory reporting between legal requirements and personal interpretations: Community Healthcare Professionals' reporting of child maltreatment. Child Abuse Negl. 2020;101:104261. https://doi.org/10.1016/j.chiabu.2019.104261.

O'Mahony C. Child protection and the ECHR: making sense of positive and procedural obligations. Int J Child Rights. 2019;27(4):660–93.

Ofsted. What is early help? Concepts, policy directions and multi-agency perspectives. 2022. Available at: publishing.service.gov.uk. Accessed 9 Apr 2022.

Palmer E, Jenkins P. Parents as partners in safeguarding children. 2014. ivisontrust.org.uk. Available at: https://ivisontrust.org.uk/wp-content/uploads/2013/11/1116_parents_as_partners_white_paper_V2_sgls.pdf. Accessed: 27 Apr 2024.

Public Health England. Making every contact count (MECC): consensus statement. 2016. Available at: Main heading. england.nhs.uk. Accessed 9 Apr 2024.

Public Health England. Rapid review on safeguarding to inform the Healthy Child Programme 5 to 19. 2018. Available at: publishing.service.gov.uk. Accessed on 9 Apr 2024.

Rolfe G, Jasper M, Freshwater D. Critical reflection in practice: generating knowledge for care. Basingstoke: Palgrave Macmillan; 2011.

Royal College of Nursing. Safeguarding children and young people: roles and competencies for health care staff. 2019. Available at: Royal College of Nursing. rcn.org.uk. Accessed 9 Apr 2024.

Royal College of Paediatrics and Child Health. Safeguarding children and young people: roles and competencies for paediatricians. 2019. Available at: safeguarding_cyp_-_roles_and_competencies_for_paediatricians_-_august_2019_0.pdf. rcpch.ac.uk. Accessed 29 May 2024.

Sinclair R, Franklin A. A quality protects research briefing: young people's participation. London: Department of Health, Research in Practice and Making Research Count; 2000.

Taylor J, Dickens J, Garstang J, Cook L, Hallett N, Molloy E. Tackling the 'normalisation of neglect': messages from child protection reviews in England. Child Abuse Rev. 2024;e2841. Available from: https://doi.org/10.1002/car.2841.

Toros K. Children's participation in decision making from child welfare workers' perspectives: a systematic review. Res Soc Work Pract. 2021;31(4):367–74.

Tufford L, Lee B, Bogo M, Wenghofer E, Etherington C, Thieu V, Zhao R. Decision-making and relationship competence when reporting suspected physical abuse and child neglect: an objective structured clinical evaluation. Clin Soc Work J. 2021;49:256–70. https://doi.org/10.1007/s10615-020-00785-6.

UK Gov. Age groups. 2023a. Available from: Age groups – GOV.UK. Ethnicity facts and figures. ethnicity-facts-figures.service.gov.UK. Accessed 14 Mar 2024.

UK Gov. Children in need. 2023b. Available from: https://explore-education-statistics.service.gov.uk/find-statistics/characteristics-of-children-in-need. Accessed 14 Mar 2024.

UNICEF. United Nations Convention on the Rights of the Child. 1990. Available at: Layout 1. unicef.org.uk. Accessed 20 Feb 2024.

United Nations. Convention on the Rights of the Child. 1989. General Assembly Resolution 44/25, UN Doc A/RES/44/25 UN. November 20.

Wilson S, Hean S, Abebe T, Heaslip V. Children's experiences with child protection services: a synthesis of qualitative evidence. Child Youth Serv Rev. 2020;113:104974.

Wilson S, Hean S, Abebe T, Heaslip V, Smith JA. The war within: emotional experiences of children in Norwegian child protection services. Child Geogr. 2023;22:1–16.

Working Together with Parents Network. The Working Together with Parents Network (WTPN) 2021 update of the 2016 good practice guidance on working with parents with a learning disability. 2021. Available at: FINAL 2021 WTPN UPDATE OF THE GPG.pdf. bristol.ac.uk. Accessed 9 Apr 2024.

World Population Review . Children in the world by country 2024. 2024. Available from: worldpopulationreview.com. Accessed 14 Mar 2024.

9 Understanding Emotional and Behaviour Control Difficulties That Can Lead to Aggression and Relationship Problems

Celeste Foster

C. Foster (✉)
Directorate of Nursing and Midwifery, University of Salford, Salford, UK
e-mail: c.m.foster@salford.ac.uk

G. Trainor, V. Heaslip (eds.), *Needs of Children and Young People Living with Complex Mental Health Difficulties*,
https://doi.org/10.1007/978-3-031-84532-1_9

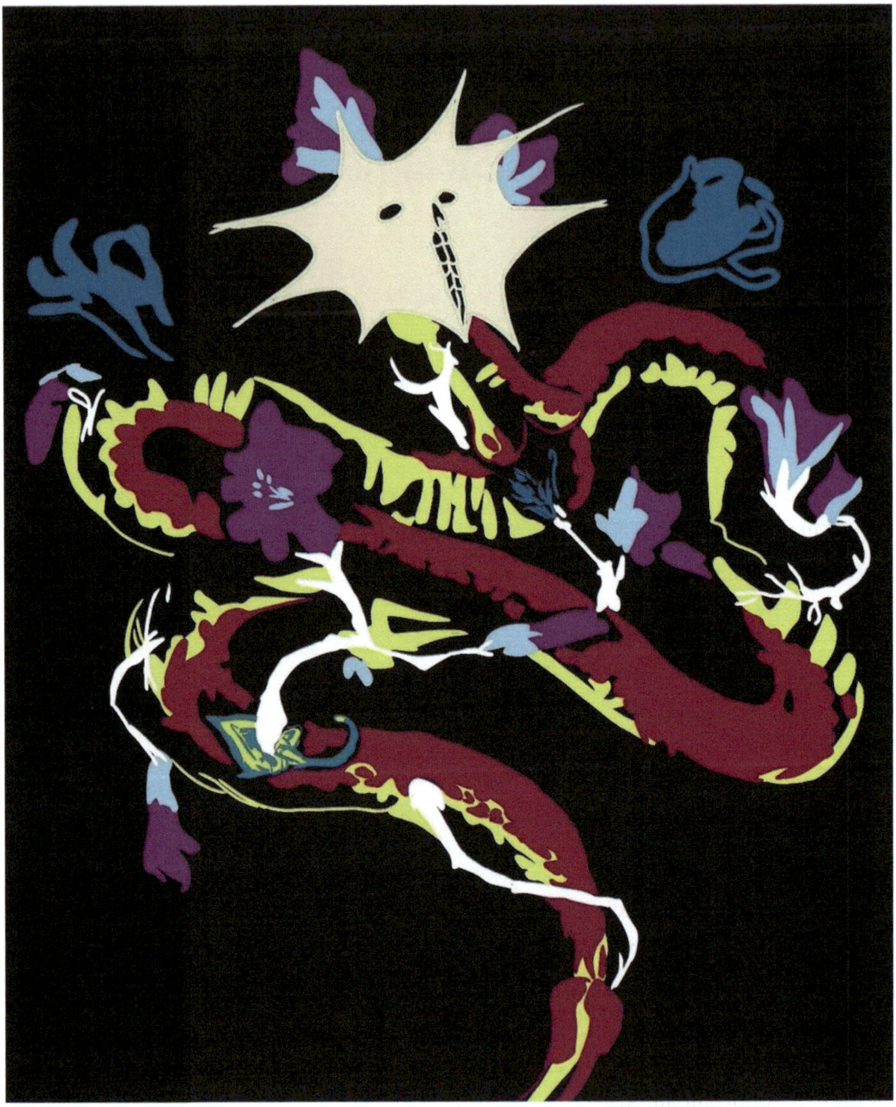

9.1 Introduction: All Behaviour Is Information

It is an almost universally accepted fact that when babies cry, scream, wriggle, and make themselves purple, they are telling us something vitally important and that it is our job to try and work out what that thing is, so we can respond to it, whilst also working to soothe the baby's immediate distress. Even though the sound of persistent baby cries can be one of the most disturbing noises—making us anxious and driving fantasies of being able to just make it stop or to pass the baby to someone else and run away—most people recognise the baby's helplessness in that moment and the need to lend one's own psychological, emotional, and physical resources to the baby, to help them out of the state that they are in.

In this way, we work to bring the baby's mind, and its awareness of what is going on inside itself, into life. We work to feel our way into the baby's place, using our own knowledge and life experience to imagine what might be going on for them and then responding to them in a way that they can take in (e.g. a bottle, or breast, for a hungry baby), so that as well as being soothed the baby can learn something about itself (I am hungry!). In child development terms, recognising and responding to this type of very primitive communication as meaningful and understanding our role to help the baby with it are referred to as emotional containment or parental holding (Bion 1962; Winnicott 1984). Over time, repeated good-enough experiences of this process produce the foundations of our mental resilience and well-being.

Over time, with the help of available and attuned adults, we gain greater awareness of our bodily states and the emotions that these denote, alongside language to communicate our needs more directly. However, the capacity to instinctively use behaviour to communicate our needs, manage difficult internal feelings, and cope with external stress never leaves us and especially re-emerges at times of stress, when our words can fail us (McCluskey and O'Toole 2019). Understanding this ordinary developmental process and the things that can disrupt it is the key to being able to respond helpfully to children and young people who are struggling to manage relationships and/or behaving in ways that are disruptive, risky, or damaging to their own life chances.

Children and young people's behaviour always has a function, no matter how maladaptive or extreme it may appear, even if it seems to be doing the opposite of what the young person intended it to do. Challenging behaviours can commonly be a way of defending against pain or vulnerability; distraction from unbearable feelings/states of mind; a concrete physical expression of something that cannot be said; an indirect way of communicating how something feels; an attempt to solve a problem; a way of gaining physical relief from emotional distress; and an attempt to regain a sense of control or to enlist our help (see Table 9.1 for specific examples).

As children get older, more self-directed, and more uniquely themselves, they require a balance between compassionate receptive appreciation of what they are trying to communicate alongside clear boundaries and expectations, to help them regulate themselves and learn pro-social behaviours. It can be hard for adults to hold on to the idea that all behaviour carries important communication. Just as teenagers can lose their way, giving into destructive and reckless impulses, adults can get caught up in power battles with young people, responding in ways that focus only on extinguishing difficult behaviour, rather than trying to make sense of it. This is particularly so when we work in jobs that require management of large groups of children and young people, where adherence to rules for the purpose of safety and learning is paramount (e.g. schools and youth clubs), or when we come into contact with young people in crisis who are bullish and defensive, behaving in ways that belie their underlying vulnerability.

Table 9.1 Understanding challenging behaviour: defence and coping responses

It is important to remember that behaviour always has a function—no matter how unhelpful or extreme it may appear or how unlikeable it is.
Challenging, reckless, and harmful behaviours can be:
Defence against pain and vulnerability
For example, joining a gang
Distraction from unbearable feelings/states of mind (mindless or unthinking states)
For example, alcohol and/or drug use
Concrete physical expression of something that cannot be said (unconscious)
For example, soiling, aggression
Communication (giving others a 'taste' of what it feels like to be us, through the things we do)
For example, behaving in ways which make others feel powerless or hopeless (bullying)
Problem-solving
For example, running away or taking an overdose to escape something that feels intolerable
Physical relief from emotional distress
For example, self-harm, sex, fighting
Regaining of control
For example, aggression, self-harm, restricting diet, using emerging sexuality to seduce
Alerting others to your need for help
For example, *confabulating or telling lies, dramatic or risky behaviour that brings you to the attention of blue light services*

Starting from a position of recognising the ordinary developmental function of using behaviour to act out and communicate one's feelings and needs and to solve interpersonal problems helps us to identify the underlying cause of a particularly challenging or risky behaviour, which in turn can help to identify actions to help address the problem. It also reminds us that we should be just as worried about children and young people who are super well behaved and never display any behaviours or acts of rebellion or assertiveness, as overly controlled behaviour can provide important clues that children and young people are living in fear of adult responses (Cook et al. 2005).

9.2 Understanding How Life Experience and Formative Relationships Positively and Negatively Influence the Way Young People Manage Internal and External Life Stressors and Future Relationships

Our ability to bear and regulate our emotions comes from us taking in our experience of our primary carers and other helpful adults, who regulate our emotions for us at times of stress whilst also showing and teaching us how to do it for ourselves. This starts at the beginning of life: how we are looked upon, handled, and touched forms the basic template upon which our sense of safety, self, worth, and ability to live comfortably within our own body is based (Lemma 2014). Looking and touching confer love (or not). In good-enough circumstances it is the experience of not just being looked at but being taken in, recognized, and reflected back by a receptive other, one that provides a kind of mirror in which the infant discovers an image of himself in relation to others and the world (Schore and Sieff 2014). As toddlers, if we are lucky, the mirror that our carers provides includes realistic acceptance of all that we are—the good, the angry, the jealous, and the naughty—enabling us to see, accept, and manage the more troubling and destructive parts of our feelings, such as spite, greed, envy, and aggression (Winnicott 1984). In early childhood and pre-puberty, our access to safe and responsive relationships and social environments supports our neurological and cognitive development, as we are helped to grapple with everyday challenges, which provides the basis for stress management, social interaction and interpersonal communication skills, and the ability to understand and regulate strong emotions (Gerhardt 2015).

The cumulative effect of these critical developmental stages produces what we often call emotional/affect regulation and interpersonal relationship skills. It is essential to remember that these skills, such as impulse control, frustration tolerance, empathy, delaying gratification, listening to, and accommodating the needs of others, are all works in progress that are slowly built and consolidated over time. These newly developing capacities are fragile and at times of stress can quickly fall through young people's hands like grains of sand.

When the delicate balance between the risk and protective factors that produces growth and resilience is disrupted, it is often by difficult events in young people's lives. These include:

- *Loss or separation*: e.g. resulting from death, parental separation, hospitalisation, loss of friendships (especially in adolescence), family conflict, or breakdown that results in the child having to live elsewhere, being taken into care
- *Big life changes*: e.g. the birth of a sibling, moving house or changing schools, and transitions from primary to secondary school
- *Traumatic experiences*: e.g. abuse, neglect, domestic violence, bullying, accidents and injuries, and traumatic incidents such as a natural disaster or terrorist attack (Department for Education 2018).

The effect of deprivation, neglect, and overwhelming or traumatic events at any life stage can be the loss or shattering of our internalised resilience, meaning that we go back to having to rely on others to regulate our emotions for us, until we can do it for ourselves again. This can be temporary or can take a long time to recover, depending on the nature and severity of the trauma (Kezelman and Stavropoulos 2018). If there are pre-existing difficulties and deprivation in our early experience of care, then our defences will be more vulnerable to being overwhelmed more easily, meaning that seemingly small stressors can be enough to produce difficult or challenging behaviours in children (Cook et al. 2005). Similarly, the earlier in our life that traumatic experiences occur, the smaller they need to be to disrupt the balance of coping, the more likely they are to impact on self-concept, learning emotional regulation, and relationship skills, and the bigger their impact over time (The Lancet Psychiatry 2022). For more detailed information about the impact of traumatic events and trauma-informed care, see Chap. 10.

9.3 Understanding the Relationship Between Underlying Mental Health Needs, Behaviour, and Interpersonal Relationships

Emotional and psychological distress and mental health needs are usually expressed by children and young people through the ways in which they act or behave. As children and young people are absolutely dependent on relationships for having their needs met, difficulties nearly always show up in their relationships with both adults, siblings, and peers. This can include observable changes in their:

- Emotional state (e.g. presenting as fearful, irritable, withdrawn, or self-berating and critical)
- Behaviour (e.g. reckless, aggressive, oppositional, or coercive controlling behaviour)
- Interpersonal behaviours (e.g. indiscriminate contact or affection seeking, excessive dependence on others, demonstrating excessively 'good' behaviour to prevent disapproval, being unable to accept support and help at times of distress, and extreme 'all-or-nothing' behaviours within peer relationships) (Department for Education 2018).

The different range of ways that children display their distress is often linked to the developmental stage that they are in. For example, toddlers learning to control their bodily functions may display behavioural difficulties around toileting (enuresis or encopresis). In early teenage years, where the primary task is adjusting to pubertal, hormonal, and body-based changes, it is more common for children to display eating problems (anorexia nervosa or binging and purging), other forms of harm to their body, and/or high levels of irritability, whereas in older adolescents where the primary task is developing one's identity in relation to others, sense of purpose, and occupational goals, problems can manifest in peer relationships, social and educational engagement, or at worst as hopelessness and suicidality.

Struggling to cope with one's own feelings, particularly in teenage years, often produces a sense of shame, which can get in the way of seeking help from adults and peers. It can lead to young people feeling desperately dependent on the help of others, as they feel out of their depth and frightened, sometimes seen as overdependence on particular adults, or it can lead to withdrawal and avoidance of help altogether. The more mindful of these barriers to seeking help the adults around young people are, the easier it is to build bridges to support young people to get out of difficult cycles of behaviour, before they become entrenched.

9.4 Defence, Coping, and Communication in Children and Young People

So far, this chapter has emphasised three intersecting principles that are fundamental to helping young people who are displaying difficulties with emotional, behavioural, and relationship management:

1. All behaviour has meaning, no matter how difficult or challenging it may be.
2. It is developmentally ordinary for children and young people to use their bodies to communicate and solve interpersonal crises. For younger children this can be because they have not yet learned the language to explain their feelings, even to themselves, so, for example, they may be more likely to report difficulties as tummy aches, pain, or sickness. For teenagers, this is because they are in the throes of puberty, which puts their body front and centre of every aspect of their experience.
3. The key to helping is being able to tune in and make sense of what is going on and enabling parents/carers and family members to do the same.

Alongside these three principles, we also need an awareness of what can trigger children and young people to become dysregulated. Whilst the specific triggers will be unique to each young person, a general understanding of the ways in which children and young people tend to perceive and respond to power imbalances and threat can be really useful to help us 'decode' difficult patterns of coping and behaviour. It is helpful to remember that children and young people are always in unequal power relations with adults and are often being judged against how they measure up to their peers, by themselves and by others (e.g. parents, teachers, school nurses, paediatricians, national curriculum tests, exam boards, friends, prospective romantic partners, sibling, etc.). Research has identified five repeated themes as the most common triggers of distress and emotional and behavioural disturbance in children and young people. These are actual or perceived:

- Physical threat
- Psychological threat
- Personal failure
- Hostility from others
- Injustice (Van Wijk-Herbrink et al. 2021; Fuggle et al. 2013)

Applying this knowledge to the individual circumstances of specific young people we are working with can often help start to unravel the puzzle of what is going on for that young person.

It is important to consider that many people can exhibit the behaviours discussed here. Table 9.2 provides you with the opportunity to reflect on your own experiences and behaviours.

Table 9.2 Reflective Activity 1

Even though it is hard to recall, nearly all of us will have at some point as young people behaved in a way that was considered by the adults around us as difficult, reckless, problematic, or challenging. Take time to reflect on your own childhood and teenage years and identify a time when you were in trouble for the way you behaved that as an adult you would now consider to be unacceptable.
Can you remember what triggered this?
What were the feelings that were underneath it?
What were you trying to achieve through your behaviour?
What do you wish that you could have explained to those around you?
What do you think you needed from adults around you at that time?
If you could go back and talk to that younger version of you, what would you like to say to them?

9.5 Helping Young People with Emotional, Relational, and Behavioural Control Problems: The Role of Non-mental Health Specialists

- *Prevention:* All children and young people, and especially those experiencing mental health problems, need a safe, calm, and secure environment and access to responsive and reliable adults. In whatever setting you are in, it is important to promote a structured day with a balance between activities and relaxation, work, and play. The role that schools play in promoting the resilience of their pupils is particularly important for children with less supportive home lives. Schools should be a safe and affirming place for children where they can develop a sense of belonging and feel able to trust and talk openly with adults about their problems (DfE 2018).
- *Early dentification and provision of early help for children and young people who are beginning to struggle with relationship and behavioural difficulties:* This includes spotting changes in young people's behaviour and intervening quickly and implementing everyday strategies to deescalate and help the young person solve the problems in their life and learn how to manage big feelings that are triggered by certain situations and relationships.
- *Identifying those young people who needs are more persistent, severe, and complex and that may need referral to specialist services*: Everyone involved in working with children and young people with behavioural and emotional difficulties should understand the criteria for when to seek more complex, intensive, and specialist mental health assessment (NICE 2015, see below for more details of how to do this).
- *Advocacy for children and young people*: Limited mental health resources and the challenges associated with young people who express their needs through externalising or challenging behaviour can mean that services are prioritised for children and young people who present with internalised difficulties (low mood/sadness, social avoidance, self-harm). Terms like conduct disorder and oppositional defiant disorder, which are used to describe young people presenting with a cluster of problematic and risky externalising behaviours, can be used to exclude or bar access to CYP mental health services. In fact, national clinical

guidelines (NICE 2017) state that there should be clear pathways for assessment and treatment for young people in this group, as if difficulties are left untreated, they can lead to lifelong mental health disorder and social impairment. Being armed with this knowledge can help us advocate for equal access to treatment for all young people, no matter the particular way that they express their distress.

9.6 Principles for Providing Effective Early Help

It is often that case that the more a young person's way of coping, relating, and behaving is difficult to manage or risky to themselves or others, the less they are involved in their care, as everyone clambers to try and gain some sort of control and reduce the chances of anyone coming to harm. In actual fact, evidence tells us that to effectively reduce or resolve challenging, risky, and harmful behaviour, we need to work even harder to involve young people in their care and any decision-making about them. NICE (2015) clinical guidelines for working with children who have learning disabilities and/or behaviours that challenge state that we *must* work in partnership with children, young people, and their family members or carers, involving them in decisions about care, working together to develop a shared understanding about the function of the behaviour that is causing concern, and support self-management and independence through providing accessible information about the nature of the person's needs and the range of interventions and services available to them.

Many children and young people struggling with emotional, behavioural, and interpersonal dysregulation have experienced adverse or traumatic life circumstances, so the basic principles of trauma-informed care should be adopted for all. This means working to create psychological safety through predictability and reliability, promoting choice and agency wherever possible (Isobel and Delgado 2018). Effective early help therefore needs to address four domains:

- Creation of an environment that is predictable and safe and limits re-traumatisation, in cases where young people have experienced prior traumatic events.
- Forging of stable attuned, steady therapeutic alliances with trusted adults that provide growth and reparation promoting experiences.
- Interventions that help young people make sense of and contextualise their difficulties and work through their experiences.
- Supporting the development of new relational and self-management skills and approaches to replace old habits (whilst understanding that old habits die hard when they might have saved your life).

New skills development should include:

- Increasing children's awareness of their own and others' emotions.
- Teaching self-control of emotional/physiological arousal and behaviour.
- Promoting a positive self-concept and good peer relations.
- Developing children's problem-solving skills (NICE 2017).

Although some of these skills may be developed through formal learning programmes, often they are most easily learnt by children and young people through relationships with adults who can model these skills for them in action. Table 9.3

Table 9.3 Top tips for successful engagement

Intervene early—changes in behaviour and ways of relating to peers and adults are always a opener for communication. Do not wait for it to get worse
Promote active engagement through structured and personalised daily activities, including adjusting the school curriculum for children and young people to help them be successful
Work hard to communicate that you are committed to trying to understand and to help, even if it is difficult
Identify triggers
Try to understand what is driving the behaviour and what the behaviour is communicating about the young person's underlying needs, worries, feelings, and concerns
Involve families and carers in working out how to respond helpfully to patterns of difficult behaviour
Try not to take it personally
Remember that knowing what you are doing is wrong/unhelpful is not the same as knowing what to do instead—children are often motivated to change but get stuck at the point of working out alternative strategies to replace their difficult behaviour
Focus as much time on working with the young person in times of calm to co-produce understanding of what helps them stay in control and alternative strategies when they are feeling triggered
Identify preventive strategies to calm the person when they begin to show early signs of distress
Set boundaries, expectations, and consequences in a planned way, rather than reactively. Make them proportionate and communicate them to the young person well in advance. Proactively implemented boundaries feel like safety, while reactively implemented consequences feel like punishment
Avoid getting caught in direct power struggles with young people wherever possible: Young people who are feeling out of control and struggling with poor self-concept are able to take far bigger risks with themselves than you, which can lead to un-winnable and counterproductive battle for control
Use interpersonal strategies that allow you to come alongside the young person, rather than head to head:
Always remains calm and show curiosity rather than judgement
Avoid leaving a young person feeling as though there is nothing to lose: offer dignified climb-downs, second chances, and guided opportunities to fix mistakes
Try not to get ahead of the young person and tell them how they are feeling or what they are thinking
Role model that it is alright not to know the answer and to make mistakes
Avoiding chronological expectations, e.g. 'they are old enough now to know better', in favour of expectations based on knowledge of individual development/life experience.
Accept where they are starting from and support them to grow from there
Remember that new ways of coping take time for young people to learn. They also need help to learn and practice new ways of coping. Using a coaching approach—where you tell, show, do with, get the young person to do, and then provide feedback and praise—can really help with this and build rapport and trust, which in itself can reduce risk of challenging behaviour even occur
Seek support and supervision—children and young people who are struggling with behavioural, interpersonal, and emotional control problems can be provocative when they feel stuck and can evoke very difficult feelings in adults who are trying to help them

provides a range of practical advice and guidance that can be implemented to increase the chances of successful engagement of young people who are struggling with emotional, behavioural, and interpersonal difficulties. For more detailed discussion of how to forge therapeutic alliances with children and young people, see Chap. 12.

9.7 Identifying More Persistent or Severe Problems

9.7.1 When to Refer to Specialist CYP Mental Health Services

The Anna Freud Centre has developed a freely available guide for professionals managing challenging behaviour in school settings, as part of their Mentally Healthy Schools website (The Anna Freud Centre 2020, see Table 9.4 for further details). They provide a helpful list of indicators that may identify that a child or young person is experiencing underlying psychological difficulty and may need further specialist assessment and help.

Children and young people who need more specialist assessment are likely to display more than one of these difficulties, and they will be present in more than one context (e.g. school as well as home). Children and young people in this group benefit from comprehensive assessment by a specialist child and young people's mental health service (CAMHS). Any young person who has additional complicating factors, such as co-existing mental health problems, a learning disability, substance misuse, or a neurodevelopmental condition, e.g. autism or ADHD, should always be referred to specialist CAMHS services (NICE 2017).

9.7.2 Assessment

It is extremely important to understand that children and young people with these symptoms are vulnerable, not just disruptive or a risk to others. Many of them will have or be experiencing adverse or traumatic life events. Therefore, young people

Table 9.4 Indicators of a more serious difficulty needing specialist assessment

A child or young person with persistent behavioural problems may:
Be argumentative, angry, uncooperative, or irritable
Have frequent tantrums and angry outbursts
Be aggressive and provoke or bully others
Be constantly defiant
Blame others for things that go wrong
Tell lies regularly
Appear cruel and lack empathy for other children
Struggle to manage the boundaries and rules within the school environment
Find it difficult to maintain attention and concentration
Seek out risky experiences without thinking about the consequences
Become involved in antisocial behaviour as they get older
Be at risk of self-harm or suicide

Anna Freud Centre (2020)

who present with significant problems with emotional, behavioural, and relational dysregulation should also trigger assessment and management of any potential risks they are facing, using usual local safeguarding procedures. This should include assessment for the presence of, or risk of, physical, sexual, and emotional abuse, self-neglect, exploitation by others, self-harm, or harm to others (NICE 2017). Assessments should also include the young person's strengths and protective factors, not just focus on risks.

9.7.3 Intervention

Young people whose difficulties are persistent and life interfering may receive a psychiatric diagnosis of conduct disorder. To be given a diagnosis, there must be evidence of core symptoms, which include (NICE 2017):

- Patterns of negativistic, hostile, or defiant behaviour in children aged under 11 years.
- Aggression to people and animals, destruction of property, deceitfulness or theft, and serious violations of rules in children aged over 11 years.
- Increased risk associated with ADHD and autism diagnosis—importance of ensuring young people are getting the right care packages for these underlying difficulties as a means of reducing the risk.

Care and interventions should include an equal focus on addressing the underlying issues, not just management of the problematic behaviour (McGorry et al. 2024). There is an increased risk of receiving a diagnosis of conduct disorder associated with ADHD and autism diagnoses, and so it is important that young people are getting the right care packages for these underlying difficulties as the primary way of reducing risk and improving outcomes. Similarly, many young people presenting with persistent conduct or emotional dysregulation and interpersonal difficulties will have experienced complex trauma. Complex trauma described the cumulative effects of threats in interpersonal relationships and life experiences. It results in young people presenting with complex deficits in cognitive, social, physiological, and emotional functioning (Maercker et al. 2022). Young people should have access to evidence-based psychological treatments for this condition, which focus on safety, psychoeducation about trauma, and psychological treatment to improve affect and interpersonal regulation, such as dialectical behaviour therapy, mentalisation-based therapy (MBT), and trauma-focused psychotherapies (Lancet Psychiatry 2022). Very occasionally, this will include prescribing of medicines that give 'respite' from severe emotional dysregulation. Medicines of this kind should only be prescribed by a specialist child psychiatrist, and it is important to understand that it is just one tool to help reduce risks and support the young person to avoid worsening of their situation whilst other interventions are being implemented. Medication is not a cure or first-line treatment for emotional dysregulation (NICE 2009).

Evidence-based interventions for conduct disorder can vary, but they are all underpinned by four themes:

1. A strong focus on working with parents and families.
2. A recognition of the importance of working with the young person's wider social system in enabling effective interventions.
3. A focus on preventing or reducing the escalation of existing problems.
4. Provision social and cognitive problem-solving programmes (using cognitive behavioural problem-solving model).

In young people with complex or severe needs, this should include a case coordinator and multi-professional plan of care and risk management, with regular review, coordination, and communication between all agencies involved, e.g. school, police, youth services, CAMHS, social services (NICE 2017). The case study of Sam, in Table 9.4, illustrates how this is done in practice. You can read more about the process of assessing and managing mental health-related risks in Chap. 11 of this book.

9.8 Whole System Responsibility to Address Intersectional Experiences of Discrimination That Can Create Barriers to Successful Intervention

Establishing working therapeutic relationships with children and young people and their parents or carers is essential for interventions to be effective. This requires everyone who comes into contact with the young person and their family to understand the intersectional forms of discrimination that families may have experienced and how this can make engagement with services much more difficult for them. We need to be mindful that the experiences of children and families that lead to emotional and behavioural control difficulties often include negative experiences of marginalisation, prejudice, and outright discrimination due to issues such as socioeconomic status, race, ethnicity, learning disabilities, mental illness, physical, sexual, and psychological abuse.

Many children and young people given a diagnosis of conduct disorder may have had poor or punitive experiences of care and be mistrustful or dismissive of offers of help as a result (NICE 2017). Those living in unpredictable environments may have honed skills in reading non-verbal interpersonal cues, the emotional temperature in the room, well beyond their years, making them highly sensitive to signs in you that indicate that you are not to be trusted with their feelings, or that you are making judgements (Foster and Gardner 2023). So the principles and tips for building helpful relationships laid out earlier in this chapter become even more important. Similarly, parents and carers of children and young people with a conduct disorder might feel blamed or have actually been blamed for their child's problems or stigmatised by their contact with services. For more detailed information about the concept of intersectional discrimination and its role in exacerbating mental health difficulties in children and young people, see Chap. 7. Table 9.5 presents the case study of Sam. After reading this, please undertake Reflective Activity 2 (Table 9.6).

Table 9.5 Case study

Sam—A Young Person in Need of Specialist Help

Sam, just 18 years old, was referred to a young person's mental health team by the youth offending team (YOT). Sam was an on a YOT order, after being found guilty of a suspected racially aggravated assault of a stranger in a park near to her supported living accommodation. Her YOT worker found Sam to be very affable and friendly and keen to try and get herself out of trouble, but in contrast to this picture, there were increasingly concerning reports about Sam behaving in aggressive ways towards strangers on the bus and in the corridors of the further education college she attended to get help with her significant literacy and numeracy needs. The contrast in these two versions of Sam made the YOT worker worry that there was an underlying problem being missed, and there were very real concerns that Sam was heading towards receiving a custodial sentence should criminal charges be brought for further acts of aggression. Sam had a difficult early life story. Both her parents struggled with drug misuse. Her mum left her at an early age in the care her dad. Her dad struggled with being in trouble with the police due to drug and alcohol-related offences throughout Sam's childhood. Sam experienced a great deal of neglect and witnessed much violence. Sam loved her dad very much and appreciated that he had tried to care for her as best he could when her mum had left the family home. Sam's dad held very strong ideas about protecting oneself by being strong, never showing weakness, and always throwing the first punch that he imparted to Sam. Sam's dad died of drug overdose when Sam was 15, meaning that Sam went into the care of the local authority in a residential children's home and then into semi-independent living accommodation. As a care leaver, Sam was expected to demonstrate independence getting to and from college, doing her shopping and managing her flat in the supported housing. However, her experience of neglect (i.e. not having anyone to show her how to do these things) and difficulties with reading and writing made this very difficult.

The multidisciplinary assessment revealed that Sam could not read facial expressions and often felt very vulnerable and frightened about other people's intention towards her. These feelings were intensified when she could not understand what people were saying (e.g. due to them speaking in a different language) or she felt trapped, for example, whilst on a bus. In these moments, if she felt under threat or was unsure if someone meant her harm, she followed her dad's advice and threw the first punch. She also felt a great deal of shame about her difficulties with doing everyday tasks, due to not being able to read or write. Sam had very low impulse control and difficulties seeing things from other people's perspectives, especially at times of stress, and struggled with intense surges of overwhelming feelings that she did not know how to manage.

Plan of Care—Clinical Guidelines in Action

Sam was allocated a care coordinator in the CAMHS team, to bring together all the professionals in her life (housing, social worker, college, YOT, police) through regular multi-professional care planning meetings, which Sam attended. As Sam did not have any close or extended family, helping her build trust in a professional group who had her best interests at heart was an important part of working to reduce her risk to others. This included developing a short-term risk management strategy in partnership with Sam—Identifying triggers and simple actions she could take to avoid these triggers or get help. She had a psychiatric assessment to see if there were underlying mental health conditions that needed treating and a detailed neuropsychological assessment to understand her cognitive difficulties with executive functioning and impulse control. Sam was assessed for neurodevelopmental conditions such as ADHD and foetal alcohol spectrum disorder. She received treatment with medicine to address her underlying social anxiety and to help at times when she was extremely emotionally dysregulated. Her care coordinator provided psychoeducation about her mental health needs and trauma, challenging her worries that her problems were a sign of weakness. She was engaged in a psychological treatment called dialectical behaviour therapy, which includes an interpersonal skills training component to help people learn new ways to cope with surging feelings (like panic or anger). For Sam this included having weekly one-to-one interpersonal problem-solving training sessions which included learning how to read and name differing states of emotion, in both herself and in the facial expressions and body language of others, and strategies to help her pause and think before acting at times when he felt frightened. Sam was allocated a support worker to help build up her confidence and skills using the bus/public transport and with shopping and paying bills. Her care coordinator also provided advice and guidance for college and her supported living staff, on the how to help deescalate Sam at times of crisis

Table 9.6 Reflective Activity 2

Getting Sam back to further education to help her build her literacy, numeracy, and social skills was identified as a very important part of reducing her risk to others and improving her life chances. However, high risk of causing others harm at times of stress remained, whilst psychological interventions took time to work. If you were working with the mental health team to help Sam get back into the classroom, what information and help would you need from the CAMHS team? Write down some ideas of what you could include in a safety plan to reduce the risk of Sam becoming aggressive towards others.

9.9 Highly Specialist Help for Very High-Risk Behaviours: Community Forensic CAMHS Services

Occasionally, young people present with such persistently high-risk, dangerous, or harmful behaviours, e.g. violence, sexually harmful behaviours, and fire setting, that they need an even more specialist assessment and management of their needs and risk. This is referred to as a forensic mental health assessment, where the risk of criminality and engagement with the justice system is high. As part of the NHS Long-Term Plan (NHS England 2019), NHS England has commissioned 13 regional community forensic CAMHS (FCAMHS) services in England and Wales, to ensure parity of access to highly specialist help and support. The aim of FCAMH services is to provide high-quality, consistent mental health support that reduces the risk of offending, or escalation in offending, and addresses health inequalities experienced by children and young people who present with high-risk, high-harm, high-vulnerability needs. These are tertiary services, meaning they are small, highly specialist multidisciplinary teams who work in support of mainstream CAMHS and youth offending (YOT) services. For example, in the case study of Sam (Table 9.5), if the package of care set out did not improve her well-being and reduce her risk to harm others over time, then a referral to the regional FCAMHS team might be considered by her care coordinator. Aside from taking direct referrals for young people already involved in CAMHS and YOT services, they should also be accessible to all agencies (e.g. social services, prisons, courts, solicitors, education, health commissioners, etc.) that may have contact with young people exhibiting risky behaviours or young people in the youth justice system who have mental health difficulties, to provide consultation, advice, and guidance.

9.10 Challenges Across the Life Course: Understanding the Relationship Between Adolescent Difficulties and Adult Psychiatric Diagnoses of Personality Disorder

The relationship between behavioural and emotional and interpersonal regulation disturbance in young people and psychiatric disorders of adulthood is complex. Many statistics point to the fact that if left without intervention, young people with emerging patterns of emotional dysregulation, problems sustaining relationships, and conduct problems are at high risk of receiving a diagnosis of borderline/emotionally unstable or antisocial personality disorder in adulthood (NICE 2017, 2009). Whilst this is no doubt true to some extent, the story underneath the statistics is complicated.

The lack of understanding of child development in the general health and social care workforce and policy framework means that young people face two related but opposite types of structural discrimination that increase their risk of receiving personality disorder labels in adulthood. In one direction there is a tendency to dismiss early behavioural indicators of distress and difficulty as either 'naughty' or just 'typical teenage behaviour', rather than an indicator of underlying distress. This means that a proportion of young people do not get access to the early help and psychological interventions that are known to prevent progression to more long-term difficulties, increasing their risk of having mental health problems into adulthood.

In the other direction, the increased emotionality and tendency to become temporarily dysregulated at times of acute stress, which is actually a developmentally ordinary part of being a young person, can be too quickly seen through the lens of 'psychiatric disturbance', leading to young people's behaviour being pathologized and them being too quickly labelled (McGorry et al. 2024). This is a particular challenge for services and professionals that only see young people for brief snapshots of time at moments of crisis, who may also not have had any training about young people's mental health, for example, emergency/blue light services and professionals working in A&E departments. Accurate assessment of young people's difficulties needs to take place over a period time, considering their presentation in a range of situations and contexts, before any decisions about potential diagnosis of a mental disorder should be made.

The situation is made more complex because the psychiatric diagnostic criteria and systems used for assessment of mental health disorders are based on presentations in adulthood and have significant limitations for young people (McGorry et al. 2024). Diagnostic criteria assume that symptoms of particular mental health disorders are stable and cluster together in particular patterns, whereas research tells us that in young people symptoms come and go and change over time as the young people themselves are in a dynamic state of change and development. Signs of distress in young people can often fall across a number of different diagnostic categories at once, without fully reaching the threshold of any one diagnosis criteria. All of this means that young people are at risk of having transient difficulties labelled as long-term entrenched problems, such as personality disorder, too quickly, or of not meeting service criteria for help, when they are clearly in significant distress (McGorry et al. 2024). Up to 70% of harmful behaviours to self and others that we see in adolescence are estimated to have stopped by early adulthood (25 years plus). This does not mean that we should leave children and young people to just get on with it with no help, but it does mean that part of our role is to try and differentiate between young people whose risk behaviours are inherently linked to navigating the adolescent life stage they are in and those whose difficulties are more likely to persist in adulthood. The Lancet Psychiatry Commission on youth mental health has identified that finding a way to respond to genuinely increasing rates of mental ill health in our young people through access to evidence-based care, whilst avoiding harm from labelling, stigmatising, or over-treating young people who are transiently distressed, is a key challenge for addressing the current youth mental health crisis, globally (McGorry et al. 2024).

One way to address the challenge is to organise services on a 'transdiagnostic clinical staging' model, based on need, that is, a model which provides a level of intervention proportionate and appropriate to the distress at the time, rather than based on diagnostic criteria. In this model, at-risk individuals who are showing signs of distress or behavioural and conduct disturbance should receive generic trauma-informed psychosocial interventions, such as mental health literacy, psychoeducation self-management, and social skills training, as set out in the first part of this chapter. If two or more clinical indicators are observed, access to specific evidence-based early intervention programmes should be facilitated, through locally commissioned mental health services. If severity increases, multidisciplinary care packages of case management, family intervention, and more intensive psychological therapies, within specialist CYP mental health services, should be considered (Lamb et al. 2018).

Most organisations and experts in the field of young people's mental health have long recognised the need for specific youth (16–25 years) mental health services that recognise and address their specific developmental needs and the particular burden of risk of mental health disorder that they face (Centre for Mental Health 2016). In the UK, the provision of CYP mental health care extending to the age of 25 years is set out as an aim in the NHS Long-Term Plan, but it is not yet a reality.

9.11 Conclusion

This chapter has explored the complex issue of supporting and enabling children and young people who are experiencing difficulties with self-concept, emotional, behavioural, and interpersonal regulation. A framework for making sense of young people's difficult behaviour has been provided. Key to this is starting from a position that children and young people's behaviour always has function and meaning and that working to make sense of it and to identify the underlying drivers is the foundation of all effective helping strategies. Persistent relationship, behaviour, and emotional management problems in children and young people are often associated with the difficult life experiences and in worst cases complex trauma. Principles of partnership and collaboration with young people and their families, seeing behaviour though the developmental life stage that children and young people are in, implementing primary and secondary prevention strategies through access to safe, reliable, and trustworthy adults and environments, and the importance of transdiagnostic, needs-led, and staged interventions that address the underlying problems have all been highlighted.

Non-mental health specialists have a pivotal role to play in early identification of vulnerable children and young people, providing early help to prevent

Table 9.7 Online resources

Guidance for managing challenging behaviour in education settings:
Anna Freud Centre Mentally Health Schools website: https://www.mentallyhealthyschools.org.uk/mental-health-needs/challenging-behaviours/
Education Endowment Foundation (2019): Improving behaviour in schools: https://educationendowmentfoundation.org.uk/education-evidence/guidance-reports/behaviour
Resources to help understand complex trauma and how to respond to it
Blue Knot Foundation (Australia): https://blueknot.org.au/product/talking-about-trauma-guide-to-conversations-and-screening-for-health-and-other-service-providers-digital-download/
National Child Traumatic Stress Network (USA): https://www.nctsn.org/what-is-child-trauma/trauma-types/complex-trauma
This is an animation from Manchester Resilience Hub about trauma and young people and how to help. It has been co-produced by young people and mental health specialists: https://thejourneyofrecovery.co.uk/

escalation of difficulties; understanding when referral to more specialist assessment and intervention may be needed; and advocating for young people and families, who may be at risk of marginalisation and exclusion. This chapter has provided principles, advice, and tips for engagement and early intervention and information about more specialist services and when to refer on, in order to support all those who come into contact with children and young people who are struggling, to contribute positively to their care and well-being. A list of online resources is available in Table 9.7.

References

Anna Freud Centre. Managing challenging behaviour in school settings. 2020. https://www.mentallyhealthyschools.org.uk/mental-health-needs/challenging-behaviours/. Accessed 22 Oct 2024.

Bion W. Learning from experience. Abingdon: Routledge; 1962.

Centre for Mental Health. 16–25 years missed opportunities: children and young people's mental health. In: Khan L, editors. Missed opportunities: a review of recent evidence into children and young people's mental health. 2016. www.centreformentalhealth.org.uk/missed-opportunities. Accessed 22 Oct 2024.

Cook A, Spinazzola J, Ford J, Lanktree C, Blaustein M, Cloitre M, Van der Kolk B. Complex trauma in children and adolescents. Psychiatr Ann. 2005;35(5):390–8.

Department for Education. Mental health and behaviour in schools. 2018. Available from: https://assets.publishing.service.gov.uk/media/625ee6148fa8f54a8bb65ba9/Mental_health_and_behaviour_in_schools.pdf. Accessed 22 Oct 2024.

Education Endowment Foundation. Improving behaviour in schools: a guidance report. London: Percipio; 2019. Available from: Https://educationendowmentfoundation.org.uk/education-evidence/guidance-reports/behaviour. Accessed 22 Oct 2024

Foster C, Gardner L. Understanding the developmental impact of domestic violence and adverse experiences in childhood across the life-course. In: Roddy J, editor. Working with client experiences of domestic abuse. Taylor & Francis (Routledge); 2023. p. 117–32. https://doi.org/10.4324/9781003253266-9.

Fuggle P, Dunsmuir S, Curry V. CBT with children, young people and families. London: Sage; 2013.

Gerhardt S. Why love matters: how affection shapes a baby's brain. 2nd ed. London: Routledge; 2015.

Isobel S, Delgado C. Safe and collaborative communication skills: a step towards mental health nurses implementing trauma informed care. Arch Psychiatr Nurs. 2018;32(2):291–6.

Kezelman C, Stavropoulos P. Talking about trauma: guide to conversations and screening for health and other service providers. Sydney: Blue Knot Foundation; 2018. Available from: https://blueknot.org.au/product/talking-about-trauma-guide-to-conversations-and-screening-for-health-and-other-service-providers-digital-download/. Accessed 22 Oct 2024

Lamb N, Sibbald S, Stirzacker A. Shining lights in dark corners of people's lives: the consensus statement for people with complex mental health difficulties who are diagnosed with a personality disorder. 2018. Available from: https://www.mind.org.uk/media/21163353/consensus-statement-final.pdf. Accessed 22 Oct 2024.

Lemma A. Minding the body: the body in psychoanalysis and beyond. London: Routledge; 2014.

Maercker A, Cloitre M, Bachem R, Schlumpf Y, Khoury B, Hitchcock C, Bohus M. Complex post-traumatic stress disorder. Lancet. 2022;400(10345):60–72. ISSN 0140-6736. https://doi.org/10.1016/S0140-6736(22)00821-2.

McCluskey U, O'Toole M. Transference and countertransference from an attachment perspective: a guide for professional caregivers. London: Routledge; 2019.

McGorry P, Mei C, Dalal N, Alvarez-Jimenez M, Blakemore S-J, Browne V, Dooley B, Hickie IB, Jones P, McDaid D, Mihalopoulos C, Wood SJ, Azzahra El Azzouzi F, Fazio J, Gow E, Hanjabam S, Hayes A, Morris A, Pang E, Paramasivam K, et al. The lancet psychiatry commission on youth mental health. Lancet Psychiatry. 2024;11:731–74.

NHS England. The NHS long term plan. 2019. https://www.longtermplan.nhs.uk/. Accessed 22 Oct 2024.

NICE. Borderline personality disorder: recognition and management. Clinical guideline [CG78]. 2009. Available from: https://www.nice.org.uk/guidance/cg78. Accessed 22 Oct 2024.

NICE. Challenging behaviour and learning disabilities: prevention and interventions for people with learning disabilities whose behaviour challenges. NICE guideline [NG11]. 2015. Available from: https://www.nice.org.uk/guidance/ng11. Accessed 22 Oct 2024.

NICE. Antisocial behaviour and conduct disorders in children and young people: recognition and management. Clinical guideline [CG158]. 2017. Available from: https://www.nice.org.uk/guidance/cg158. Accessed 22 Oct 2024.

Schore AN, Sieff DF. On the same wave-length: how our emotional brain is shaped by human relationships. In: Understanding and healing emotional trauma. Hove: Routledge; 2014. p. 111–36.

The Lancet Psychiatry. Editorial: responding to childhood trauma. Lancet Psychiatry. 2022;9(10):759. https://doi.org/10.1016/S2215-0366(22)00316-9.

Van Wijk-Herbrink MF, Lobbestael J, Bernstein DP, Broers NJ, Roelofs J, Arntz A. The influence of early maladaptive schemas on the causal links between perceived injustice, negative affect, and aggression. Int J Forensic Ment Health. 2021;20(2):133–49.

Winnicott D. The maturational processes and the facilitating environment studies in the theory of emotional development. London: Routledge; 1984.

Trauma-Informed Care

10

Justine Rothwell and Nicola Curran

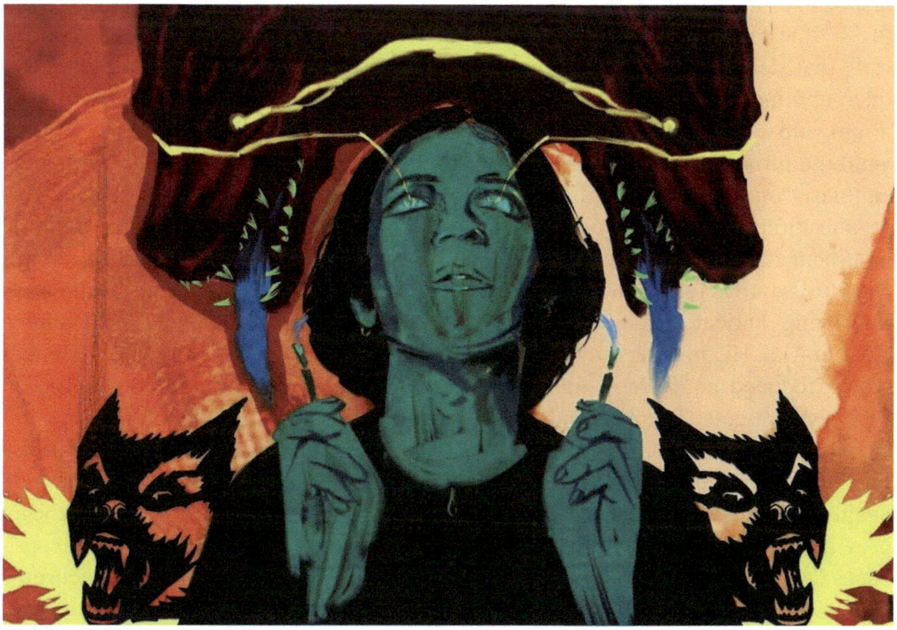

© Robyn Heaslip

J. Rothwell
Meadows Care, Rochdale, UK
e-mail: justinerothwell@meadowscare.co.uk

N. Curran (✉)
Meadows Psychology Service, Rochdale, UK
e-mail: nicolacurran@meadowspsychologyservice.co.uk

G. Trainor, V. Heaslip (eds.), *Needs of Children and Young People Living with Complex Mental Health Difficulties*,
https://doi.org/10.1007/978-3-031-84532-1_10

10.1 Introduction

Trauma-informed care (TIC) is a strategic framework and growing social movement for providing quality of care to survivors of individual, interpersonal, collective and structural trauma (Elisseou 2023). TIC can be broadly described as a move to offer support in a way that incorporates an understanding of the lived experiences of trauma. TIC is based on the understanding that we need to explore how one's life experiences impact their current psychological presentation. It is often described as shifting the focus from 'what is wrong with you' to 'what has happened to you'. In other words, it is moving away from an understanding that locates difficulties within the person (i.e. anxiety as a mental health problem) and places difficulties within the context of their experiences, thus leading to the need to offer support in a way that understands that context and offered by people who are trauma informed and trauma responsive. It recognises we need to have a comprehensive picture of the person's life so that the best intervention can be provided. It also prioritises the wellness of staff that deliver interventions, acknowledging that in order to provide effective interventions, those delivering them need to be regulated, calm and have the ability to empathise and emotionally connect to others. TIC also aims to reduce burnout and high turnover which in turn leads to poor care and increasing costs by placing emphasis on supporting staff well-being. Evidence suggests (Hales et al. 2019) organisations that implement TIC improved engagement, adherence to intervention/treatment and better outcomes. Additionally, implementing TIC can result in significant cost savings for healthcare organisations by reducing healthcare utilisation and improving patient outcomes. For instance, a study conducted by the Camden Coalition of Healthcare Providers demonstrated that implementing TIC practices led to reduced emergency room visits and re-hospitalisations among high-cost, high-risk patients. This, in turn, resulted in substantial cost savings for the healthcare system (Levins 2015). Additionally, research highlights that TIC can optimise outcomes for complex trauma survivors by addressing the root causes of high healthcare utilisation. By focusing on trauma-informed practices (TIPs), healthcare providers can mitigate the long-term health impacts of adverse childhood experiences (ACEs), which are closely linked to increased healthcare costs due to chronic illness and other health issues (Lovell et al. 2022).

TIC and trauma-informed practice (TIP) gradually are being implemented through a broad section or services (mental health, social care, education, justice systems, police and crisis services). There is an increase in recognising, and a greater understanding, of the impact of trauma and the frequency of adverse childhood experiences. 'Trauma informed' is an approach to health and care interventions which is grounded in the understanding that trauma exposure can impact and individuals neurological, biological, psychological and social development. A trauma-informed model of care is highlighted as central to any organisation working with those who have experienced trauma, particularly those working with children and adolescents, and is more increasingly being applied into universal services with a recognition that a large proportion of society will have experienced some form of trauma, and services need to be offered in a way that avoids re-traumatisation.

This chapter will provide an overview of the principles of trauma-informed work and how they are applied, different types of trauma, intersectionality in trauma, signs symptoms and presenting behaviour, intervention approaches and a framework for service delivery including the evidence base, and we will provide a case study to illustrate and example of TIC.

10.2 Definition of Trauma

To set the context and to aid the delivery of weaving TIC into the fabric of the system or organisation, it helps to understand what trauma is and the different types presented. Trauma is a broad and rich topic, and it is beyond the scope of this chapter to provide the depth required for a thorough understanding of the topic. There are many variations and ideas on definitions of trauma and adversity. The most common definition used across the literature has been developed by The National Chid Traumatic Stress Network (Substance Abuse ad Mental Health Services Administration (SAMHSA) 2014):

> Individual trauma results from an event, series of events, or set of circumstances that is experienced by an individual as physically or emotionally harmful or life threatening and that has lasting adverse effects on the individual's functioning and mental, physical, social, emotional, or spiritual well-being.

However, inherent in the definition is the context of the individual and the sense they make of their lived experience. Their perspective on trauma plays a significant role in enhancing understanding and providing an intervention that is tailor-made to meet their individual needs. It has been named the 'Three E's: An event, an experience of the event and the effects' (SAMSHA 2014). It is important here to note the role resilience plays in trauma experience. Resilience studies have found that resilient trauma survivors show specific characteristics (hardness, self-enhancement, optimism) (Zhou et al. 2016) and that resilience can provide a buffering role in the relationship between trauma experience and psychological outcomes. There is also a developing evidence base on the experience of post-traumatic growth, which refers to the enduring positive psychological change that one experiences as a result of adversity, trauma or highly challenging life circumstances (Jayawickreme et al. 2020) leading to identification of ways in which we can support trauma survivors more effectively. It is beyond the scope of this chapter to explore the evidence base on resilience or post-traumatic growth.

Later in the chapter we will discuss cross-sectional perspectives on trauma and how trauma is influenced by wider contexts (cultural, political, etc.). These factors must be considered when thinking about trauma as the definition is not simplistic; it is multi-layered and complex. A word commonly used alongside trauma is that of adversity and adverse childhood experiences (ACEs); these are frequently discussed when considering TIC and will be highlighted in the chapter. When considering the different types of traumas, it is essential to understand the additional perspective of adversity. Likewise, it is important to hold in mind the individual and their unique experience as a concept or label can be reductive and invalidating of their experience and journey (Spence et al. 2019; Straussner and Calan 2014).

10.3 How Prevalent Is Trauma and Adversity?

For an organisation to become more trauma sensitive and trauma informed, it is helpful to highlight how widespread and pervasive the problem is. From the extensive research, evaluations and lived experience accounts, we know there is a wide-ranging occurrence of trauma and adversity. Bessel van der Kolk published his early work on developmental trauma in the mid-1980s which laid the foundation for understanding how early trauma affects brain development and psychological functioning (van der Kolk, The Psychological Consequences of Overwhelming Life Experiences, 1987) following up with an influential paper in 1994 'The Body Keeps the Score: Memory and the Evolving Psychobiology of Posttraumatic Stress' (van der Kolk 1994). In 1998, Felitti et al., published one of the most well-known and impactful study relating to trauma and its effects reporting the association between adversity in childhood and poor outcomes in adulthood (Felitti et al. 1998). It highlighted an adult who experiences a greater number of ACEs was at greater risk of negative health outcomes later in life. Studies in the UK (Bellis et al. 2014) were consistent in their findings that four or more ACEs are strongly associated with both physical and psychosocial problems, mental health, substance use, risk-taking, interpersonal violence and self-harm (Björkenstam et al. 2017; Hughes et al. 2016, 2017). This was echoed in the Dunedin longitudinal studies (Poulton et al. 2015). Many studies acknowledge there is an overrepresentation of those who have experienced trauma and adversity in the looked after and criminal justice system, homeless population and out of education or employment resulting in them being the most vulnerable in society (Buhrich et al. 2000; Sundin and Baguley 2015; Bromley et al. 2015). It is likely these studies are an underestimation due to methodological limitations (self-report questionnaires that are not adequate measures to capture the complexity of the issue and the fact trauma is often hidden, misunderstood and invalidated). Understandably people then underreport or are resistant to sharing their experiences.

It is important to note that while the ACE literature has gained significant attention for its contributions to the understanding and impact of childhood trauma, it also faces several criticisms: that it offers a reductionist perspective; that is has an over-focus on quantitative measures often excluding protective factors; that it can stigmatise and label people; that it offers an oversimplification in policy and practice; and that it presents with ethical concerns related to screening a history of ACEs. We need to keep these criticisms in mind (Kelly-Irving and Delpierre 2019).

There is no question, however, that there are far reaching impacts of trauma and adversity which highlights the need for practice, care and interventions that can reduce the impact of the adverse early life experiences and promote more positive outcomes into adulthood. It is helpful for services to look beyond ACEs and integrate the cross-sectional perspectives; they need to have a deeper understanding and consider and include the wider factors such as poverty, exclusion, oppression and racism (Kelly-Irving and Delpierre 2019). To highlight the unique needs of individuals and to reduce the risk of re-traumatising, organisations and practitioners need to consider and understand the multi-layered complexity of trauma and adversity and respond proactively.

10.4 Different Types of Traumas

It is important to reflect and highlight different types of trauma when organisations are implementing TIC to ensure there is a thorough understanding of the complexities of trauma experiences and the intersectionality of the experiences of trauma (The National Child Traumatic Stress Network (NCTSN)). There could be a whole chapter to describe the different types of traumas, so this is an overview of the most common, and this not a fully comprehensive list nor is it prescriptive.

10.4.1 Single-Event Trauma

This is related to a single, one-off event such as a car accident, sexual assault or burglary. Equally experiencing significant loss can be traumatic, for example, the death of a loved one, miscarriage or suicide (The National Child Traumatic Stress Network (NCTSN)).

10.4.2 Developmental Trauma

This is experienced by being exposed to significant neglect, sexual abuse and or physical abuse in childhood, impacting on critical windows of development. It is likely to have an effect on all the stages of development (brain, physical, cognitive, speech and language, social and emotional, identity, moral and psychosexual) (Hughes et al. 2017; Liming and Grube 2018). It can go on to disrupt personal attachments and compromise relational security which leads to another trauma type.

10.4.3 Relational, Interpersonal, Complex and Attachment Trauma

Those who experience complex and relational trauma can experience a disrupted attachment bond with their primary caregivers. They can then experience interpersonal challenges crucial for psychosocial development. The primary caregiver struggles to hold them in mind as they are too busy surviving this and then interferes with the child developing emotional and behavioural regulation skills, empathy and a difficulty in understanding others' needs and motivations often driven by a lack of trust. Their age-typical pro-social skills necessary to support learning are interrupted, and they have a profound fear and expectation of neglect and abandonment. The strategies they then adopt for survival to confirm safety may not be well understood and can lead to many challenges with relationships in early adulthood. It can lead to difficulties setting boundaries and how you relate and understand yourself, such as problems with self-esteem and a sense of self (Berthelot et al. 2015; Pat-Horenczyk et al. 2017).

10.4.4 Community and Collective Trauma

This occurs when there is exposure in a community to violence that is intentional and interpersonal. As with all the types of traumas, there is a broad and overlapping range that impacts on the different generations in the community (e.g. bullying, youth group violence, civil wars, school shootings, stabbings, bombings and terrorism). Several are woven into the fabric of the community and can be anticipated, but others can happen suddenly without warning, e.g. the experience of a significant event such as a tsunami or civil war and unrest. Many live in communities with high numbers of homicides, sexual assaults and robberies. This can lead to families and children often living in heightened fear.

10.4.5 Abuse and Violence

This describes trauma that can happen throughout the lifespan: childhood, adolescent and adulthood. It includes:

- Neglect and physical, sexual, and emotional abuse.
- Intimate partner violence and relational abuse.
- Financial, online, organisational, system or cultural trauma.
- Criminal and sexual exploitation, trafficking, slavery, honour-based violence and child labour.

10.4.6 Organisational and System Trauma

Organisational trauma examines how an organisation, system or team around the person can re-traumatise the people it is there to help by not understanding trauma, how it presents and how you approach it. This lack of training and understanding for organisations and teams can also lead to traumatising staff and increase burn out; this will be considered closely in this chapter. An example is residential childcare.

If the staff do not understand the whys around the behaviour, their responses can increase shame and trauma for the child. The trauma can be reinforced by the systems themselves. An example is victim blaming/shaming in cases of child sexual exploitation where sometimes the systems, police and court can be trauma inducing and not reducing (Treisman 2024).

10.4.7 Peer Victimisation or Bullying Trauma

This is a premediated and unwelcome action that occurs with the intent of inflicting social, emotional, physical and/or psychological harm to someone who often is perceived as being less powerful (NCTSN 2022). This is typically repeated and prevents someone from continuing their daily life without stress or harassment. It can be in the home, school, community, workplace or online via cyberbullying (texts/messages that are hurtful). The recent Online Safety Act (2023) has recognised the increase in severity of this and has introduced criminal offences.

10.4.8 Traumatic Grief, Loss and Bereavement

Many children and adults experience daily ongoing challenges after the death of a loved one. An individual can experience a traumatic reaction after a death. If this impacts on daily functioning, then the individual is experiencing traumatic grief. Greif is not only in response to the death of a loved one, but there is disenfranchised loss and grief (Treisman 2024).

10.4.9 Intergenerational Trauma

This can also be referred to as transgenerational, multigenerational or inherited trauma. Individuals experiencing this trauma experience symptoms, reactions, patterns, coping styles and cycles experienced by previous generations and are not limited to parents and grandparents. Fraiberg et al. (1975) described the psychological, emotional and social 'chains of pain', unresolved trauma and loss. It could occur if a parent experienced ACEs and then the cycle of their trauma impacts on their parenting. It can include racial trauma where the result of oppression or systemic oppression impacts on the individual and community. In addition to the cycles and patterns of emotional and psychological experiences passed down is the biology. Epigenetics describes how your behaviours and environment can cause changes that affect how your genes work. These changes can appear across both physical and psychological aspects of health, for example impacting the digestive system alongside psychological impacts such as depression and anxiety (Treisman 2024).

Reflective Questions

- Why is it important to consider the different types of traumas?
- This list was not exhaustive. Are there other traumas you would consider?
- What is your understanding of the other types of traumas and how would this inform your practice?
- Which trauma do you work with most, and are there some not as acknowledged?
- How does your understanding of trauma impact the services you deliver?

10.5 Intersectionality in Trauma: Understanding the Complexity of Experiences

As discussed, trauma is a multifaceted phenomenon that can manifest in various forms, ranging from individualised experiences to collective community traumas. However, it is crucial to recognise that these different types of trauma often intersect, intertwining with various aspects of an individual's identity and social context. This concept is known as intersectionality (Collins and Bilge 2016) (see Chap. 7). Intersectionality acknowledges that individuals hold multiple social identities, such as race, gender, sexuality, socioeconomic status and ability that intersect and interact to shape their experiences and vulnerabilities. When examining trauma through an intersectional lens, it becomes evident that no single aspect of identity exists in isolation; rather, these identities intersect to influence the nature and impact of traumatic events. For example, consider the experience of bereavement. While the loss of a loved one is inherently traumatic, the grief experienced by an individual may be compounded by other intersecting factors. A person's cultural background, religious beliefs, socio-economic status and familial support network can significantly shape their experience of bereavement and grief. Furthermore, systemic inequalities and social injustices may exacerbate the trauma, particularly for marginalised communities who may face additional barriers to accessing support and resources (Lee and Hughes 2021; Brown and Green 2020).

Similarly, developmental trauma, which stems from adverse childhood experiences, can intersect with various factors such as family dynamics, socio-economic status and community environment. Children growing up in marginalised communities or in households affected by poverty, substance abuse or violence may be at heightened risk of experiencing developmental trauma. Moreover, intersecting identities such as race and ethnicity can influence the availability and effectiveness of interventions and support systems for these children. Furthermore, single-event traumas, such as accidents or assaults, are not experienced in a vacuum; they occur within broader social contexts that can exacerbate or mitigate their impact. For instance, an individual's gender identity may intersect with their experiences of sexual assault, influencing their likelihood of seeking help, the societal response to their trauma and the availability of culturally competent support services.

By recognising the intersectionality of trauma, organisations and professionals within them can adopt a more holistic and inclusive approach to support those who access services. It is essential to acknowledge the diverse identities and experiences of individuals affected by trauma and to address the intersecting factors that shape their recovery journey. Only by addressing the complex interplay of social, cultural and structural factors can we provide a comprehensive and effective support to those who have experienced trauma. By embracing an intersectional perspective, we can work towards creating more inclusive and equitable systems of support for all individuals affected by trauma (Sokoloff and Dupont 2017; Crenshaw and Wane 2019).

10.6 Signs, Symptoms and Presenting Behaviour

Understanding the signs, symptoms and behaviours associated with trauma experiences is crucial for recognising and responding to trauma-related issues effectively. Trauma can manifest in various ways, and its effects will differ depending on individual experiences and coping mechanisms. Here are some broad common signs and symptoms associated with trauma.

- Emotional dysregulation
- Flashbacks and intrusive memories
- Avoidance behaviours
- Hyper- or hypo-arousal
- Physical symptoms
- Social withdrawal
- Cognitive distortions
- Maladaptive coping strategies

10.7 Trauma-Informed Care

As discussed, TIC is a framework that emphasises on understanding and responding to the impact of trauma on individuals' lives. At its core are the four Rs developed by SAMSHA (2014):

- Realisation—understanding trauma and how it can impact people
- Recognition—being able to recognise the signs and symptoms of trauma experience
- Response—having a system which can respond and offer effective interventions for those who have experience trauma
- Resisting re-traumatisation—ensuring that an organisation is set up in a way that does not re-traumatise those who access support or those who deliver support

Operationally, embedding trauma-informed care and practice is complex and requires a whole system to support this process. Trauma-informed care is not just about the way of working with children, young people and anyone who uses services, rather it is a whole organisation approach that may require cultural, structural and process change at every level and department. It is as much about how those who are employed in an organisation experience TIC as well as those who use the service (Treisman 2024). Embedding TIC approaches requires working in a relational way, centring relationships at the heart and centre of organisations. Karen Treisman (2024) noted:

> we are relational creatures, and each person comes into the work with their own relational and attachment history, life experiences, ghosts, and angels of the past and these will colour, and shape our lens, our responses, our values, and our team role.

This is particularly true in services working to support care-experienced children where there is a high percentage of those in caring industries having early experiences of trauma (Whitfield et al. 2003). We also know that trauma travels through systems, so traumatised children can have a significant impact on those who support them, who if they are trauma informed might not understand the impact the work is having, leading to challenges in management and so on. TIC is about making explicit how trauma impacts systems.

Using the 4 Rs can be a helpful way to think about embedding TIC

- Realisation
  The NICE guidelines (NICE 2015) recognise the impact of trauma on children in care and the need for trauma-informed training, providing practitioners working with children in care a greater understanding of developmental trauma and behaviour as a trauma response and a form of communication and for them to be able to recognise trauma responses and have a deeper understanding of attachment and loss to help them strengthen connection and provide relational security. NICE recognises self-care for carers and professionals in the system is central to prevent burnout and high staff turnover in all organisations. This is not done through a singular training, rather this is an ongoing programme and provides opportunities for learning in the organisation, offering reflective practice and ensuring the opportunities are there for people to consider and think about the impact of trauma.
- Response
  The idea that 'every interaction can be an intervention' is useful to keep in mind when working to embed TIC. Effective evidence-based interventions to support those who have experienced trauma are key but so are having an approach that focuses on improving relationships and connections. If we can foster an ethos of curiosity, reflectiveness, empathy and compassion, we can ensure that every interaction within an organisation can support people to feel safe, heard, validated and understood, whether employees or service users (Bryson et al. 2017).
- Recognise
  Recognise the signs and symptoms of trauma in children, staff and the whole system.

- Resisting re-traumatisation
  TIC recognises the impact of trauma on a child and young person's day-to-day living and the need for trauma-aware staff who can provide safe containment and reduce the likelihood of re-traumatisation (Cannon et al. 2020). Emphasis is on the importance of staff well-being. The old adage 'you can't pour from an empty cup' is key in ensuring that those who look after some of the most vulnerable children and young people are well supported and regulated, able to emotionally connect and empathise with those who have experienced significant trauma.

Organisations providing TIC need to create a safe space, empower service user involvement and voice, identify trauma-related needs at individual and systemic levels, nurture a culture of well-being and resilience for individuals and the organisation as a whole and work with a 'whole systems' approach, supporting cross-agency collaboration and integrated communication (Dermody et al. 2018; Wilson et al. 2013).

Effective trauma-informed care faces several barriers, hindering its full integration into various systems and practices. Some of the key barriers include limited understanding and awareness, resource constraints, resistance to change, misconceptions about TIC, inadequate training and education, systemic inequalities and measurement and evaluation challenges. Particularly to care-experienced children, coordinating care between health, social care and education can impact on the delivery of TIC/TIP. Manging these wider systems and holding the complex needs of children and young people in mind while considering the needs of a staff team can be a challenge (Robinson and Brown 2016). It is often reported that working with such complexity and balancing competing demands of the social economic climate are a strain on resources and can lead to gaps in providing a high standard of trauma-informed care. Many practitioners attend trauma-informed training but due to high caseloads and complex cases do not have the time or capacity to deliver the model (Hummer et al. 2010).

10.8 The Evidence Base

There is a real gap in the literature around effectiveness and evidence-based interventions in these settings. Measuring what works and the different models of care for children and young people across all services and settings is problematic. Recently there has been a review of some intervention approaches (Clarke 2011; Macdonald et al. 2012). However, there is a lack of larger-scale, robust research and longitudinal controlled studies. A paucity of standardised sensitive measures within this group is also challenging when implementing research design. This results in a poor understanding of the mechanisms of change, and all this contributes to not being able to make any meaningful comparisons between the different models of care presented in the literature. There is some evidence of good practice and promising findings, but it has been acknowledged that further practice base evidence is required through more rigorous and robust research. The difficulties in design and delivery of research in these settings seems to reflect the complexity of the children within these services. (Roberts et al. 2016). In Australia a study emphasised it was important there was trust and safety central to the care experienced. However, it was acknowledged there are many unavoidable inconsistencies and unpredictabilities in residential care (hight staff attrition and shift patterns) (Moore et al. 2018).

There are several models of care and flexible frameworks that can support practitioners working with children and young people who experience developmental and relational trauma, such as attachment, regulation and competency (Blaustein and Kinniburgh 2018), sanctuary model of care (Bloom and Yanosy 2008) and CARE (Holden et al. 2010), though this list is not exhaustive. The foundations of all these models are grounded in attachment-based theories and practice and an understanding of developmental and relational trauma and focus on developing emotional connection, emotional warmth and safety in the child-caregiver relationship. These models allow practitioners to adapt and continue to use their valuable experience and skills already embedded in their organisations. The evidence-based interventions recommended complimenting and integrating well within these models of care (e.g. dyadic developmental psychotherapy (DDP), dialectical behaviour therapy (DBT) and eye movement desensitisation reprocessing (EMDR)) and using playfulness, acceptance, curiosity, empathy (PACE) approaches. The models described are continuously developing and evolving to keep up with the ever-growing knowledge base and understanding of trauma.

Here we will elaborate on the ARC model of trauma-informed therapeutic care.

10.9 Attachment, Regulation and Competency (ARC) Model of Care (Blaustein and Kinniburgh 2018)

The ARC framework is grounded in trauma, attachment and child development theories: a flexible, components-based intervention developed for children and adolescents who have experienced complex trauma, along with their caregiving systems. Implementation has been in several varied settings in the USA and the UK (residential, community, group and inpatient). The focus is on the flexibility of the social systems and contextual frameworks. The ARC model recognises the complexity and need for individualised and tailored approach and an understanding that 'one size does not fit all'. All trauma models focus on developing safety in the child-caregiver relationship. ARC's foundation is built upon four key areas of study: normative childhood development, traumatic stress, attachment and risk and resilience. Drawing from these areas, ARC identifies important childhood skills and competencies which are routinely shown to be negatively affected by traumatic stress and by attachment disruptions and which when addressed predict resilient and positive outcomes. A wide range of therapeutic modalities fits within and compliments the framework, e.g. DDP and PACE, psychodynamic, systemic family therapy, sensory and body-based strategies, cognitive behavioural therapy and EMDR (Table 10.1).

Table 10.1 Case study of Ashley

Case Study: A Trauma-Informed Lens on Child Sexual Exploitation

Child sexual exploitation (CSE) and human trafficking are when victims are taken advantage of for someone else's gain (DfE 2017). Adults and children from diverse populations, all ages and genders are vulnerable to exploitation in multiple ways. Those exposed to adverse childhood experiences have increased vulnerabilities to exploitation for a whole range of reasons (connection, inclusion and a sense of belonging, promises of financial security and a better life)

When working with the victims of CSE, it is important that the professionals involved all have a solid understanding of trauma. It is believed if professionals have a deeper understanding of trauma, then they can provide a more empathic, compassionate and non-judgemental approach to children and young people who are sexually exploited or trafficked

Trauma-informed care is based on safety, trust, choice, collaboration and time invested in connecting with the young person. Providing relational security and safety aims to disrupt the exploitation and promote disclosures. The attuned, responsive and nurturing relationships are the intervention itself

Meet Ashley. She is 15 Years Old

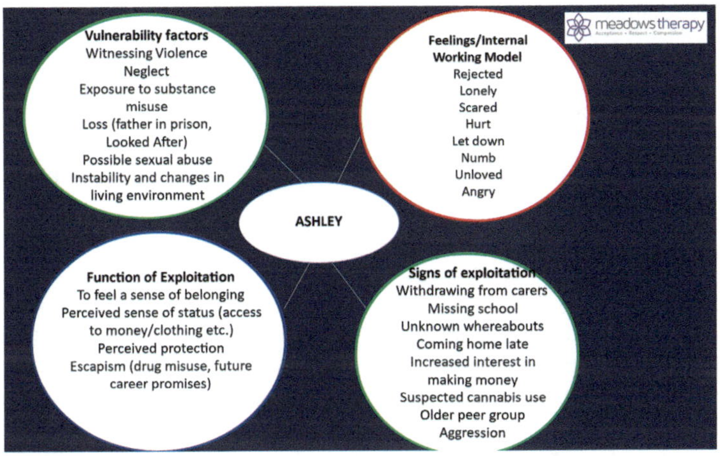

Trauma-Informed Approach

Central to disrupting this exploitation is providing relational security for Ashley, offering her responsive and nurturing care and connecting with her so she wants to be at her current home. The registered manager and her team of support workers are skilled at risk management to help keep her safe. There is an individualised safety plan, developed in collaboration with Ashley, so she has coping skills she can use when she has the urge to go missing and gravitate to risky relationships. The team is attuned to her needs and will offer positive activities and distractions to reduce the opportunities of her leaving the home. Constantly her free time is negotiated, and Ashley is given a sense of agency and control over this and over other aspects of her life when appropriate. For Ashley a pull to going missing, increasing her vulnerabilities, is feel controlled by the limited setting in residential care. Her care team uses their relationships to have these conversations and increase the positive connection. When Ashley goes missing, they follow the risk assessment that has been agreed in the multi-agency meetings with the team of professionals involved in her care, e.g. the residential home, therapist, school, police from complex safeguarding, substance misuse worker and any other professionals around her. Her mother will be invited to these meetings as inclusion of the family is important as they can be key to help disrupt the exploitation

Her care team and the police will be aware of locations she may be residing at and will be proactive at trying to find her. The police work collaboratively sharing current intelligence and knowledge of the local areas. On her return her team is sensitive to her needs. No matter what the time of night, they are available to pick her up, and they offer a compassionate approach, settling her with favourite foods and providing her with comforts agreed on her safety plan. They will use their relationship to explore the locations she has been frequenting and sensitively encourage her to attend the sexual abuse referral centre (SARC). Ashley will have been informed of the return home procedures, so she is aware of what to expect. Education will reach out and encourage her to attend school; they also have a sound understanding of her formulation and will use their relationships to encourage attendance as large gaps of free time and school exclusion are a risk factor for exploitation

A strategy meeting will be held if there are three or more missing or a significant incident occurs. In this meeting all professionals will attend, and it is led by the police to ensure everything has been implemented to keep Ashley safe. The risk assessments and safety plans are reviewed, intelligence discussed and how the exploitation can be disrupted always using a trauma-informed approach and holding Ashely and her formulation in mind

https://www.gov.uk/government/publications/child-sexual-exploitation-definition-and-guide-for-practitioners

Case Study and Infographic: Meadows Psychology Service

10.10 Putting Theory into Practice: Actionable Steps for Trauma-Informed Care

This final section provides some practical guidance for parents, carers and professionals who are supporting children and young people impacted by trauma. Recognising the critical role that caregivers and professionals play in the healing journey, we offer strategies to prioritise safety, build trusting relationships and promote resilience. By empowering both caregivers and professionals with practical tools and insights, we aim to foster environments that nurture healing, growth and well-being for trauma-impacted individuals.

Prioritise Safety and Stability

- Create a safe and predictable environment for children and young people.
- Establish consistent routines and boundaries to provide a sense of stability and security.
- Ensure access to safe spaces where children can express their emotions and feel supported.

Build Trusting Relationships

- Foster trusting and supportive relationships with children and young people based on empathy, respect and understanding.
- Listen actively to their experiences and validate feelings without judgement or criticism.
- Be patient and consistent in your interactions, demonstrating reliability and dependability.

Promote Healing and Resilience

- Provide access to support services tailored to the individual needs of children and young people.
- Encourage the use of coping strategies and self-care techniques to manage stress and regulate emotions.
- Empower children and young people to identify their strengths and resources, fostering a sense of agency and resilience.

For Parents and Caregivers

- Create a nurturing and supportive home environment that prioritises emotional safety and open communication.
- Educate yourself about trauma and its effects on children's development, seeking guidance from professionals as required.
- Practice self-care and seek support for you own well-being to better support your child's healing journey.

For Professionals

- Advocate for trauma-informed policies and practices within your organisations or community, emphasising the importance of prevention, early intervention and holistic support.
- Collaborate with community resources to ensure comprehensive and coordinated care for children and young people affected by trauma.
- Invest in ongoing training and professional development in trauma-informed approaches, staying informed about emerging research and best practice.

We would like to end with 'every interaction is an intervention' (Treisman 2024). If we can pass on one piece of advice, it would be this. To keep in mind that every interaction with someone who has experienced trauma can be healing, by engaging with people from a position of acceptance and empathy, we can offer someone a different relational experience than they may have had previously. The smallest interaction can be meaningful to a person.

References

Bellis MA, Hughes K, Leckenby N, Perkins C, Lowey H. National household survey of adverse childhood experiences and their relationship with resilience to health-harming behaviors in England. BMC Med. 2014;12(1). https://doi.org/10.1186/1741-7015-12-72.

Berthelot N, Ensink K, Bernazzani O, Normandin L, Luyten P, Fonagy P. Intergenerational transmission of attachment in abused and neglected mothers: the role of trauma-specific reflective functioning. Infant Ment Health J. 2015;36:200. https://doi.org/10.1002/imhj.21499.

Björkenstam C, Kosidou K, Björkenstam E. Childhood adversity and risk of suicide: cohort study of 548 721 adolescents and young adults in Sweden. BMJ. 2017:j1334. https://doi.org/10.1136/bmj.j1334.

Blaustein M, Kinniburgh K. Treating traumatic stress in children and adolescents: how to foster resilience through attachment, self-regulation, and competency. 2nd ed. New York: Guilford Press; 2018. https://doi.org/10.1007/978-3-319-46138-0_14.

Bloom SL, Yanosy S. The sanctuary model of trauma-informed organizational change. Reclaiming Child Youth. 2008;17(3):48. Available at: ProQuest One Academic

Bromley E, Mikesell L, Jones F, Khodyakov D. From subject to participant: ethics and the evolving role of community in health research. Am J Public Health. 2015;105(5):900(8). https://doi.org/10.2105/AJPH.2014.302403. (Accessed 4th May 2024)

Brown A, Green C. Grief, intersectionality, and marginalized identities: understanding the complexities of loss. Death Stud. 2020;44(7):438–54. https://doi.org/10.31887/DCNS.2012.14.2. PMID: 22754284; PMCID: PMC3384440

Bryson SA, Gauvin E, Jamieson A, Rathgeber M. What are effective strategies for implementing a trauma-informed care? A review of the literature. Can J Commun Ment Health. 2017;36(2):37–60. https://doi.org/10.7870/cjcmh-2017-002.

Buhrich N, Hodder T, Teesson M. Lifetime prevalence of trauma among homeless people in Sydney. Aust N Z J Psychiatry. 2000;34(6):963–6. https://doi.org/10.1080/000486700270.

Cannon LM, Coolidge EM, LeGierse J, Moskowitz Y, Buckley C, Chapin E, Warren M, Kuzma EK. 'Trauma-informed education: Creating and pilot testing a nursing curriculum on trauma-informed care', Nurse Education Today. 2020;85:104256. Available at: https://doi.org/10.1016/j.nedt.2019.104256. (Accessed: 15th April 2024).

Clarke A. 'Three therapeutic residential care models: The Sanctuary Model, Positive Peer Culture and Dyadic Developmental Psychotherapy and their application to the theory of congruence', Children Australia, 2011;36(2):81–7. Available at: https://doi.org/10.1375/jcas.36.2.81. (Accessed: 15th April 2024).

Collins P, Bilge S. Intersectionality. 2nd ed. Cambridge: Polity Press; 2016.

Crenshaw K, Wane N. The role of intersectionality in trauma-informed care: enhancing inclusivity and equity in support services. J Trauma Dissociation. 2019;20(2):115–34. https://doi.org/10.1186/s12913-017-2463-1. PMID: 28784138; PMCID: PMC5547533

Department for Education. Children looked after in England (including adoption), year ending 31 March 2017. [online] Available at: https://assets.publishing.service.gov.uk/government/uploads/system/uploads/attachment_data/file/664995/SFR50_2017-Children_looked_after_in_England.pdf. (Accessed: 15th 2024).

Dermody A, Gardner C, Davis S, Lambert S, Dermody J, Fein M. 'Resilience in the face of trauma: Implications for service delivery', Irish Probation Journal. 2018;15:161–78.

Elisseou S. 'Trauma-informed care: A missing link in addressing burnout', Journal of Healthcare Leadership, 2023;15:169–73. Available at: https://doi.org/10.2147/JHL.S389271. (Accessed May 2024)

Felitti V, Anda R, Nordenberg D, Williamson D, Spitz A, Edwards V, Marks J. Relationship of childhood abuse and household dysfunction to many of the leading causes of death in adults: The Adverse Childhood Experiences (ACE) Study. Am J Prev Med. 1998;14(4):245–58. https://doi.org/10.1016/s0749-3797(98)00017-8.

Fraiberg S, Adelson E, Shapiro V. Ghosts in the nursery. A psychoanalytic approach to the problems of impaired infant-mother relationships. J Am Acad Child Adolesc Psychiatry. 1975;14(3):387–421. https://doi.org/10.1016/s0002-7138(09)61442-4.

Hales T, Green S, Bissonette S, Warden A, Diebold J, Koury S, Nochajski T. Trauma-Informed Care Outcome Study. Res Soc Work Pract. 2019:529–39. https://doi.org/10.1177/1049731518766618.

Holden MJ, Izzo C, Nunno M, Smith EG, Endres T, Holden JC, Kuhn F. Children and residential experiences: a comprehensive strategy for implementing a research-informed program model for residential care. Child Welfare. 2010;89(2):131–49.

Hughes K, Bellis MA, Hardcastle KA, et al. Relationships between adverse childhood experiences and adult mental well-being: results from an English national household survey. BMC Public Health. 2016;16(1). https://doi.org/10.1186/s12889-016-2906-3.

Hughes K, Ford K, Williams W, et al. The effect of multiple adverse childhood experiences on health: a systematic review and meta-analysis. Lancet Public Health. 2017;2(8):e356–66. https://doi.org/10.1016/s2468-2667(17)30118-4.

Hummer VL, Dollard N, Robst J, Armstrong MI. Innovations in implementation of trauma-informed care practices in youth residential treatment: a curriculum for organizational change. Child Welfare. 2010;89(2):79–95. PMID: 20857881

Jayawickreme E, Infurna F, Alajak K, Blackei L, Chopik W, Chung J, Park C. Post-traumatic growth as positive personality change: challenges, opportunities and recommendations. J Pers. 2020:145–65. PMID: 32897574; PMCID: PMC8062071

Kelly-Irving M, Delpierre C. A critique of the adverse childhood experiences framework in epidemiology and public health: uses and misuses. Soc Policy Soc. 2019;18(3):445–56. https://doi.org/10.1017/s1474746419000101.

Lee J, Hughes D. The intersections of grief: socioeconomic status, cultural, and familial factors. J Soc Pers Relat. 2021;38(3):456–73.

Levins H. The cost saving potential of trauma-informed primary care. Penn LDI, Leonard Davis Institute of Health Economics; 2015. Available at: https://ldi.upenn.edu/our-work/research-updates/the-cost-saving-potential-of-trauma-informed-primary-care/. Accessed 4th May 2024

Liming KW, Grube WA. Wellbeing outcomes for children exposed to multiple adverse experiences in early childhood: a systematic review. Child Adolesc Soc Work J. 2018;35(4):317–35. https://doi.org/10.1007/s10560-018-0532-x.

Lovell R, Greenfield D, Johnson G, Eljiz K, Amanatidis S. Optimising outcomes for complex trauma survivors: assessing the motivators, barriers and enablers for implementing trauma-informed practice within a multidisciplinary health setting. BMC Health Serv Res. 2022; https://doi.org/10.1186/s12913-022-07812-x.

Macdonald G, Millen S, McCann M, Roscoe H, Ewart-Boyle S. Therapeutic approaches to social work in residential child care settings, London. 2012. Available at: https://www.scie.org.uk. Accessed: May 2024.

Moore T, McArthur M, Death J, Tilbury C, Roche S. Sticking with us through it all: the importance of trustworthy relationships for children and young people in residential care. Child Youth Serv Rev. 2018;84:68–75. Available at:. https://doi.org/10.1016/j.childyouth.2017.10.043.

National Child Traumatic Stress Network. Trauma types. 2022. Available at: www.nctsn.org/what-is-child-trauma/trauma-types. Accessed: 12 June 2024.

National Institute for Health and Care Excellence. Children's attachment: attachment in children and young people who are adopted from care, in care or at high risk of going into care. NICE guideline NG26. 2015. Available at: https://www.nice.org.uk/guidance/ng26. Accessed: 22 May 2024.

Online Safety Act. UK Parliament. 2023. 27 October 2023. Retrieved 30 April 2024. https://www.legislation.gov.uk/ukpga/2023/50

Pat-Horenczyk R, Cohen S, Ziv Y, Achituv M, Brickman S, Blanchard T, Brom D. Stability and change in posttraumatic distress: a 7-year follow-up study of mothers and young children exposed to cumulative trauma. J Trauma Stress. 2017;30(3):1–10. https://doi.org/10.1002/jts.22177.

Poulton R, Moffitt TE, Silva PA. The Dunedin Multidisciplinary Health and Development Study: overview of the first 40 years, with an eye to the future. Soc Psychiatry Psychiatr Epidemiol. 2015;50(5):679–93. https://doi.org/10.1007/s00127-015-1048-8. Epub 2015 Apr 3. PMID: 25835958; PMCID: PMC4412685

Roberts L, et al. Improving well-being and outcomes for looked after children in Wales: a context sensitive review of interventions. Adoption Fostering. 2016;40(4):309–24. https://doi.org/10.1177/0308575916675563.

Robinson LR, Brown A. Coordinating care for children with complex health needs in the context of trauma. Pediatr Clin N Am. 2016;63(1):135–50. https://doi.org/10.1016/j.pcl.2015.09.012.

Sokoloff N, Dupont I. Intersectionality and trauma: addressing complex needs in mental health services. Traumatology. 2017;23(3):277–85. https://doi.org/10.1192/bja.2018.29. PMID: 30174829; PMCID: PMC6088388

Spence R, Kagan L, Bifulco A. A contextual approach to trauma experience: lessons from life events research. Psychol Med. 2019;49(9):1409–13.

Straussner S, Calan A. Trauma through the life cycle: a review of current literature. Clin Soc Work J. 2014;42(4):323–35. https://doi.org/10.1007/s10615-014-0496-z.

Substance Abuse and Mental Health Services Administration (SAMHSA). Trauma-informed care in behavioural health services, Treatment Improvement Protocol (TIP). Rockville: SAMHSA; 2014.

Sundin EC, Baguley T. Prevalence of childhood abuse among people who are homeless in Western countries: a systematic review and meta-analysis. Soc Psychiatry Psychiatr Epidemiol. 2015;50(2):183–94. https://doi.org/10.1007/s00127-014-0937-6.

Treisman K. Trauma informed healthcare: a reflective guide to improving care and services. London: Jessica Kingsley Publishers; 2024.

van der Kolk B. The psychological consequences of overwhelming life experiences. In: Psychological Trauma; 1987. p. 1–30. https://doi.org/10.1176/appi.books.9781615376520.lg01.

van der Kolk BA. The body keeps the score: memory and the evolving psychobiology of posttraumatic stress. Harv Rev Psychiatry. 1994;1(5):253–65.

Whitfield CL, Felitti VJ, Anda RF, Dube SR. The enduring effects of abuse and related adverse experiences in childhood: a convergence of evidence from neurobiology and epidemiology. Eur Arch Psychiatry Clin Neurosci. 2003;253(6):381–91. https://doi.org/10.1007/s00406-003-0440-8.

Wilson C, Pence DM, Conradi L. Trauma-informed care. In: Courtois CA, Ford JD, editors. Treating complex traumatic stress disorders in children and adolescents: scientific foundations and therapeutic models. New York: The Guilford Press; 2013. p. 124–42.

Zhou X, Wu X, An Y. Understanding the relationship between trauma exposure and depression among adolescents after earthquake: the roles of fear and resilience. Front Psychol. 2016;7(204) Viewed 30 June 2024, https://www.frontiersin.org/journals/psychology

Assessing, Formulating, and Responding to Mental Health-Related Risks

11

Andrew Sweetmore and Shelley O'Connor

A. Sweetmore (✉)
Department of Nursing Science, Bournemouth University, Bournemouth, UK
e-mail: asweetmore@bournemouth.ac.uk

S. O'Connor
Department of Nursing and Advanced Practice, Liverpool John Moores University, Liverpool, UK
e-mail: S.B.OConnor@ljmu.ac.uk

G. Trainor, V. Heaslip (eds.), *Needs of Children and Young People Living with Complex Mental Health Difficulties*,
https://doi.org/10.1007/978-3-031-84532-1_11

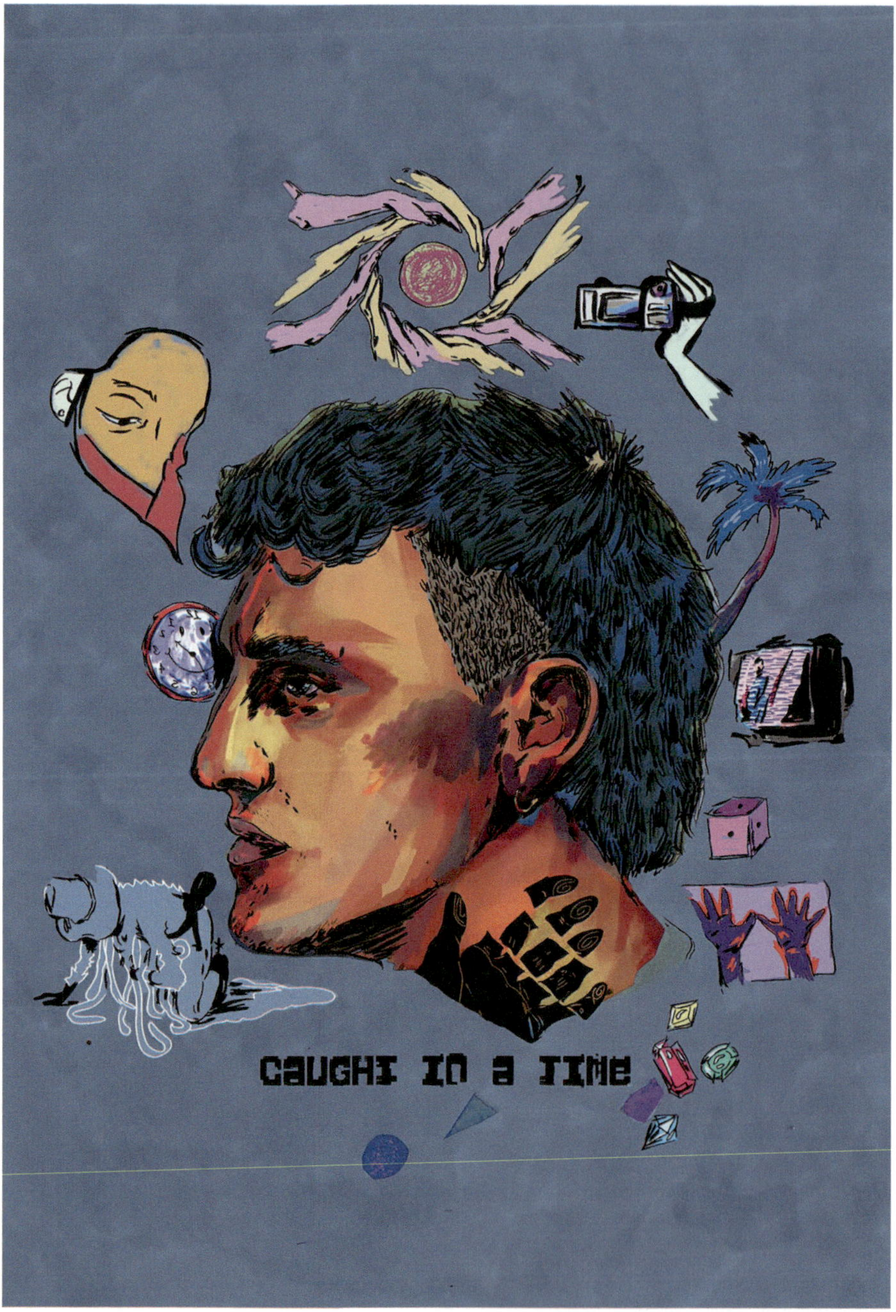

© **Robybn Heaslip**

11.1 Introduction

The occurrence of mental health issues among children and young people (CYP) is on the rise, with estimates suggesting that one in five individuals aged 8–25 years exhibits symptoms indicative of probable mental disorders, such as anxiety, low mood, and self-harm (Xiao et al. 2022). Given this significant prevalence, mental health is now a public health priority, necessitating a comprehensive and immediate response not only from specialised mental health services but from all organisations that work or interact with CYP (Harris et al. 2022).

Whilst many mental health problems begin in adolescence, they can develop much earlier in childhood and are even seen in preschool children. Despite this, the majority of conditions are not diagnosed until adulthood, which can delay effective intervention and potentially lead to the development of worsening mental health (Wlodarczyk et al. 2017). This can have a wide-ranging consequence, negatively affecting their general health and educational attainment and also lead to significant impairments later on in life, such as underemployment and relationship difficulties (NSPCC 2024).

A dynamic interplay of risk and protective factors influences and determines a child's mental health, which, if identified, can be modified to potentially mitigate adverse outcomes. These determinants are a combination of factors which include the individual, their environment, their relationships, and wider societal context (Savolainen et al. 2023). Consequently, it is important for all professionals who work with or interact with children to be aware of the risk and protective factors, as this awareness is crucial for timely intervention and support, which can significantly mitigate potential adverse effects on the child's mental health, now and in the future (DHSC 2024).

Recognising that the mental health of a child is largely determined by the presence or absence of protective and risk factors, this chapter acknowledges that risk assessment is not an exact science which can accurately predict what may occur but a continually evolving practice that requires adaptability, curiosity, and a relationship with the young person, however short that may be in the context of a professional interaction. Consequently, central to the discussion is the prioritisation of the young person's perspective in all decision-making processes concerning their well-being, advocating for strategies that not only reduce disparities in childhood but also sustain any protective factors. This approach asserts that all services should prioritise maintaining these protective factors as part of their role working with children.

11.2 Assessing Mental Health-Related Risks

To understand how best to support CYP, we need to look at the prevalence of mental health difficulty among CYPs. As described in other chapters, CYPs in England alone represent a third of the population, and improving their health and well-being is viewed as a national priority, with a recent report into the mental health of CYP in England identifying a rise in mental health-related disorders between 2017 and 2023 (Children's Commissioner 2024; Newlove-Delgado et al. 2023) (see Table 11.1).

Table 11.1 Mental health of CYP in England, between 2017 and 2023 (based on Newlove-Delgado et al. 2023)

Variables	Age of CYP 8–16 years old	Age of CYP 17–19 years old	Age of CYP 17–25 years old	Age of CYP 20–25 years old
Rise in MH disorders	20.3%	23.3%		21.7%
A parent who could not afford outside school activities	26.8%			
CYP not able to afford to socialise or pay for activities			26.1%	
Bullied in person	36.9%			
Bullied online	10.8%			
Worried about impact of climate change			54.8%	
Optimistic about having enough money			Female (38.5%) Male (60.5%)	
Optimistic about their health, mental health, and well-being			Female (51.4%) Male (67.8%)	
Identified eating disorders	2.6% (11–16-year-olds) Female (4.3%) Male (1.0%)	12.5% Female (20.8%) Male (5.1%)		5.9% No differences in gender

The interplay between the determinants of mental health and well-being is inextricably linked (Trainor and O'Connor 2023). Well-being encompasses an individual's thoughts, emotions, and actions and can include the CYP's ability to form relationships with peers, family members, and other members in society, impacting on their education, hobbies, activities, and decision-making, whereas the determinants of mental health can include the CYP's social environment (see Table 11.2) (WHO 2022; Astier 2023). With these two factors at play, the mental state of the CYP may be threatened.

Mental health risks can emerge throughout a child's life. Traumatic events, whether single or prolonged, can disrupt their sense of security and trust, leading to attachment issues in adulthood, such as poor relationships and trust problems (Colizzi et al. 2020). Adverse childhood experiences (ACEs) affect both physical and mental health, potentially causing conditions like cardiovascular disease, cancer, diabetes, anxiety, depression, and PTSD and increasing the risk of experiencing or perpetrating violence (Manchester university NHS Hospitals 2024). Therefore, supporting children and young people (CYPs) requires considering their childhood experiences, family dynamics, caregiver responses, and their interactions with caregivers (Young Minds 2018) (Box 11.1).

Box 11.1: Some CYP At-Risk Groups (Based on SBRI Healthcare 2021)

- Children with a learning disability.
- Children with a physical impairment/illness.
- Children with a mental illness.
- Children with a parent who has a mental illness.
- Looked after children.
- Children as carers.
- Young males in custody.
- Homeless young people.
- Those with low socio-economic status.
- Some Black and minority ethnic groups.
- Those with limited English proficiency and non-English speakers.
- LGBTQ+.
- CYP with difficult temperament, inflexibility, impulsivity, and poor concentration.
- Drug and alcohol users.
- Chemsex users.
- Those being groomed.
- Those with self-harm practices.
- Those with previous suicide attempt.
- Those facing academic pressures.
- Those who are bullied.
- Those who are in bereavement.

Table 11.2 Determinants of mental health (WHO 2022; Astier 2023)

Level	Adverse	Factors	Protective
Individual	Genetic factors: prevalence of mental and physical health problems	⟷	Resilience, health literacy
	Substance use	⟷	Physical health fitness
	Poor communication skills	⟷	Communication skills
	Absent mental health literacy	⟷	Mental health literacy
	Inability to manage stress	⟷	Healthy coping mechanisms
	Experience trauma	⟷	Manage experiences
	Experience/witness violence	⟷	Open dialogue on experience. Avoid learned behaviours
	Rejection due to sexuality	⟷	Healthy stress response
	Absent parent	⟷	Open dialogue on reasons
	Harsh parenting (including physical abuse and bullying)	⟷	Educate and build resilience

(continued)

Table 11.2 (continued)

Level	Adverse	Factors	Protective
Environmental	Poor, unsafe communities	⟷	Safe communities/ community cohesion
	Poor education (including truancy)	⟷	Quality education
	Poor, inadequate living conditions	⟷	Government/local council addresses housing issues
	Poor or negative social networks	⟷	Stronger social networks in person/online
	Economic downturns	⟷	More investment
	Disease outbreak	⟷	Investment in medical science/improvements in public health
	Humanitarian emergencies and forced displacement	⟷	Strengthening systems and resilience and education
	Climate change crisis	⟷	Protect the environment/ understand causes
	Government instability	⟷	Economic stability/ parliamentary democracy
	Discrimination/prejudice	⟷	Educate and enforce legislation

Additional factors contributing to risk include parental factors, peer factors (such as peer rejection) poor academic achievement, and community factors (such as adversity and poverty).

Long waiting times for assessment and treatment, coupled with poor early identification of mental health risks, lead to negative outcomes for children and young people (CYPs). Factors contributing to poor recognition include a lack of knowledge in identifying mental health symptoms, inadequate information sharing, and not using active listening and participation skills with CYPs and their families. Improving risk identification can start in schools and homes and with frontline responders and General Practitioners (GPs). Developing accurate early identification tools and providing education and training on their use can enable timely support for CYPs, potentially reducing the rising trend of mental health crises (Colizzi, et al. 2020; Young Minds 2018). Yet not one size fits all, and responses to mental health risks must be multi-layered and tailored to the individual. Strategies can include early recognition and prevention of childhood traumas, psychosocial development, legislative action to protect the vulnerable and poorer members of society, and promotion of their rights.

The next section of this chapter helps you to identify risk factors, understand, and apply risk assessment and management of CYPs using case formulation examples.

11.3 Formulating an Understanding of Risks

Risk assessment is the systematic gathering and examining of information to identify (potential) risks that may cause someone (or others) harm. In managing these risks, a risk management plan is created to identify a traffic light system of measures (green, amber, red) of low, medium, and high risk, to reduce any likelihood of an untoward event happening. Although it cannot eliminate risk-taking behaviours, it can be used as an early warning indicator to reduce the likelihood of risks and keep CYPs safe. It is important not to just quantify risk but to conduct a thorough psychosocial assessment, as NICE guidance (2020) advises that risk assessment tools should not be used on their own.

11.3.1 What Is Case Formulation?

Following a thorough risk assessment, a case formulation can be drawn up. Case formulation is a case-specific plan that identifies the unique problems, issues, and needs of the CYP, and interventions are tailored to their specific needs, and this is addressed in detail in the chapter on self-harm and elsewhere in the book. One could address the problem through interventions, for example, cognitive behavioural therapy (CBT), family-focused therapy, or pharmacological input if necessary (antidepressants in CYP suffering with moderate to severe depression) (National Institute for Health and Care Research 2020). However, involving CYPs and their families/care givers is crucial in the process of developing a formulation for it to be a success. Risk is a vital part of the formulation, and this can be addressed using the four Ps as indicated below.

- **Predisposing** *(why me?)*
- **Precipitating** *(why now?)*
- **Perpetuating** *(why does it continue?)*
- **Protective factors** *(what can I rely on?)*

This focuses on gathering information, past and present presentations, thus shaping the plan for the CYP (Fig. 11.1).

To support you in case formulation, you could ask the following questions:

1. *Are you able to share your [CYP] experiences with me, so that I can better understand your perspective?*
2. *Can I ask your parent/carer to give their perspectives of what has happened?*

Predisposing	Precipitating	Perpetuating	Protective factors

Fig. 11.1 The four Ps

3. *What do we need to find out more about?*
4. *Tell me, what has worked well in the past that might be helpful to us now?*
5. *What do you want to happen to you and your care?*

11.3.2 Question: What Other Questions Could You Ask? (Table 11.3)

Task 11.1
To highlight the importance of understanding the individual's context, including family, school, and community environments, carefully read through the following case studies, their formulation plans, and survey of historical and current risks and attempt to answer the questions.

Table 11.3 An illustrated example of using the four Ps and the biopsychosocial model (based on Astier 2023)

	Biological	Psychological	Social
Predisposing	Genetic predisposition inherited by parents, challenges during pregnancy and birth, brain injury	Attachment disorders, characteristics that form a person's character, confinement, lack of confidence, overwhelming worry someone will leave you	Abuse and violence in the home, destitution, hardship, instability at home, spousal estrangement
Precipitating	Sleep disturbances, substance dependency	Bereavement and grief, worry, fear of being left alone	School anxiety, loss of companionship, saying goodbye to your home
Perpetuating	Treatment resistant, continued pain and neurological issues	Key features of characteristics and personality, defence mechanism to cope with adverse events, self-reliance, and confidence in others	Stigma in accessing treatment, financial instability
Protective factors	Enough sleep, good diet, genetics, exercise, resilience, emotional intelligence	Showing a deep understanding, how to conduct yourself around others, deal effectively with something difficult	Common characteristics, partnerships, wider support, family, religious beliefs, financial assistance where needed, health services

Case Study 11.1
Daisy (not her real name), an 11-year-old girl, over the summer holidays began using a free online chat website that allowed her to socialise with strangers. The site randomly paired users in one-on-one sessions where they could message anonymously without registering their details. Unfortunately, Daisy was coerced into sending indecent images and videos of herself to males overseas, in return for money. Her mother, Carol, recently discovered the abuse on Daisy's mobile phone and tablet and broke down in tears. Carol blames herself for Daisy's actions. Both Daisy's parents work shifts, her mother works nights, and her father works days, they are both exhausted. Daisy's parents in recent months have had to use food banks just before pay day, due to the cost-of-living crisis. And the community youth club closed the year before, due to no council money being allocated to youth centres. Because of this, Daisy was spending more time indoors and on her tablet and mobile phone. Daisy felt embarrassed by what she had sent but felt trapped and scared fearing she would get into trouble. Carol had thought that she had practised good online safety measures by setting parental controls and limiting time on devices but stated that at times, this was overlooked due to feelings of guilt for not always being around for her children or being too tired to interact with them.

Question *What are your initial thoughts here?*

Before you move onto the formulation and risk assessment plan, write down the key issues you would unpick from Case Study 11.1.

11.3.3 Formulation

- Daisy is an 11-year-old girl with *some vulnerability factors*, which interact to predispose her to her current difficulties.
- Daisy is at risk of sexual and criminal exploitation. Daisy's mother and father were working shift work and had not been able to take Daisy or her siblings on holiday or on family outings. This has had a significant impact on her emotional and mental health development.
- Daisy was suffering from online bullying via a social media platform, for not having fashionable clothing or an expensive mobile phone.
- A lack of adult supervision both online and in the real world has had an impact on Daisy's social, behavioural, communication, and interpersonal functioning.
- Daisy's family are on the poverty line, and Daisy is increasingly vulnerable to criminal gangs, affecting her social and environmental experiences, through online predatory means.

- Daisy did not at first realise she was being exploited, and sending indecent pictures for money seemed like a quick fix for Daisy.

11.3.4 Risks

Daisy is at risk of exploitation, and this could have a lasting effect on her emotional and mental health development. Without support through individual counselling or therapy and family-focused therapy, it is highly likely that this may escalate to family conflict or Daisy developing a mental health problem. Therapy and counselling should be offered to Daisy as a child with experience of online abuse and exploitation, giving her a chance to rebuild her life. Both the police service and social services involvement should also be considered, both short and long term, to support both Daisy and her family.

Question *Would you have approached the formulation and assessment of risks any differently? What questions would you ask Daisy? What questions would you ask Carol?*

Task 11.2
Using the four Ps and the biopsychosocial approach, unpick the case study below and allocate each significant key issue to each box as in Table 11.3.

Case Study 11.2
Bobby, a 13-year-old boy, growing up witnessed regular domestic violence in the household from both his father and mother. He was physically abused himself by both parents, who often stated that he was a burden on them, more so his mother, when his father was sent to prison. Whilst in custody, his father committed suicide by hanging, and this affected Bobby. Subsequently, Bobby's behaviour at school suffered, and after multiple fights with his peers and assaulting a teacher, he was excluded from secondary school. His mother has a diagnosis of borderline personality disorder. She also drinks alcohol daily where she would often drink to excess and forget to pick up Bobby's twin sisters from primary school, which caused issues with the school, and safeguarding referrals were made, resulting in a family social worker to support the family. Since his father's death and expulsion from school, Bobby has been associating with older males around the community where he lives and has been engaging in drug taking and criminal activity. He has adopted a recent fascination with knives and has recently been arrested for carrying a knife. When frustrated Bobby will also wish himself dead and talks about his father's death.

Question *What are your initial thoughts here?*

Before you move onto the formulation and risk assessment plan, write down the key issues you would unpick from Case Study 11.2, and create your own formulation and risk.

11.3.5 Formulation

- Bobby is a 13-year-old boy with *several vulnerability factors*, which interact to predispose him to his current difficulties and presentation.
- Bobby has endured several traumas in his childhood which appear to have had a significant impact on his emotional and mental health development.
- Bobby has significant difficulties coping with the demands in relation to social, behavioural, communication, and interpersonal functioning. This is potentially a result of being exposed to and experiencing significant amounts of domestic violence.
- Bobby has low frustration tolerance and finds it difficult to regulate his emotions. He lacks impulsive control, as seen by the events leading up to his exclusion from school, associating with older males, drug taking, and arrest by the police and further negative social and environmental experiences through witnessing aggression being used to gain control.
- Subsequently, Bobby has learnt how to demand his needs through aggressive behaviours. These inconsistencies in Bobby's life have compounded these problems and appear to have contributed to the unpredictability of his behaviour. As a result, Bobby finds it difficult to engage in friendships with peers in his own age due to his difficulties.
- The main consistent figure in Bobby's life has been his mother. This has resulted in Bobby becoming extremely attached to his mother which can result in violence towards her, physically and verbally when he feels his needs are not being met. Similarly, Bobby will often direct his violence towards his twin sisters to convey his emotional needs at the time.

11.3.6 Risks

Bobby exhibits volatile behaviour that poses a risk to others, manifesting both at home, in school, and in the community. Without multi-agency support and a stable environment, his behaviour is likely to escalate, increasing the risk of further criminal activity and exploitation. Bobby's impulsivity also makes him a danger to himself, as indicated by comments about self-harm. Whilst Bobby has not received a formal diagnosis, concerns persist regarding potential mood disorders or depressive illness, raising fears of self-harm through misadventure or communication of dissatisfaction with his life. Involvement from the youth offending team is necessary to coordinate support from various agencies, including police, probation, schools, and social services, to mitigate Bobby's risk of engaging in criminal behaviour.

Question *Would you have approached the formulation and risk assessment any differently? Can you think of anything that may be supportive to Bobby's plan?*

11.4 Evidence-Based Approaches for Managing Different Types of Risk Factors

The next section of this chapter helps outline evidence-based approaches for managing the different types of risk factors and discusses strategies for enhancing protective factors and resilience, including promoting positive relationships, skill building, and access to resources. It also provides guidelines for crisis management and when to escalate concerns to higher levels of care.

11.5 Responding to Mental Health-Related Risks

Mental health can change over time, and it can be difficult to recognise when a CYP needs support with their mental health issues, especially if the CYP finds it difficult to communicate their issues. It is therefore crucial to recognise the signs and symptoms of [deteriorating] mental health and have the knowledge to appropriately support and/or signpost the CYP to the correct services. Consent should be sought and should include the young person and their families' narratives.

11.5.1 Recognise, Respond, and Know Where to Signpost

How would you distinguish between a mental health issue and deterioration in mental health presentation or a developmental tantrum? Why is the CYP not able to communicate, due to disability or not knowing how to communicate?

Recognise *Identify distress in CYP by noticing mood swings, self-harm, sleep and eating changes, weight fluctuations, exercise extremes, and social withdrawal*	**Respond** *Proactively engage CYP, listen supportively, create safe environments, and promote mental health through shared activities and routines. Avoid arguments*
Signposting *Discuss plans with CYP, follow school policies, involve pastoral support, and inform CYP of necessary escalations to maintain trust*	***Support services*** *Seek GP advice and referrals to CAMHS or counselling services but be aware of potential delays. In emergencies, contact 999 or take CYP to safety immediately*

11.5.2 Safety Management Plan

Where feasible, implementing a safety management plan for identified risks is crucial to mitigate the potential for adverse events. Such plans are cooperative efforts involving the child or young person (CYP), their family or friends, and healthcare professionals and can be effective for a broader audience when properly adhered to.

For instance, in Case Study 11.2 featuring Bobby, who has expressed suicidal thoughts and engaged in self-harm, a safety management plan is pertinent. To aid Bobby, it is necessary to pinpoint and evaluate the issues, engage him with open-ended inquiries about his feelings of anger and frustration, and formulate a supportive strategy. With Bobby's agreement, involve his mother in the plan, setting clear goals and identifying evidence-based interventions. It is also advisable to include professionals from the police, social services, youth offending teams, and educational institutions to coordinate support efforts for Bobby.

Key points to consider when supporting a CYP with a safety management plan: this is described more fully for young people who self-harm in Chap. 2.

1. What information do you already have about the CYP?
2. Ensure you are communicating effectively and actively listening.
3. Develop a rapport and discuss confidentiality, consent, and safeguarding.
4. Explore the factors affecting the CYP and what risks the plan is focussed on, e.g. exploitation.
5. Assess their current mental state and ask them if they are experiencing, e.g. suicidal thoughts, feeling out of control, or wanting to run away.
6. Evaluate all risks, low, medium, and high, and put them in a hierarchy of low to high.
7. Create the safety plan and decide what services will be needed to support them and ensure the CYP and their family are involved in all decisions.
8. Ensure it is written in a child-friendly way.
9. Share, with the young person's consent, with relevant people in their lives who can support them.
10. Consider historical risk-taking and concordance.
11. Is there anything that is likely to occur that would change the risk?
12. Include factors that may stop the young person acting on impulses.

Question *Before reading on, can you identify what the risks are? Write down what you consider to be the risks to be for that young person.*

11.6 Balancing Risk and Protective Factors

There are a variety of factors that impact a child's mental health, and not one single risk or protective factors can be identified that will solely determine the mental health of young people or predict the development of a mental disorder (Wilhelmsen et al. 2023). It is the combined effects of these various determinants which influence the mental well-being of children, and it is a combined approach from professionals, non-professionals, and across professions—balancing the need to mitigate risk against protective and resilience factors—which is required to ensure the health and well-being of the young person (DHSC 2024).

Not all of these factors will significantly impact a child's mental health immediately or have long-term negative effects; indeed, adversities may serve as catalysts for positive motivation in a young person's life (Gartland et al. 2019). It is important not to make assumptions about the potential impacts of these factors on any individual child or to become complacent, as it is often the accumulation of additional risk factors later in life, particularly when combined with those experienced in early childhood, that may precipitate a decline in a person's mental health (DHSC 2024). Conversely, an overly protective approach can also hinder a young person's development by preventing them from acquiring essential life skills, therefore promoting problem-solving skills which can help modify any adverse experiences they may go through subsequently in life. Risk cannot be eliminated but can be assessed, managed, and mitigated.

What is required then is a balanced and genuinely collaborative approach with the young person and their family to understand the various factors that influence their mental health. This will require input from other sources, such as other family members, teachers, or healthcare professionals, as well as the young person, to build a picture of what is occurring in their life (Wright et al. 2013).

11.7 Building Trusting Relationships with Young People

Building a trusting relationship is fundamental to effective risk management, serving as the initial step in engaging the young person. Establishing rapport may occur quickly, but for children who have experienced trauma, trust can be more difficult to build, and in some cases, it may not develop at all (Dianiska et al. 2024). Even if a child is reluctant to engage in a dialogue, this does not preclude the possibility of support. Paramount in these interactions is inquisitiveness and a genuine curiosity about the young person's life and experiences. Establish eye contact and make it clear that you value their opinion. Do not prejudge behaviour or make assumptions. Above all, be honest, explaining the purpose of your meeting with them and how it may help.

Whilst there is no specific formula which can be used to engage a young person and build a rapport with them, there is a broad consensus on what has been shown to be helpful. The manner in which professionals conduct challenging conversations and establish rapport not only influences the success of their interactions but also serves as a role model for young people, demonstrating what a trusting relationship with an adult should entail.

11.8 Case Studies and Practical Examples

11.8.1 Weighing Up the Risk and Protective Factors

Upon establishing a rapport, however tenuous, we then need to identify and contextualise the risk and protective factors that may influence a young person's mental health. This assessment is essential to ascertain that the individual is not in imminent danger nor suffering from acute physical or mental health conditions necessitating urgent intervention. Once it is determined that there is no immediate risk requiring emergency response, we will now need to weigh up these factors in order to inform our decision-making.

Considering the impact of child abuse on a young person's mental health, and their resilience, a safe and supportive home environment and a nurturing relationship with a caregiver capable of ensuring safety emerge as critical protective factors (Gartland et al. 2019). These elements are fundamental in sustaining mental health and bolstering a child's resilience. Indeed, these protective factors can be viewed as primary conditions in the balance between risk and protective factors, providing a crucial foundation for a child's emotional and psychological development.

To assess these primary protective factors, the following inquiries should be considered:

- Do you consider the young person's home environment to be safe and caring?
- Does the young person maintain a trusting and communicative relationship with a caregiver?
- Does the caregiver acknowledge the risks the young person faces, do they take these risks seriously, and are they capable of ensuring the child's safety?
- Does the young person feel safe at home and/or with their primary caregiver?

Discussions with the primary caregiver are essential, and the outcomes of the dialogue between the young person, caregiver, and professional will determine the subsequent actions required, potentially involving further discussions with other agencies such as local authority child safeguarding teams.

Although a young person may possess numerous protective factors, the absence of a safe, caring environment, and a positive relationship with a caregiver can significantly hinder their ability to maintain resilience and mental health. When evaluating these conditions, it is important to avoid making assumptions or judgements based on one's own moral and cultural values, which may differ from those of the young person and their family. This caution is necessary to ensure an unbiased assessment of risks and protective factors.

11.8.2 Does the Young Person Feel Safe?

Insight into the young person's perceptions of their risks and protective factors, and understanding how they perceive their own safety, is critical for robust decision-making, so it is necessary therefore to ask the young person whether they feel safe as they are in that moment and at home and in any other relevant contexts, such as at school or with friends.

Actively listening to and validating the perspectives of young person are essential, yet it is equally important to recognise that they may not always express their true thoughts openly, whether due to circumstance, reluctance, or communication difficulties. Therefore, employing alternative methods of communication, such as written questions or conversing via text message, might prove beneficial in eliciting more open and reflective responses from them.

11.8.3 What Resources Do They Have Available to Support Resilience?

One approach we can take in assessing the presence of protective factors, and what resources the young person has available to them to remain resilient, is by using the Child & Youth Resilience Measure-Revised (CYRM-R). The CYRM-R is a tool designed to measure resilience in children and adolescents by assessing how effectively they can access and utilise personal, familial, and community resources to overcome adversity and sustain their well-being (Jefferies et al. 2019).

For our purposes the CYRM-R can be used for both initial assessments and as a measure to assess a young person's resilience within the context of identified risk and protective factors. By incorporating the CYRM-R in assessments, practitioners can gauge how these factors balance against each other, factoring in discussions with the family and other professionals. This process will require strategising ways within this network to mitigate risks whilst enhancing or maintaining protective factors, acknowledging that changes in one can significantly influence the other; subsequently, consideration will need to be given as to how these factors may interplay and the consequences discussed with the young person and their caregiver.

It may be the case that decision-making is limited to the young person, a family member, and just one other professional; it thus becomes a case of reaching a consensus within this group and planning a safe way to proceed. This requires focused collaboration to effectively balance the identified risk and protective factors, again focusing on what can be done to safely reduce risk factors whilst promoting resiliency. This emphasis on a unified approach highlights the principle that child safety is a collective responsibility, necessitating coordinated efforts from all available stakeholders to safeguard the child's well-being.

11.8.4 Setting the Scene

When having potentially sensitive discussions with young people, the first thing to consider is the setting, where practical a calm, quiet, and private environment is ideal. Such settings minimise distractions and create a safe space where young individuals can focus, process information, and express themselves without the fear of being overheard or misunderstood. This is particularly important for those with sensory processing issues who may be easily overwhelmed by noise and activity. A private setting also assures confidentiality, which is fundamental to building trust. Trust, in turn, encourages openness and honesty during discussions, allowing for more effective communication and support.

11.8.5 Approaches to Take

Once we have found an appropriate place to talk in private, we can start the conversation and build a rapport with the young person. Begin by clearly explaining the purpose of the discussion, offering reassurance about the nature of the conversation, and explaining any rules around confidentiality and sharing information. It is helpful to maintain transparency about your intentions and avoid setting specific expectations or making promises about resolving issues. Using simple, child-friendly language often works best.

Effective communication in interactions with young people is grounded in the principles of active listening, empathy, and maintaining a non-judgemental demeanour. Active listening entails a deep engagement with what the young person is saying and validating what they express. Empathy extends beyond simple understanding to embodying a genuine sensitivity and compassion towards the challenges the young person faces, attempting to view situations from their perspective. Furthermore, adopting a non-judgemental approach creates a secure environment where young individuals feel safe to express their thoughts and emotions without the fear of facing criticism or harsh judgment.

When guiding the conversation, it is advisable to use open-ended questions that encourage the young person to describe their experiences in their own words, such as asking, "Tell me about what has happened," or "Can you explain what happened today?". Dianiska et al. (2024) suggest that using open-ended questions along with mutual self-disclosure can be effective in building rapport, for example, sharing our own experience of discussing sensitive topics with a professional, which can make the young person feel more understood and less isolated. However, this approach should be used judiciously; any anecdote needs to be innocuous and not dominate the conversation, as we must remain mindful of maintaining professional boundaries and the potential power imbalance in these interactions.

Further into the conversation, closed questions may be necessary to gather specific details but should be used sparingly. It can be helpful to feedback what the young person has said as you go along, as it not only clarifies the discussion but also shows that you are listening. Conclude conversations by thanking the young people for their participation, summarising the key points discussed, and clearly outlining any agreed actions and responsibilities. This ensures clarity and mutual understanding, reinforcing the importance of their contributions and setting a clear direction moving forward. Chapter 12 provides an in depth discussion on the therapeutic use of self and reflective practice can promote engagement.

11.9 Recap

11.9.1 Tips for Building Rapport and Effective Communication

- Where practical, a quiet and calm environment should be used.
- Consider any potential communication challenges.
- Clearly explain purpose of discussion.
- Utilise simple and easy to understand language.
- Adhere to the principles of active listening, empathy, and maintaining a non-judgemental demeanour.
- Ask open-ended questions. Where appropriate, you can use personal anecdotes.
- Use closed questions to confirm details.
- Feedback what the young person says as you go along.

Thank the young person for their time and confirm any plans or actions before ending the conversation.

11.10 A Case Study Example

Case Study 11.3

Adam (not his real name), a 13-year-old boy, was discovered by police officers loitering at a train station late at night. CCTV footage captured him standing close to the platform's edge, appearing upset. In his possession was a backpack, which he initially refused to allow the officers to inspect. Upon examination, the backpack was found to contain drug paraphernalia, although no drugs. Adam claimed the backpack was not his, explaining that older boys had told him to use the train to meet someone at the station, which he had done. Lost and unable to find his way home, Adam could recall his address, mentioning that he lived with his grandmother in a different town. Adam said he got on well with his grandmother and that they had a close relationship. Adam clarified that he was looking down the tracks in anticipation of an approaching train and did not have thoughts to harm himself. Adam appeared mature, articulating his thoughts coherently and demonstrating a level of thoughtfulness. He did not appear overly upset; however, Adam was unable to stand still and had difficulty following the conversation as he was easily distracted. Adam also mentioned he had not eaten throughout the day and that he was hungry.

We will now identify the main risk and protective factors and use the above advice to address them:

Risk and protective factors	Potential solutions
Adam found loitering at train station, seemingly upset and at risk.	Move Adam to a safer location; assess his physical and emotional state for immediate risks.
Establishing trust and communication with a minor.	Officers should introduce themselves and explain their purpose. Offer reassurance and use non-judgemental and empathetic communication to build rapport and encourage openness.
Unclear circumstances regarding the backpack and interaction with older boys.	Use open-ended questions to let Adam explain the situation in his own words, avoiding confrontational or accusatory language. They should use active listening and validate Adam's experiences. Focus on what Adam says, reflect his statements, and ask clarifying questions to demonstrate genuine interest and understanding.
Clarify context about Adam's life and current situation.	Inquire about his home life, family dynamics, and any immediate needs to understand broader risk and protective factors. Use mainly open-ended questions and use closed question to confirm details.
Identify immediate needs that may affect his well-being.	Help with contacting his grandmother and offer safe transportation home. Will then be able to assess the home situation and speak with the grandmother.
Ensuring Adam's long-term safety and well-being beyond the immediate interaction.	Formulate all the information, balancing risks and protective factors. Consider further actions involving child safeguarding services and plan follow-up care or check-ins from partner services.

In the above scenario, Adam, an adolescent found late at night in a potentially unsafe situation, is initially perceived to be at risk of harming himself. However, it soon becomes evident that he might be exploited and involved in a county lines drug operation. Living with his grandmother suggests complex family dynamics, which necessitates verification of his guardianship and a discussion around whether she knew of Adam's whereabouts. Although Adam denies any intention of self-harm, this assertion has yet to be evaluated by a mental health professional, indicating a need for cautious interpretation. His articulateness and confidence are positive indicators of his ability to communicate effectively, though his difficulty in remaining still and following conversations could suggest neurodiversity, anxiety, or drug use.

This situation underscores the concern that Adam was potentially exploited and without supervision and is in a vulnerable position. Immediate steps should include further discussions with his grandmother and potentially involving local authority child safeguarding teams to assess his safety comprehensively. The presence of positive factors, such as his resourcefulness and strong relationship with his grandmother, provides a counterbalance to the risks; however, these factors are overshadowed by the immediate concerns. Engaging with his grandmother could lead to interventions that mitigate the risk of exploitation, illustrating the dynamic interplay between risk and protective factors in assessing and responding to Adam's needs.

A Practice Case Study
Zainab (not her real name) is a 15-year-old girl who lives at home with her mother and father. Zainab was slow to start talking and was seen by a speech and language therapist at the age of 4. By the time she commenced secondary school, her speech issues had resolved, although she remains quiet and reserved, with a small circle of friends. Being the only Muslim student in her school, Zainab has faced bullying and discrimination from her peers, notably derogatory remarks about her wearing a hijab. Academically, Zainab excels and is predicted to perform well in her exams, though she has shared her fears of failing with her favourite teacher, Ms. Jones. On one occasion, Ms. Jones observed Zainab disposing of her lunch in the bin, citing a lack of appetite. A few weeks later Ms. Jones found Zainab exercising in the classroom during the lunch break and once again did not eat her lunch. Ms. Jones is growing increasingly concerned for Zainab's well-being and is looking for ways to offer support.

11.10.1 Exercise

How should Ms. Jones approach the situation? (See Chap. 3 on eating disorders for further information.)

Can you identify three main risk factors and three main protective factors within this case study?

11.11 Conclusion

This chapter explored the combined role of risk assessment and formulation which is an understanding of what the potential risks are and when they may be present, what triggers and indicates, and how often and how serious they are. An important aspect of risk management is the role of protective factors which can act as a buffer for some of the risk factors. Additionally, risk should be viewed a constant changing phenomenon, when thinking about historical and current presentations of risks.

Moreover, risk factors at both the individual level (genetic, biology, affect behaviour, and cognitions) and wider systemic level (school, family, community) can interact and affect the mental health of CYPs. Therefore, prevention of mental health conditions requires multi-level interventions that address risk and protective factors. Therefore, all adults involved in supporting CYPs must focus on encouraging positive adjustment and promote healthy communities within their home and school, to reduce the likelihood of risk factors. Those supporting the CYP from all levels need to address elevated adversity and craft ways to encourage the CYP to adopt healthier ways to cope with challenges and stressors of everyday life. By familiarising with and adopting the evidence-based approaches and exercises found within this chapter, and wider book, you will equip yourself with the necessary tools to support CYPs and manage their mental health-related risks and practices.

References

Astier A. The 4P factor model and its purpose in psychological medicine. 2023. https://www.andreasastier.com/blog/the-4p-factor-model-and-its-purpose-in-psychological-medicine. Accessed 21 Apr 2024.

Children's Commissioner. Children's mental health services 2022-23. 2024. Available from: https://www.childrenscommissioner.gov.uk/resource/childrens-mental-health-services-2022-23/. Accessed 29 Apr 2024.

Colizzi M, Lasalvia A, Ruggeri M. Prevention and early intervention in youth mental health: is it time for a multidisciplinary and trans-diagnostic model for care? Int J Ment Heal Syst. 2020;14(23) https://doi.org/10.1186/s13033-020-00356-9. Accessed 2 Apr 2024

Department of Health and Social Care. Improving the mental health of babies, children and young people: a framework of modifiable factors. 2024. Department of Health and Social Care. Available from: https://www.gov.uk/government/publications/improving-the-mental-health-of-babies-children-and-young-people/improving-the-mental-health-of-babies-children-and-young-people-a-framework-of-modifiable-factors#introduction. Accessed 10 Mar 2024.

Dianiska RE, Simpson E, Kim S, Lyon TD, Quas JA. Building rapport in interviews with adolescent trafficking victims. Child Abuse Rev. 2024;33(2):e2864. Available from: https://doi.org/10.1002/car.2864. Accessed 25 Apr 2024.

Gartland D, Riggs E, Muyeen S, et al. What factors are associated with resilient outcomes in children exposed to social adversity? A systematic review. BMJ Open. 2019;9:e024870. Available from: https://doi.org/10.1136/bmjopen-2018-024870. Accessed 14 Apr 2024.

Harris LM, Huang X, Funsch KM, Fox KR, Ribeiro JD. Efficacy of interventions for suicide and self-injury in children and adolescents: a meta-analysis. Sci Rep. 2022;12(1):12313. Available from: https://doi.org/10.1038/s41598-022-16567-8. Accessed 20 Apr 2024.

Jefferies P., McGarrigle L, Ungar M. The CYRM-R: a rasch-validated revision of the child and youth resilience measure. J Evid-Based Soc Work. 2019;16(1):70–92. Available from: https://doi.org/10.1080/23761407.2018.1548403. Accessed 19 Mar 2024.

Manchester University NHS Hospitals. Adverse childhood experiences and attachment. 2024. Available from: https://mft.nhs.uk/rmch/services/camhs/young-people/adverse-childhood-experiences-aces-and-attachment/#:~:text=Adverse%20Childhood%20Experiences%20%28ACEs%29%20are%20%E2%80%9Chighly%20stressful%2C%20and,security%2C%20trust%20or%20bodily%20integrity.%E2%80%9D%20%28Young%20Minds%2C%202018%29. Accessed 18 Apr 2024.

National Institute for Health and Care Research. NIHR Evidence; Antidepressants for children and teenagers: what works for anxiety and depression? 2020. https://doi.org/10.3310/nihrevidence_53342. Accessed 11 Apr 2024.

National Society for the Prevention of Cruelty to Children (NSPCC) (2024) Child mental health: recognising and responding to issues I NSPCC Learning.

Newlove-Delgado T, Marcheselli F, Williams T, Mandalia D, Dennes M, McManus S, Savic M, Treloar W, Croft K, Ford T. Mental health of children and young people in England, 2023. NHS England, Leeds. 2023. Available from: https://digital.nhs.uk/data-and-information/publications/statistical/mental-health-of-children-and-young-people-in-england/2023-wave-4-follow-up. Accessed 29 Apr 2024.

Savolainen O, Sormunen M, Turunen H. Promotive and risk factors for children's mental health—Finnish municipal policymakers' and leading officeholders' views. Health Promot Int. 2023;38(2):daac111. Available from: https://doi.org/10.1093/heapro/daac111. Accessed 26 Mar 2024.

SBRI Healthcare. 2021. https://www.sbrihealthcare.org/media/pages/competitions/sbri-healthcare-competition-19-mental-health-inequalities-in-children-and-young-people/20ba9f6753-1688551994/SBRI-Competition-19_CYP-Mental-Health_Brief_Final_230821.pdf. Accessed 5 June 2024.

Trainor G, O'Connor S. Mental health intervention skills for the emergency services. Springer; 2023.

Wilhelmsen T, Røysamb E, Lekhal R, Brandlistuen RE, Alexandersen N, Wang MV. Children's mental health: the role of multiple risks and child care quality. J Appl Dev Psychol. 2023;86:101546. Available from: https://doi.org/10.1016/j.appdev.2023.101546. Accessed 17 Apr 2024

Wlodarczyk O, Pawils S, Metzner F, et al. Risk and protective factors for mental health problems in preschool-aged children: cross-sectional results of the BELLA preschool study. Child Adolesc Psychiatry Ment Health. 2017;11:12. Available from: https://doi.org/10.1186/s13034-017-0149-4. Accessed 10 Apr 2024.

World Health Organisation. Mental health. 2022. Available from: https://www.who.int/news-room/fact-sheets/detail/mental-health-strengthening-our-response#:~:text=Individual%20psychological%20and%20biological%20factors%20such%20as%20emotional,make%20people%20more%20vulnerable%20to%20mental%20health%20problems. Accessed 16 Apr 2024.

Wright MO, Masten AS, Narayan AJ. Resilience processes in development: four waves of research on positive adaptation in the context of adversity. In: Goldstein S, Brooks R, editors. Handbook of Resilience in Children. Boston: Springer; 2013. Available from: https://doi.org/10.1007/978-1-4614-3661-4_2. Accessed 16 Apr 2024.

Xiao Q, Song X, Huang L, Hou D, Huang X. Global prevalence and characteristics of non-suicidal self-injury between 2010 and 2021 among a non-clinical sample of adolescents: a meta-analysis. Front Psychiat. 2022;13. Available from: https://www.frontiersin.org/journals/psychiatry/articles/10.3389/fpsyt.2022.912441. Accessed 10 Apr 2024.

Young Minds. 2018. Understanding trauma and adversity. Available from: https://www.youngminds.org.uk/professional/resources/understanding-trauma-and-adversity/. Accessed 18 Apr 2024.

Therapeutic Use of Self and Reflective Practice for Engaging Young People and Their Families

12

Lisa Fairclough and Celeste Foster

L. Fairclough
BUPA, Manchester, UK
e-mail: Lisa.fairclough@bupa.com

C. Foster (✉)
Directorate of Nursing and Midwifery, University of Salford, Salford, UK
e-mail: c.m.foster@salford.ac.uk

G. Trainor, V. Heaslip (eds.), *Needs of Children and Young People Living with Complex Mental Health Difficulties*,
https://doi.org/10.1007/978-3-031-84532-1_12

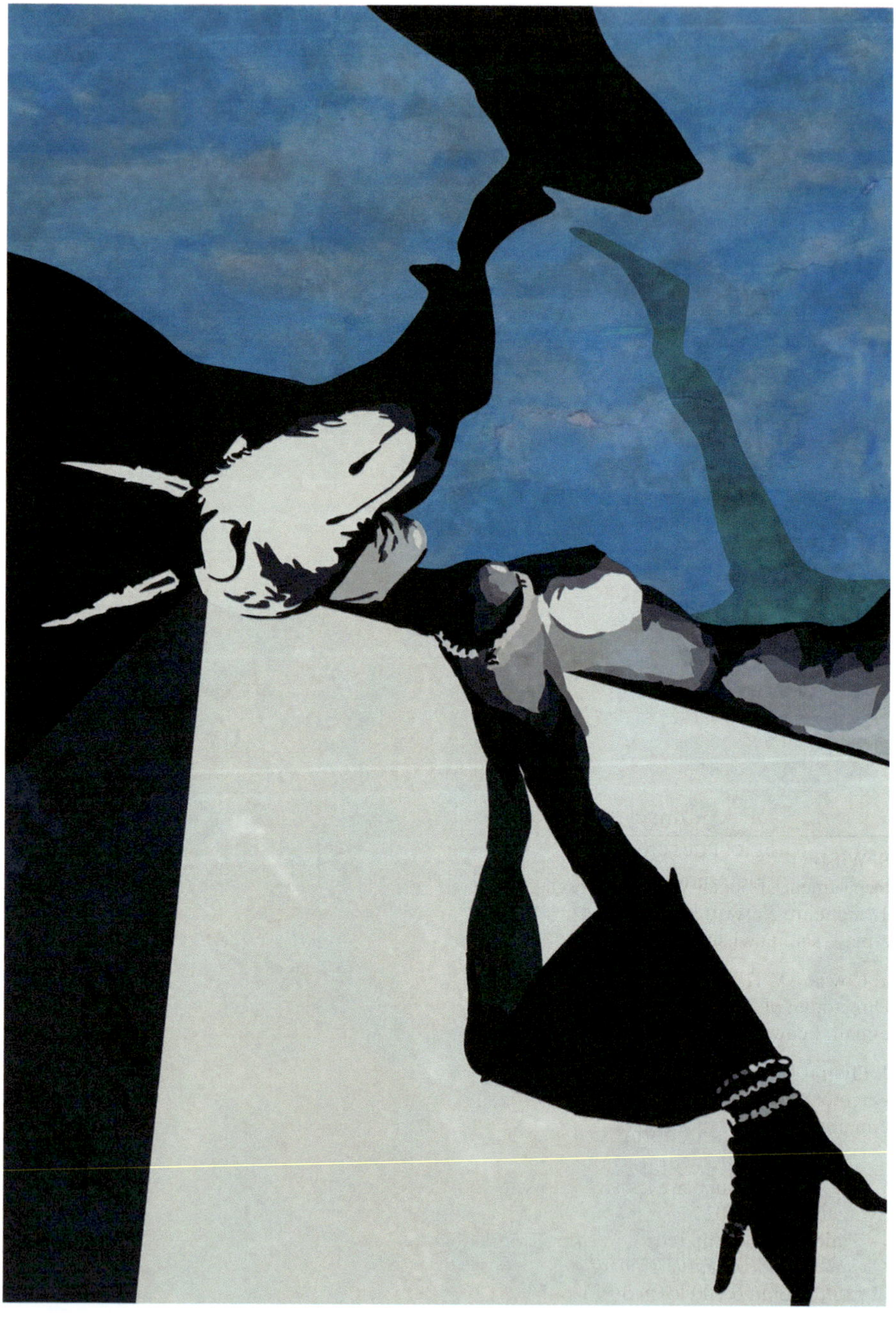

12.1 Introduction

The previous chapters of this book have laid out the various psychological, biological and social challenges that young people face, as they navigate the business of growing up into themselves and making the transition to adulthood. One of the most important things that any professional can do to promote good mental health and prevent or intervene helpfully in mental health problems is to hone their relationship building, interpersonal and engagement skills with children and young people. Having a foundational understanding of the developmental tasks of different stages of childhood and adolescence, the impact of adverse childhood experiences and the common challenges that young people face all help us consider and refine our communication and engagement approaches. It is the foundation for understanding how, as adults, we can work collaboratively with young people to understand their perspective and give them an experience of being heard and having their needs met.

12.2 Why Are Adult Relationships and Engagement So Important for Improving Mental Health Outcomes of Children and Young People?

From birth to adulthood, attachment and interpersonal relationships with the adults that children come across in their everyday life are the primary vehicle for ordinary growth and development (Seigel 2012). Even when things are going well, children and young people are reliant upon on relational environments that confer safety, belonging and legitimacy, and that works to keep stress hormones at bay and support neurological development, learning, emotional regulation and problem-solving skills and understanding of our self and others (Sunderland 2016). So it follows that relationships with helpful adults are the most active agent for positive change, when a young person is facing challenges to their mental health.

Many psychological and mental health difficulties in children and young people emerge in response to overwhelming life stressors (e.g. bullying, living through a pandemic, discrimination, marginalisation, grief, physical illness, parental ill health) or the cumulative impact of adverse childhood experiences (ACEs) and trauma. In other words, the difficulties the young person is experiencing outstrip the understanding and coping skills that they have gained from their life experience so far or temporarily collapse their newly developing and fragile internal resources and resilience, meaning that they need adults to help in ways that can sometimes echo earlier stages of development.

The availability of helpful, attuned and consistent adults, who can give us space to validate and work through our experiences, can help assuage psychological distress, reduce vulnerability and address gaps in skill development (Delaney et al. 2017). Positive attachment relationships with primary carers, wider family and adults in their community are also known to serve as a protection against the negative impacts of some ACEs, helping children to feel safe, to bounce back and to understand what has happened to them. In addition, evidence tells us that how a young person experiences the first contact they have with an adult, when they disclose concerns about their mental well-being, goes a long way towards deciding whether young people will engage with other helping services (Mboweni and Sumbane 2019). This is particularly true in relation to issues where children may be worried about adults having negative attitudes and responses (e.g. self-harm or struggles with alcohol and/or drug misuse) (see Chap. 11).

Puberty and adolescence bring very specific challenges that can get in the way of usual engagement and communication process, making it much harder for young people to take the first steps and increasing the likelihood of miscommunication and conflict within family relationships (Zapf et al.,2024). This means that adults have to be equipped with the knowledge and the commitment to overcome these barriers and step forward in a very active way to build a bridge between them, the young person and their family.

12.3 Developmental Considerations for Getting Communication and Engagement Right

Adolescence is characterised by dynamic brain development in which the interaction with the social environment shapes the capabilities an individual takes forward into adult life. The only other period on the life course when our brains are subject to such a rapid and high level of neurological change is infancy (Patton et al. 2016).

Advances in neurodevelopmental science mean that we now have good evidence to suggest that teenage decision-making processes differ from those of either adults or children. In particular, adolescent brains are primed for rapid change and to respond quickly to the challenges in front of them. This can make it harder for them to slow down and consider all information before they act. The biological imperative of puberty can make it difficult for young people to conceptualise longer-term impacts and consequences, as their brains are wired to prioritise short-term factors when weighing up the balance of risks and benefits. Meanwhile, the presence of peers is now understood to significantly affect the way in which young people process social information, with heightened sensitivity to the perceived impact of decision-making upon reputation, over and above other priorities (such as impact on health). Adolescence is the stage of highest emotional complexity, occurring at a time when young people do not yet have the verbal language to fully express it (Patton et al. 2016).

Repeated research studies have highlighted that teenagers hold specific fears about talking with adults about their emotional health needs and that these are tied into their developmental issues. If these fears are addressed, research also suggests that the majority of young people are then motivated to access help (Hollidge 2013). To help with this, it is useful to remind ourselves of the developmental tasks of puberty and adolescence (see Table 12.1).

Table 12.1 Psychosocial tasks of adolescence

Integration of body-based changes of puberty into self-concept
Separation from parent/family
Independence
Identity formation—Individual, group, sexual
Mourning childhood in order to move towards adulthood
Managing the increased intensity of emotional and aggressive impulses that come with puberty, within in a body that has newly developed power to act on them and not yet developed language skills to express complicated feelings verbally
(Based on Waddell 2018)

The experience of psychological distress, physical or mental illness and needing others directly challenges the key developmental task of learning to be more self-reliant and independent. This can trigger feelings of vulnerability, shame and fear (that something is terribly wrong), which in turn can sometimes prompt anger and aggression or attempts to manage these difficult feelings by avoiding/denying the problem or adopting an all-knowing/all-powerful position (Waddell 2018).

As a result, young people will not always approach you when they are struggling with their emotions. Recognising the need for help at a time when you are trying to master the idea of independence can be difficult, and ambivalence about accessing help is to be expected (Foster and Gardner 2023). When they do approach for help, their window of tolerance to exploring their feelings and being supported by adults can be small. Being prepared to follow the young person's lead, working from a position of collaboration and expecting everything to take longer than you imagine can all help to ease the initial interactions with young people about whom you are worried.

Communication is two-way dynamic and engagement between adults and young people always involves trying to bridge the gap between two different perspectives, developmental standpoints (particularly in terms of power) and cultural contexts. It is just as important to consider and manage the adult-focused barriers to therapeutic engagement, as it is those that are located in the developmental tasks of being a young person.

12.4 The Problem of Adultism and Power

A consistent concern of young people is that they are not really listened to or taken seriously by adults (Coyne et al. 2015) or that the listener will have a negative judgement or attitude towards their concerns.

The natural and logical thing to do as an adult is to draw on one's own experience of childhood/being a teenager, as a means of trying to empathise with young people and see things through their eyes. However, the sociocultural context in which young people are growing up in 2024 is radically different to most of our experiences of being teenagers several decades earlier. The impact of access to digital technology, social media and 24-h rolling news reporting means that young people are continuously connected to each other and the world around them in ways that are far more complex and unfiltered than most adults experienced during their own childhood. This is freighted with both risk and opportunity. Social media and the Internet offer important connections and community. However, they can find it difficult to disconnect, and instant access to large amounts of information can be overwhelming. Global climate and financial and health threats form an ever-present backdrop to most young people's lives that were not so prescient for most of us.

The triple whammy of adult's tendency to draw on their own childhood experiences, the struggle for adults to really remember what the 'felt' experience of being a teenager was like and the tendency to operate on a paternalistic model of interaction (knowing what is best), produces adultism, i.e. adult behaviours and attitudes based on the assumption that adults are better than young people, know more than them and are entitled to act upon and for young people without their agreement (Liebel 2014). At best this can result in young people's mental health needs being minimised, but at worse it results in systemic oppression and marginalisation of young people which can and actually worsen their mental health difficulties. See Reflective Activity 1.

Reflective Activity 1 Using Reflection in Action to Deepen Communication, Empathy and Engagement with Young People

How do you demonstrate an attitude of acceptance, curiosity and a non-judgemental stance to a young person in practice, especially if their communication style and behaviour are difficult to comprehend?

- *Step 1* is being aware of and using your body language to send a very clear non-verbal intent that you are here to listen (Delaney et al. 2017).
  - Write down three ways you could do this.
- *Step 2* is sometimes referred to as reflection in action (Redmond 2017). This involves noticing your initial emotional reactions to the young person and then using reflective questions to have an internal dialogue that helps re-focus your attention on the young person. For example:
  - What am I focusing on most right now?
  - What else should I be paying attention to in this situation?
  - What is the young person's underlying emotional state?
  - What does he or she need?
  - How is the young person viewing me, my approach and my non-verbal communication?
  - What are the power dynamics at play in this conversation?
  - How is this affecting the way they are interacting with me?
  - What could I do to improve this?
- *Step 3 is* crafting a response using the new insights developed from the reflective questions to decide the best way to respond that will communicate to the other person that you have heard and are responsive to their needs in that moment.

Make a commitment to practise this strategy for enhancing communication with someone in your work or personal life. Make a note of anything you learn from being intentional in your communication in this way.

12.5 Facilitators of Successful Engagement with Young People

The good news is that there is also really good understanding of what factors facilitate therapeutic engagement and successful communication with young people. Repeated studies with children and young people highlight the same key principles again and again. These are:

- Access to quality relationship with attuned, reliable and helpful adults, who help young people feel important and heard.
- Promoting choice and autonomy.
- Reducing stigma and shame through validation and normalisation of distress and modelling how to cope with difficult feelings.
- Taking an egalitarian and non-judgemental stance.
- Adopting a collaborative approach to solving problems.
- Giving information and education (promoting mental health literacy).
- Creating private and accepting spaces where young people feel safe to express feelings.
- (Roberts et al. 2022; Peach et al. 2018; Hollidge 2013)

These universal principles for all young people need to be considered alongside the specific communication needs of young people with additional challenges, particularly those who are neurodivergent (see Chap. 5: Learning Disabilities and Neurodiversity) and those who have experienced discrimination or marginalisation on the basis of protected characteristics (see Chap. 7: Social Exclusion, Intersectionality and Discrimination).

12.6 So How Can you Approach a Young Person When you Suspect Something Is Not Right?

When preparing to engage young people, it is not always straightforward. As we have already outlined, young people often do not have the words easily available to explain their feelings. We have to consider the range of direct and indirect ways that they may communicate or open up to about their internal thoughts and struggles. This requires us to notice and take in a combination all of their verbal, non-verbal and behavioural cues and to see behaviour (even difficult behaviour) as containing important information and clues. This is often referred to as attunement (Delaney et al. 2017).

12.6.1 Catching the Moment

If a young person approaches you of their own volition, maintaining engagement is key! This might be the first time they have opened up to someone. This is the most difficult and vulnerable time for the young person. Your response matters as it will set the tone for all future helping interactions.

12.6.2 Managing Oneself

Implementing self-awareness to think about how you come across to the young person can make a big difference. Adult/professional interpersonal style and approach are directly associated with improving the working alliance and the health outcomes for children and young people (Ryan et al. 2023). Or as the young people who helped co-produce the 'Just a Thought' communication model, to help adults talk to children about difficult things, put it: 'Don't just think about what you want to ask us, also think about how you are letting us know that you are someone we can talk to' (Peach et al. 2018). Specifically, use positive body language, remind them it is okay to talk at their own pace, directly ask about any worries and see them as partners in finding solutions.

12.6.3 Setting the Environment

Finding a quiet comfortable private space in which to talk to young people, away from peers or worries about being overheard, can make a big difference. Taking steps to reduce the power differential can also help set the context. Work undertaken for the 'Just a Thought' project highlighted that making young people feel comfortable, respected and equal is essential to building rapport and trust (Peach et al. 2018). Think about where you are going to sit (behind a desk? On the biggest chair?); what else is this room used for? (detention? being in trouble?).

12.6.4 Listening with all of your Senses

- ***Verbal***—What is being said?
  Unlike adults who are more likely to tell you about symptoms and problems in a more medicalised way, children often express their difficulties by telling you how they feel somatically, i.e. through their body. For example, 'I have a sore tummy' or 'feel sick' or a 'headache'. In pre-pubertal developmental stages, cognitive and language development is often not developed sufficiently for children to be able to translate the physical sensations attached to troubling emotions into words. Older teenagers often express their emotional difficulties through stories about their interpersonal relationships with peers that can sometimes feel to the adult listener to be a bit irrelevant. Examples can include interpersonal conflicts with friends, worries about social events or extensive machinations about potential romantic partners. The developmental phase of mid-late adolescence is dominated by the task of developing one's identity in relation to one's peers, and so difficulties with emotional well-being are seen, experienced and reported through

this lens. In both cases, what is important is to listen carefully to the stories and hear the repeated themes, triggers and feelings behind the story that emerge as children and young people narrate their bodily or social experiences (e.g. anxiety, self-doubt, irritability). This is sometimes referred to as chasing the affect (Foster 2021).

- ***Non-verbal***—What is not being said?
  Where are the silences and gaps? What might these tell you? It also important to link verbal responses with how the young person present themselves visibly, i.e. do they have a closed body posture? Does their affect (emotional state) match their verbal responses? This is known as congruence and incongruence, e.g. if a young person is telling you that things are 'fine', but they are pacing about the room as they tell you this. Taking time to notice your own feelings in the encounter can also give important clues to what is going on, especially if you notice yourself having strong emotional response, that are uncharacteristic for you. For all of us our first communication strategy as a baby is to instinctively behave in a way that stirs up a strong feeling in our carers (think about the panic that rises when a baby will not stop crying!). This fundamental communication enables us to mobilise others to help and to give others a taste of how it feels to be us when we do not have the words to explain. For example, teenagers who feel out of control can sometime behave towards adults in ways that are dismissive and can feel derisive and condescending, leaving the adults feeling powerless, out of control and frustrated. Behaving in this way can instinctively offer the young person a moment of respite from their underlying feelings whilst also communicating something important about their 'felt' experience. Rather than reacting to one's own frustration, it can be really helpful to pause and notice, as these feelings often provide a glimpse of what it feels like to be in that young person's shoes.
- ***Behaviour***—What are they doing? What can you see?
  Your role is not to question what you see but to draw on what you see as information. Can you work to make sense of it or ask about it in a respectful way? Demonstrating a commitment to the idea that behaviour has meaning and showing an interest in understanding the child's behaviour can help to promote a trusting therapeutic relationship.
- ***Appearance***—How do they look?
  Their condition, not their behaviour. Can you let the young person know what you see, as a way of making a connection? For example, I notice you seem to look sad or anxious or tired. What clues are in their physical appearance? For example, are there signs that they are not looking after themselves or being looked after? Do they look as though they are eating or sleeping sufficiently?

12.6.5 Making Links Between All of the Above

Developing the cognitive capacities, skills and knowledge to be able make complex links between how we feel on the inside and what is happening in the world around us, our thoughts, feelings and behaviours is a work in progress that takes at least the first two decades of life to complete and needs the support and help of adults to notice and share possible links. The cognitive abilities to think in an abstract and symbolic way and to generalise across domains are neurodevelopmental achievements that emerge in adolescence, but they take time to bed in, and are fragile, temporarily disappearing at times of stress (Rahdar and Galván 2014). Do not assume that young people can or have made the link between life stressors in one part of their life (e.g. impact of a bereavement) and emotional difficulties in another (e.g. irritability in social situations with peers).

12.7 Getting the Conversation Started

Table 12.2 provides helpful tips on how you can start off a conversation with a young person about their mental health, maintain the conversation and keep the lines of communication open for the young person to come back and talk with you.

If you suspect a young person is struggling with mental health difficulties and they might need signposting or a referral to another agency, you will need to gain more structured information about their current difficulties and risks to facilitate

Table 12.2 Starting conversations with a young person about their mental health (Developed from Royal College of Psychiatry 2024; Young Minds 2024; AYHP 2024; and authors own clinical experience)

Ask! Are you OK? Has something happened? I've noticed that you're not yourself, and I am worried you might be sad? Try not to use example that may shut the conversation down. Would you like to talk about it? Can I help? If you can't tell me, is there anyone else you would like to talk to?	**Validate** That must feel really bad or I'm sorry you feel like this It's OK not to be OK I believe you I don't know how you feel, but I really want to understand. Can you tell me a little more? This is tough, you're doing really well Take your time, I'm here to listen I'm here if you need me
Do Thank them for sharing: Sharing thoughts and feeling is hard Be clear about the limits of confidentiality Tell them to take their time, go at the young person's pace Strike a balance between problem and strength-based talk. Be curious Wonder about the reasons why young people behave in the way they do, encourage them to be curious about themselves Use clear, age-appropriate language in a straightforward way	**Don't** Assume you know how the young person feels. Telling the young person that you know how they feel may shut down the conversation Pursue direct questioning The young person may shut down the conversation or feeling like they are being tested, putting them on the back foot Shy away from tricky subjects or use vague or euphemistic language Blame or use inflammatory language Bring your own feelings into the conversation. This can trigger a guilt response Instead show that you can imagine how it *might* feel to be them: When you say that "I can imagine that it might feel XX for you"

this process. This is often a source of worry for non-mental health professionals, due to worries about asking the wrong thing and making the situation worse. The following questions and prompts have been devised to help non-mental health specialists undertake an initial triage collaboratively with young people and to help them think with the young person about next steps:

- **Meaning**: Can you help me understand the reasons that have led to you feeling this way?
- **Wider problems**: Are you having any problems in:
  - School life? Family life? With friends or other relationships?
- **Safeguarding:** Has/is anything unwanted, frightening or harmful been happening to you?
- **Mental health:** Look out for/ask about feelings of hopelessness, loss of enjoyment and repetitive, intrusive or disturbing worries in the young person's narrative—these can be indicators of anxiety and depression.
- **Identifying risks**: Sometimes when people feel down/worried/angry, they can also have thoughts of wanting to hurt themselves, lash out at others or to end their life. Have you ever experienced this? (Do not be frightened to ask more details about this. If the person says yes, it is often a relief for young people to be able to talk about these feelings.)
- **Internal triggers:** Be curious about the way the young person feels about/sees themselves.
- **Resilience and self-help**: Ask questions about strengths and usual ways of coping.
- **Collaboration:** What do you think might help/we should do next?

(adapted from Foster et al. 2016)

12.8 A Systemic Approach to Thinking about Engagement and Communication with Children and Young People

The paediatrician, Donald Winnicott, famously said 'There's no such thing as a baby…. there is a baby and someone' (Winnicott 1984). This quote refers to the idea that children and young people do not exist in isolation and are always located in a family context—even if they do not live within that family context or they are at a stage of life where they are trying to separate and differentiate their identity from that of their family. Considering parents, carers and the wider family system to which young people belong is an essential component of effective therapeutic engagement.

From the onset of puberty (average age of 10 years), young people operate in a unique position that has been coined by Briggs (2008) as 'temporary outsidership'. It describes the range of ways in which adolescents, and those who care for them, need to be able to flexibly span the boundary of inside/outside in relation to self and other family and social groups, without getting stuck on either side, in order for the essential tasks of adolescent development to be achieved. The task of working towards independence means young people have a vital need for their own space, privacy and the right to access support for psychological distress without being in the company of their primary carers. Yet at the same time, they remain absolutely dependent on their carers for love, for support, for boundaries to keep them safe and for material care. They are trying to renegotiate the proximity and relative autonomy/power between them and their family members, not separate from them entirely. Therefore, communication with children and young people is always as tripartite process—even if the young person is old enough to request to speak with you in private and competent to request that you do not share information, understanding the family system that the young person is part of is essential. Wherever possible, it is good practice to engage children and families together and as a minimum keep parents of teenagers onboard and informed (Waid and Kelly 2020).

This balancing act requires that you understand the legal framework and basic rules pertaining to competence and confidentiality. The Children Act (1989/2004) and the UN Convention on the Rights of the Child (UNRC 1989) set out the basis for a Gillick competent child's right to safe, private space in which to discuss their worries and to have requests for information not to be shared taken seriously and considered carefully. The Children Act (1989/2004), combined with the Human Rights Act (1998), also sets out parent's right to information that is essential for them to meet their responsibility to keep their children safe. Working Together to Safeguard Children (HM Govt 2023) operationalises these legal instruments to provide guidance on when information sharing for the safety of the young person is essential and the process for doing this in a way that still attends to the young person's wishes and personhood.

When there are concerns about a young person's mental health, emotions are often understandably high, and there can be tension and difficulty in young people's family relationships and communication (Zapf et al. 2024). Developmentally ordinary emotionality, followed by a rapid wish to move on from problems without looking back, and a tendency to see things in black and white can leave parents and carers of young people in a whirlwind of worry and distress. It can also make it harder for professionals to maintain a neutral stance, as they are pushed and pulled into a more paternalistic role or conversely over-identifying with the young person's position at the risk of excluding parents and carers (Foster 2021).

A good rule of thumb is to not be drawn in to taking sides with either the young person or parent/carers position but instead to recognise, summarise and validate the differing perspectives and experiences of both. However, this is not always easy. Using structured frameworks for shared decision-making can be really helpful for managing these tensions. The Anna Freud Centre has developed a specific framework for shared decision-making between young people, families and professionals in relation to mental health issues (Liverpool et al. 2021) and a range of freely available resources which you can find in Table 5.

12.9 Case Example

This case (see Table 12.3) example highlights the need for flexible and attuned communication skills when talking with young people in distress. It also highlights the importance of balancing the needs of young people and parents. Communication and engagement strategies for supporting parents will be developed in the next section.

Table 12.3 Case study of Emily

Case study: Emily's story A school nurse has received a referral from A&E, regarding an incident that occurred with Emily, a 14-year-old pupil, over the weekend. The nurse has arranged to see Emily to discuss the incident and check on their Well-being. Before she gets to the appointment, she receives a call from Emily's parent that they are very distressed. They are angry with Emily for putting herself in such a risky position and also very worried about her because she will not talk to them about what happened. They ask the nurse to contact them after the appointment, to tell them what Emily says and to give them advice about what to do next
The A&E referral states that Emily had gone to a party over the weekend at her boyfriend's house. Emily attended with her friend, without the permission of her parents. Reports were that Emily was seen drinking neat vodka and there was some concern that she had also taken illicit substances. Subsequently, Emily became seriously intoxicated, and friend and peers at the party became worried about her. Emily was violently sick and then passed out on the bathroom floor. Emily's friend attempted to rouse her, but she was unresponsive. It was at this point that her friend decided to call 999 to get an ambulance. When the paramedics got to the scene, Emily was a little more responsive, but she was incoherent, distressed and crying. The paramedics felt it was important to take her to A&E to be medically assessed. Emily's friend told the paramedics that Emily had had an argument with her boyfriend at the party and they had split up. Her ex-boyfriend was later seen with another girl. The friend provided the paramedics with Emily's parent contact details, and the paramedics contacted the parents at the scene, advising them of the situation and that they were taking her to A&E. The parents made their way to A&E. After a medical assessment and few hours of observation, Emily was deemed medically fit and was subsequently discharged from A&E back into the care of her parents
When Emily arrived at her appointment with the school nurse, she was extremely upset and embarrassed. She stated that her parents had grounded her indefinitely, and this was made worse because her parents are strict, her mother is still being difficult with her and her father is not speaking to her. Emily stated that she felt like she had lost everything, her boyfriend and the trust of her parents and now feels alone and that she does not want to be here. Emily asks the school nurse not to share information about what happened at the party or about how she is feeling with her parents, as she worries it will make things worse
Reflective Activity 2 The school nurse now must engage with Emily. From the information provided, how should school nurse engage and navigate the discussion? Using your learning from this chapter, consider the following: What are the key themes from the case study? What are the developmental touch points that need to be considered? Emily has referred to 'not wanting to be here'. How would you deal with this? How can the nurse balance Emily's wish for privacy and her parents need for information and support?

12.10 Supporting Parent/Carer-Child Communication

The importance of supporting child-parent/carer communication at times of emotional distress cannot be overstated. Parents act as models for communication, shaping children's communication style and their ability to express needs and emotions. Parent-child communication is also known to affect self-esteem, school performance and their ability to manage conflict in other relationships (Zapf et al. 2024). The degree to which parent-child communication can be supported and maintained as children grow and move through transitions that tests their relationships can be a both a protective and risk factor for onset or mental health problems in young people. Professionals therefore have an important role in trying to support and enable parents and carers to listen and respond helpfully to their young people and also to helping young people effectively express themselves and communicate their needs to parents-carers.

If we think about Emily's story, it is helpful to consider the differing needs being expressed by Emily and her parents, respectively. Emily is worried about being in trouble; she is also having understandable feelings of embarrassment and worries about being judged. She feels alone and needs help to work out how to repair the ruptures in her relationships, whereas Emily's parents are worried about whether Emily is safe and want advice about how to help or take care of their child, after this frightening event. By considering the different focus of each party's communication needs, it is often possible to provide help and support for both young person and parent. Young people need to have their experiences, heard, felt and validated. This often involves listening to and appreciating detail. Parents and carers are often much less interested in the detail and want advice and guidance. It is possible to provide general guidance about helpful ways forward in the situation, based only on what the parents already know (obviously this would need to be renegotiated with Emily, if she disclosed risks to herself during the appointment).

This can include generalised information about the problem at hand (in this case excessive alcohol intake and emotional distress after a breakup) and signposting parents to mental health resources (see Table 12.4). Providing parents with advice about changing developmental dynamics in mid-adolescence (i.e. greater focus on peer relationships, higher levels of emotionality and short-term decision-making) and the impact of these on emotional health and behaviour can help parents to avoid conflict and blaming language when talking with their child, reducing the risk of young person withdrawing or act out. Remember that parents are negotiating the changes of adolescence too. Both young people and parents benefit from being supported with dignified climbdowns following a frightening event or a period of conflict. It is possible in this case to support parents to think about strategies for reopening the lines of communication—making it easier for their child to approach them and know they are available to help—without breaching Emily's request for privacy.

General conversations and advice about principles for resetting boundaries in adolescence can also be very helpful. Boundaries are of course important as they provide containment and promote responsibility, and sanctions and consequences

Table 12.4 Additional resources

Tips for engaging children and young people:
Royal College of psychiatry
https://www.rcpch.ac.uk/resources/engaging-children-young-people
Young Minds:
https://www.youngminds.org.uk/professional/resources/how-to-be-a-good-listener/
Association for Young People's health
https://ayph.org.uk/engaging-with-young-people
Talking with young people about their mental health
Young Minds:
https://www.youngminds.org.uk/professional/resources/how-to-have-a-conversation-with-young-people-about-mental-health/
University of Salford/ Pennine care NHS trust—Not just a thought
https://www.salford.ac.uk/research/care/research-groups/cyp@salford/accordion/not-just-a-thought-a-communication-model
Mental health of young people resource for parents and carers:
MindEd for families:
https://mindedforfamilies.org.uk/young-people/
Tips for promoting shared decision-making with young people and parents/ families:
The Anna Freud Centre
https://www.annafreud.org/resources/children-and-young-peoples-wellbeing/shared-decision-making/

for unwanted behaviours are a natural logical step for parents, to try and avoid repetition of risky behaviour. However, boundaries and sanctions without an exit strategy or room for negotiation can have the opposite effect. The length and scope of any sanction need to be proportionate to the event, and the young person needs something to work towards and a guide for how they can make amends or reparation. It can be difficult when there is nothing to lose and may promote further unwanted behaviours. These ideas seem logical and obvious when it is not your child and all is calm, but when you are distressed and worried, it can be easy to lose sight of such principles without the chance to talk it through with someone else.

For Emily, validating and taking her concerns seriously and exploring whether there are any other underlying mental health concerns are an important first step. Supporting her with practical problem-solving and collaborating with her on strategies for repairing her relationships and communicating her needs to her parents will reduce her feelings of hopelessness and by definition any risk associated with these feelings. Modelling an ability to see both sides and helping Emily to comprehend the source of her parents initial anxiety and defensiveness, so she feels less attacked, can help her manage her reaction and work through a strategy to talk to them about her needs (Brown 2020).

12.11 Conclusion

This chapter has explored the evidence for why engagement and relationships with trustworthy, responsive and attuned adults are so important in improving mental health outcomes for children and young people. Using a developmental approach, focusing on the neurodevelopmental and psychosocial tasks of childhood, puberty and adolescence, we have tracked the ways in which engaging young people and creating an environment in which they can be open about their concerns can be interpersonally challenging but also effectively overcome. Considering the communication barriers we present as adults, applying strategies to address young people's fears and using self-awareness to bridge the gap between adult and adolescence cultural contexts can be a central intervention in mental health difficulties in and of itself.

Engaging young people requires us to be active, open and curious to what is being communicated and to what is not being communicated, responding flexibly in our thinking and undertaking deep critical reflection to help temper our reactions, in order that we hear what young people are really trying to tell us. Engaging directly and respectfully with young people as partners, and helping them and their families find solutions, has the potential to significantly contribute to reduction in conflict, episodes of mental distress and mental illness and vulnerability. This will also support self-reliance and resilience and improve the quality of life for both young people and their carers.

References

Association for Young People's Health. 2024. Engaging with young people.. Available from: https://ayph.org.uk/engaging-with-young-people

Briggs S. Working with adolescents and young adults: a contemporary psychodynamic approach. Macmillan International Higher Education; 2008.

Brown J. Engaging with parents in child and adolescent mental health services. Aust N Z J Fam Ther. 2020;41(2):145–60.

Children Act. Available from: Children Act 1989 (legislationgovuk). 1989.

Children Act. Available from: Children Act 2004 (legislationgovuk). 2004;

Coyne I, McNamara N, Healy M, Gower C, Sarkar M, McNicholas F. Adolescents' and parents' views of child and adolescent mental health services (CAMHS) in Ireland. J Psychiatr Ment Health Nurs. 2015;22(8):561–9.

Delaney K, Shattell M, Johnson M. Capturing the interpersonal process of psychiatric nurses: a model for engagement. Arch Psychiatr Nurs. 2017;31(6):634–40.

Foster C. Children living with long term conditions – child and adolescent mental health: the nursing response. In: Glasper A, Richardson J, Randall D, editors. A textbook of children and young People's nursing. 3rd ed. Elsevier; 2021.

Foster C, Gardner L. Understanding the developmental impact of domestic violence and adverse experiences in childhood across the life-course. In: Roddy J, editor. Working with client experiences of domestic abuse. Routledge: Taylor & Francis; 2023. p. 117–32. https://doi.org/10.4324/9781003253266-9.

Foster, C., Birch, L., Allen, S., Rayner, GC., 2016 Enabling practitioners working with young people who self-harm. J Ment Health Train Educ Pract, 10(4), 268–280.

HM Government. Working together to safeguard children 2023: a guide to multi-agency working to help, protect and promote the welfare of children. 2023. Available from: https://assets.publishing.service.gov.uk/media/669e7501ab418ab055592a7b/Working_together_to_safeguard_children_2023.pdf. Accessed 8 Apr 24.
Hollidge C. Adolescents' perceptions of the factors that enhance the therapeutic relationship: a qualitative study in school-based health settings. Adolesc Psychiatry. 2013;3(3):277–87.
Liebel M. Adultism and age-based discrimination against children. In: Kutsar D, Warming H, editors. Children and non-discrimination. Interdisciplinary textbook. Children's Rights Erasmus Academic Network, University Press of Estonia; 2014. p. 119–43.
Liverpool S, Hayes D, Edbrooke-Childs J. An affective-appraisal approach for parental shared decision making in children and young people's mental health settings: a qualitative study. Front Psych. 2021;12:626848.
Mboweni RF, Sumbane GO. Factors contributing to delayed health seeking behaviours among adolescents. Global J Health Sci. 2019;11(13):67.
MindED Consortium. MindED for families. Department of Health & health education England. 2019. Available from: https://mindedforfamilies.org.uk/young-people/. Accessed 8 Apr 24.
Patton GC, Sawyer SM, Santelli JS, et al. Our future: a lancet commission on adolescent health and wellbeing. Lancet. 2016;387(10036):2423–78.
Peach, D., Rowland, A., Bates, D., Long, A., Cook, D., Cooper, L., … Smith, S., 2018. Not just a thought: a communication model - learning with children, young people and young adults about how we can keep them safe. ISBN: 9781912337064. https://www.salford.ac.uk/research/care/research-groups/cyp@salford/accordion/not-just-a-thought-a-communication-model
Rahdar A, Galván A. The cognitive and neurobiological effects of daily stress in adolescents. NeuroImage. 2014;92:267–73.
Redmond B. Reflection in action: developing reflective practice in health and social services. Routledge; 2017.
Roberts M, Jones J, Garcia L, Techau A. Adolescents' perceptions of barriers and facilitators to engaging in mental health treatment: a qualitative meta-synthesis. J Child Adolesc Psychiatr Nurs. 2022;35(2):113–25.
Royal College of Psychiatry. 2024. Engaging with children and young people. Available from: https://www.rcpch.ac.uk/resources/engaging-children-young-people. Accessed 8 Apr 24.
Ryan R, Berry K, Hartley S. Therapist factors and their impact on therapeutic alliance and outcomes in child and adolescent mental health–a systematic review. Child Adolesc Mental Health. 2023;28(2):195–211.
Siegel D. The developing mind: how relationships and the brain interact to shape who we are. 2nd ed. New York: The Guildford Press; 2012.
Sunderland M. What every parent needs to know. Love, nurture and play with your child. London: Penguin Random House; 2016.
The Human Rights Act. 1998. https://www.legislation.gov.uk/ukpga/1998/42/contents
United Nations. Convention on the rights of the child. 1989. General Assembly Resolution 44/25, UN Doc A/RES/44/25 UN November 20.
Waddell M. Adolescence inside stories. London: Karnac Books; 2018.
Waid J, Kelly M. Supporting family engagement with child and adolescent mental health services: a scoping review. Health Soc Care Community. 2020;28(5):1333–42.
Winnicott D. The maturational processes and the facilitating environment studies in the theory of emotional development. London: Routledge; 1984.
Young Minds. How to have a conversation with young people about mental health. 2024. Available from: https://www.youngminds.org.uk/professional/resources/how-to-have-a-conversation-with-young-people-about-mental-health/. Accessed 8 Apr 24.
Zapf H, Boettcher J, Haukeland Y, Orm S, Coslar S, Fjermestad K. A systematic review of the association between parent-child communication and adolescent mental health. JCPP advances. 2024;4(2):e12205.

Internet Use Amongst Young People and Its Influence on Mental Health

13

Elizabeth Harlow, Laura Hales, Isobel McMillan, and Gemma Trainor

E. Harlow (✉) · L. Hales
Manchester University NHS Foundation Trust, Manchester, UK
e-mail: Lizzie.Harlow@mft.nhs.uk; Laura.Hales@mft.nhs.uk

I. McMillan
Directorate of Nursing and Midwifery, University of Salford, Salford, UK
e-mail: i.m.mcmillan@salford.ac.uk

G. Trainor
Mental Health Nursing, Directorate of Nursing and Midwifery, University of Salford, Salford, UK
e-mail: gemma.trainor@outlook.com

G. Trainor, V. Heaslip (eds.), *Needs of Children and Young People Living with Complex Mental Health Difficulties*,
https://doi.org/10.1007/978-3-031-84532-1_13

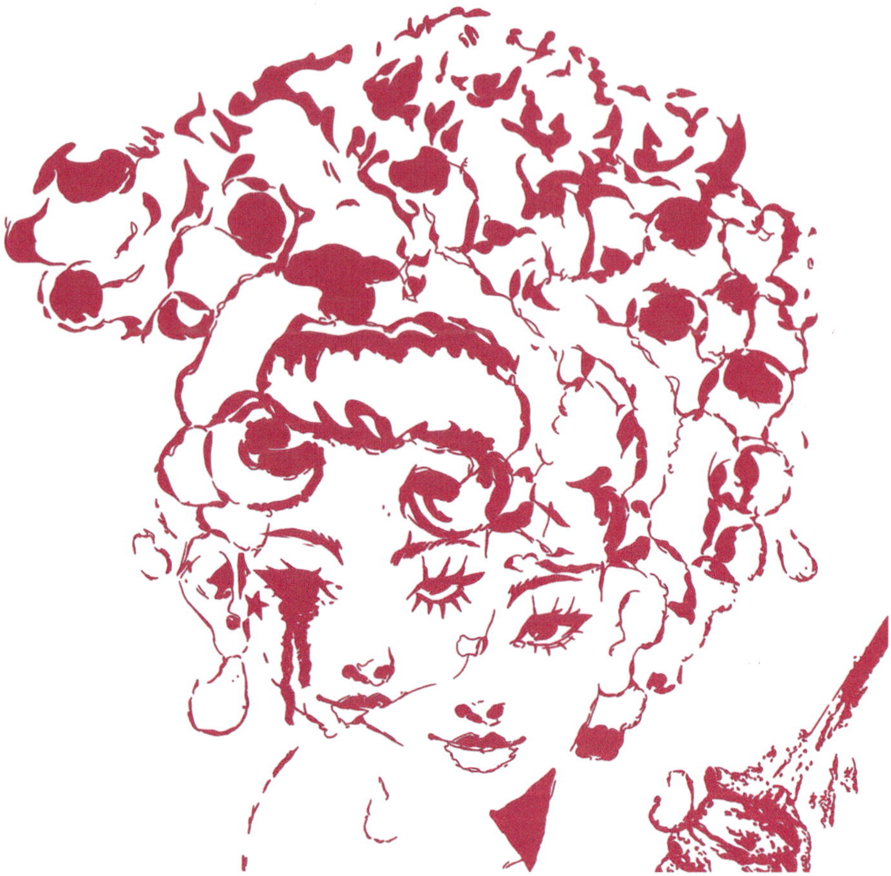

© Robyn Heaslip

13.1 Introduction

The internet is defined as a worldwide public computer network that gives users access to a variety of platforms, such as communication services, gaming servers, entertainment sites, news platforms, etc[1]. The internet is accessible in various ways including via a computer, mobile phones, digital TV, games consoles and more.

Everyone is online; however, it is an integral part of young people's lives and often far from adult scrutiny. According to a report by Global West Index (2018), people aged 16–24 across the globe spend an average of 3 hours 1 minute each day on a variety of social media platforms. This was also found for the UK with the Online Harms White Paper (Gov.uk 2019), reporting that 99% of 12–15 year-olds are online. The United Nations (UN 2023) further this, and highlight that 75% of 15–24-year-olds are online compared to 65% of the rest of the global population. Young people have been described as the drivers of online culture and therefore can be considered skilled and knowledgeable in social media (Goodyear et al. 2019).

"Social media" is an umbrella term which describes various online platforms that allow for activities such as blogging, photo sharing, social gaming and more (Aichner and Jacob 2015). Social media includes applications such as, Facebook, WhatsApp, Twitter, YouTube, LinkedIn, Pinterest and Instagram (Greenwood and Gopal 2015). The applications focus on user-generated content which can be highly influential to anyone accessing it (Greenwood and Gopal 2015).

Alongside internet use and the impact it may have on young people are the concerns regarding young people's mental health. The Mental Health of Children and Young People in England 2023 report found that approximately 1 in 5 children and young people have a "probable mental disorder" (Newlove-Delgado et al. 2023). The report noted that the rates of probable mental disorders were similar between boys and girls aged between 8 and 16 years old; however, the rates in young women aged between 17 and 25 years old were twice as high compared to young men of the same age (Newlove-Delgado et al. 2023). The report investigated possible links between these rates of probable mental disorders with sleep, loneliness, activities and health behaviours (Newlove-Delgado et al. 2023). These links have also been found between positives and negatives of internet use which will be explored further.

Adolescents who spend more than 3 hours a day using social media may be at risk of heightened mental health problems (Riehm et al. 2019). Additionally, it has been suggested that associations do exist between Internet use and mental health well-being (Kardefelt-Winther 2017). The Royal College of Paediatrics and Child Health (RCHCP 2019; Dubicka and Theodosiou 2020) supports this further by noting that young people with higher screen times have been found to have more depressive symptoms, a less healthy diet, a higher energy intake and more pronounced indicators of obesity. Recently, pressure has grown for action to be taken regarding online harm and young people when, for the first time in Britain, a coroner ruled that a 14-year-old schoolgirl, Molly Russell, had accessed online content that had contributed to her death (Dyer 2022). Although many negative aspects of Internet use have been highlighted, there are also positives. Findings have shown that young people also use the internet to explore their identity, experience independence, gain social support, find peer acceptance, connect with others and increase self-esteem (Gonzales and Hanock 2011; Radovic et al. 2017).

Due to this significant increase in Internet use, alongside growing concerns regarding young people's mental health, professionals need to understand the full impact of a young person's online behaviour, in order to to identify risk and protective factors. It has been suggested that clinicians that work with young people with mental health issues need to be engaging in discussions about their internet use (Marchant et al. 2017). Therefore, as digital technologies are here to stay, it is essential for professionals to adopt an approach that reduces risk without restricting the benefits of social media.

This chapter will explore the harmful and helpful effects on young people who experience mental health difficulties in relation to their internet use.

13.2 Harmful

13.2.1 Problematic Internet Use and Mental Health

The growth in internet use has paralleled with the growth in concerns around its use and young people's mental health. It has been found that moderate and healthy internet use is generally beneficial to those accessing it (Przybylski et al. 2019). However, not all experiences are positive, as unhealthy internet use over large amounts of time has been defined as problematic internet use (PIU). PIU can be described as Internet use which can lead to psychological, social, academic and occupational difficulties (Beard and Wolf 2001), and PIU has been recognised as a global social issue (Spada 2014). Other terms such as "Internet addiction" (Brenner 1997) are also prevalent amongst research, and the different terms are highly debated amongst the scientific community (Fernandes et al. 2019).

There has been an increase in evidence that Internet use may be impacting young people's mental health (Lavis and Winter 2020; Kelly et al. 2018). Studies have found that young people are accessing and/or experiencing content online such as cyberbullying, pornography, content promoting self-harm, suicide, eating disorders, violence and more, and consequently these have been having negative effects on mental health (Hudson et al. 2022). Research by Ofcom (2020) found that half of 12–15-year-olds said they have seen something they consider "hateful" online. Similarly in a sample of 14,944 young people aged between 11 and 16, 1 in 4 had seen content regarding suicide in their life (Katz and Aiman n.d.-a, -b). Further research analysed 314 websites targeted at young people and found suggestive images of self-harm in 21% of them (Marchant et al. 2017). Research has found that young people hospitalised for suicide attempts or ideation have reported both positive and negative impacts of social media sites (Weinstein et al. 2021; Nesi et al. 2019). Both studies reported that young people said they received positive support online but also accessed harmful content which was described as "encouraging" harmful behaviour and experienced online bullying or teasing.

> "I think obviously you'll have incidents in schools where there'll be like a girl or something who's like has self-harmed and like they would have posted about it" — Young person 2

This increase in evidence is further supported by Molly Russell's passing and the coroner's inquest. The inquest found that Molly Russell had viewed around 12 posts a day which related to suicide, self-harm and depression and that these were a contributing factor to her death. The coroner reported that the Internet had "affected her mental health in a negative way and contributed to her death in a more than minimal way" and that she had "died from an act of self-harm while suffering from depression and the negative effects of online content" (Dyer 2022).

> "I think Twitter for harmful content takes the takes the title"—Young person 1

13.2.2 Suicide Pacts

The internet is often unregulated, meaning that young people have access to forums and conversations they may not normally have access to (Mok et al. 2015). Research has found an increase in online suicide pacts (Lee and Kwon 2018). It acknowledged that online suicide pacts account for a small proportion of overall suicides; however, this number is rising, specifically in Eastern Asian countries for young people. These pacts are referred to as "cybersuicide pacts" and allow strangers to contact each other online and agree to end their lives by suicide. The first recorded online suicide pact in Japan took place in 2000 (Lester 2009); however, these "cybersuicide pacts" have been recorded across Western populations too, with the first recorded in the UK taking place in 2005 (Naito 2007). It should be acknowledged that due to the vast amounts of unmonitored chat rooms and forums, these pacts are easier than ever to make, and identify, however currently there is little evidence to assess the true involvement of the internet.

13.2.3 Physical Health

Not only are there mental well-being concerns, but there are also concerns regarding young people's physical health and the quantity of time they spend on the internet. It has been found that an increase in internet use amongst adolescents has led to an increase in obesity, reduced physical activity and consequently an increase in health concerns (Rosen et al. 2014). Research has also shown that internet use has impacted young people's sleep quality, with many young people getting less sleep therefore having negative effects on their daily functioning (Pirdehghan et al. 2021).

13.2.4 Cyberbullying

Lastly, over half of young people aged 12–15 have experienced a form of bullying in the last year, including cyberbullying (National Bullying Helpline 2022). Further reports found that 7 in 10 young people experience cyberbullying, and 37% of these young people describe it to be on a frequent basis (RSPH 2017). Having access to the internet and social media has provided various ways for young people to connect with others, and this means there is the potential for cyberbullying. Children aged

11–16 years old with a probable mental disorder were five times more likely to be bullied both in person and online, with rates of 10.8% of online bullying for those with a disorder compared to 2.6% of young people without a mental health disorder (Newlove-Delgado et al. 2023). Cyberbullying has been highlighted by the UK government as a risk for young people accessing the internet.

> "I've been added to like, I think in year nine there was like a huge, like massive group chat on Snapchat with like a lot of people in my year in, and then they would just be nasty to this one girl"—Young person 3

13.2.5 Algorithmic Monitoring of the Internet

Algorithms can be defined as "a sequence of instructions or commands that a computer can work through to solve a task" (Perez Vallejos et al. 2021). Algorithms are used to programme and monitor social media sites, with the intention to make these processes more efficient and less dependent on human monitoring. Algorithms can be independent from human input and become an almost automatic process.

Algorithms allow for personalisation of the information that young people are accessing online (Perez Vallejos et al. 2021). For example, if a young person searches a keyword on a social media site, the following content will be individualised to their searches, and they will continue to see this content. Research suggests that approximately 20% of young people aged 11–16 years old had accessed harmful online content related to topics like eating disorders, self-harm and harmful drugs (Livingstone et al. 2019). It could be suggested that the use of algorithms on social media websites may then impact the likelihood of young people seeing harmful content again after the initial search, making accessing harmful content online even easier and more likely for young people. In one study, young people reported that it was "easier" and "quicker" to access content online with the implementation of algorithmic processing on social media sites (Perez Vallejos et al. 2021). These findings suggest that even though the content young people referred to in the study may not be harmful, it could be implied that harmful content is just as quick and easy to access (Perez Vallejos et al. 2021).

Algorithms are not only used for the personalisation of content on social media sites but also used to monitor and regulate sites. Algorithmic regulation refers to systems use of algorithms to monitor and govern sites by algorithmic decision-making, rather than solely human decision-making (Yeung 2017). Despite the use of these algorithms, the use of "algospeak" and the vast amounts of uncensored online content, harmful online content can go unmonitored. Algospeak is understood to be the abbreviation, misspelling or substitution of specific words, for example, anorexia can be @norexia, and this is not always picked up on by platforms; therefore, content violating the guidelines may not be removed (Steen et al. 2023; Curtis 2022). Both Instagram (Mosseri 2019) and Facebook banned images that showed self-harm, such as images of cutting in a self-injurious context; however, such images are still accessible to young people. The aforementioned case of Molly

Russell highlights this, as it was reported that Molly had accessed images of self-harm before her suicide (Smith and Cipolli 2021). They found that since the banning of these images from Facebook and Instagram, the number of images has reduced. However, it was identified that algorithmic monitoring and regulation missed "muted" words that may have been harmful, and the use of "algospeak" makes the identification of such content even more difficult.

> "There's a lot more promoting it, like saying you can do this, or you can do that and like, saying this is what you should eat If you don't wanna eat too many calories and then it's obviously like promoting people to eat less and less, it will just be like for your dinner have cucumber and some water"—Young person 3

Algorithms may promote accessibility to harmful content by increasing the likelihood of images reappearing on young people's social media feeds. Algorithmic regulation can also be criticised, as social media users can censor or rephrase harmful content which is then missed by such algorithms. Suggestions have been made to use a combination of algorithms and human moderators in order to increase online safety and prevent young people seeing harmful online content (Leaver 2022).

> "Even if you say I don't like it, sometimes I've said I don't like a video when it's been graphic or something like a car crash for example. I don't know. I don't like seeing stuff like that, but I've still seen them, even though I clicked that I didn't want to see content like that"—Young person 1

13.3 Helpful

Although there is harmful content that young people can access, there is also content on the internet/social media that is considered to be helpful and positive.

13.3.1 Accessibility, Information and Support

A literature review found various positive effects that accessing the internet can have on young people. The internet is a key source by which young people can access information, services and support (Burns et al. 2010). When considering the wealth of knowledge the internet holds, findings show that there was a range of content on social media which promoted positive norms about mental health and well-being (Burns et al. 2010; Swist et al. 2015). The accessibility of the internet has in turn increased young people's access to mental health and well-being information, which has included peer support and communities of care and professional services (Swist et al. 2015). Further to this, the Royal Society for Public Health (RSPH 2017) reports that nearly 7 out of 10 teens expressed that they received support on social media during challenging times. Approximately 76.9% of young people reported using the Internet in order to connect with other young people (Burns et al. 2010).

> "I think it's good for socialising and like, talking to people and also like, I think if you don't have many friends as well, like online, you can like maybe start making friends"—Young person 4

13.3.2 Identity, Community and Creativity

It has been found that the internet can help to foster identity formation, community building and creativity amongst young people (Swist et al. 2015). It has been found that young people developing an online identity reported that this helped them to increase their self-esteem (Swist et al. 2015). The internet has been found to be an effective platform for self-expression, with young people being able to personalise content, be creative, explore how they identify with the world and engage in topics such as politics (University of Minnesota 2015; Orehek and Human 2016).

The community building element to social media has also been found to support young people in finding others similar to themselves to talk to. Groups that may be considered minorities such as those in the LGBTQ+ community can build online safety networks which can provide connections and a sense of community (McInroy et al. 2019; Hampton et al. 2011; Russell and Fish 2016). Approximately 16.6% of children aged 11–16 years old with a probable mental health disorder felt lonely often or always, comparatively to a much lower percentage of 0.8% for children without a probable mental disorder (Newlove-Delgado et al. 2023). A similar trend was found with young people aged 17–22 years; research found 29.5% of young people with a probable mental health disorder felt lonely often or always, compared to 5.2%, respectively (Newlove-Delgado et al. 2023). The ability to build a community and interact with others similar to yourself has allowed adolescents to use the internet to engage in activities which in turn aids their development of identity, belonging and sense of connection when these areas in the offline world may not be as easy for some (Bannon et al. 2015). This has been found to help support young people who may feel lonely through making new friends in these domains (Cipolletta et al. 2020).

13.3.3 Mental Health

The ability for young people to express themselves on the internet has been linked to positive mental health with an increase in self-belonging, being able to overcome shyness and increase the young person's potential to self-disclose (Cipolletta et al. 2020; Vaingankar 2022). Self-disclosing has been found to be associated with positive feedback from others and enhance social support and community involvement, in turn having a positive impact on the young person[29]. The ability to self-disclose in an online community has been found to validate self-harm alongside providing support in managing and coping with it; this has been considered another benefit to internet use (Thorn et al. 2023).

Similarly, young people self-disclosing and accessing support have been found in other studies including in semi-structured interviews which found that TikTok users who have a history of non-suicidal self-injury (NSSI) explored NSSI content in order to share their experiences, support others, share stories of recovery, find humour and normalise discussions around NSSI (Vera 2023).

Moderated online mental health forums often provide a space for young people to disclose and discuss issues they may find embarrassing telling someone face to face (Hanckel and Morris 2014). Online mental health support has also been found to reach clients who may not be likely to seek help in person, as well as supporting people to access help earlier. This online support has developed into 24-hour support and without the geographical or logistical constrictions in-person support may have (Rickwood et al. 2005).

13.3.4 Education and Skills

Internet use has also been linked to having a positive influence on development (Fitton et al. 2013). Young people have discussed that access to the internet has led to increases in skills and independently recognising and researching information, leading to advances in their knowledge. In turn, it is acknowledged that young people accessing the internet and learning to develop their digital literacy skills support them in preparation for their future work life (Internet Matters n.d.).

> "Go on like a hike or walk, I'll Tik-Tok what people have done, or if we go to bars like when we went to Barcelona on holiday, I'll TiKToK what people have done there, and I get more ideas from that than I ever would from Google"—Young person 1

Further to this, it is has been found that playing video games can enhance spatial perception, mental rotation and spatial visualisation (Uttal et al. 2013). Not only does internet access allow for development of these skills, it also believed to contribute to better learning outcomes and success in school (Kuhlemeier and Hemker 2007). Further support for internet use has been found in research which showed that the internet empowers learning and provides young people with further education (Buckingham 2008).

Access to the internet has allowed young people to further their education and access it during the COVID-19 pandemic where online learning was adopted during school closures (Richardson 2020). It has also been shown to support young people's understanding of what is happening in the world, as supported by 70% of young people in a recent survey (UK Safer Internet Centre 2019).

> "You can get like news as well, I guess. Like there's Snapchat news, Instagram, you get more of that too"—Young person 2

13.4 Internet Safety

As the Internet has become a key part of young people's lives with influences both helpful and harmful, there is a clear need for safety measures to be created and implemented. The risks associated with children's engagement with online content have been broadly categorised into four types of risk, referred to as the CO:RE 4 Cs (Jang and Ko 2023; Livingstone and Stoilova 2021). These 4 Cs encompass the different dimensions of risks that children may encounter when navigating the digital landscape. The 4 Cs Include:

- **Content:** Content risks refer to the type of content that children could encounter. This type of content could include harmful or age-inappropriate material such as violence, sexually explicit images or hate speech.
- **Contact**: Contact risks refer to potential interactions and communications that a child might have or receive online. This could include communication with individual's unknown to the child and those who may have malicious intent and are predators or cyberbullies.
- **Conduct**: Conduct risks refer to risks relating to the actions and behaviours of the child while they are online. Risks within this category include cyberbullying, online harassment and engaging in illegal activities.
- **Contract/Commerce**: Contract/commerce risks refer to risks to children in relation to online transactions and financial activities. Risks within this category could include falling victim to online scams, making purchases without parental consent or sharing personal data.

Examples of each of the 4 Cs can be found in Fig. 13.1 ('the 4Cs: classifying online risk to children') (Livingstone and Stoilova 2021).

In an effort to try and mitigate some of these risks, countries worldwide have started to pass or are in process of passing legislation which aims to protect children online (Song and Holzer 2023). The UN has also been involved in numerous initiatives which aim to combat risks and promote internet safety on a global scale (Song and Holzer 2023; UN 2023). These include but are not limited to the UN International Children's Emergency Fund's (UNICEF) work, aiming to tackle cyberbullying, the UN Educational, Scientific, and Cultural Organization's (UNESCO) work aiming to combat human trafficking and the UN's Office on Drugs and Crime (UNODC) work to promote and improve internet security (Song and Holzer 2023). In addition to these initiatives, the UN and UNICEF have also developed policies and legislation, such as the Convention on the Rights of the Child (UNCRC) (UNICEF 1989), which discusses children's rights more generally but also specifically states the ways that young people and children should be treated and how their rights should be protected online and in the digital world.

The UN provides general advice to policymakers, tech companies, parents and educators and sees the issue of online safety for children as a global issue which requires collaboration and cooperation between all involved (ITU 2021). This includes the need for better awareness and education around internet safety and

CO RE	Content Child engages with or is exposed to potentially harmful content	Contact Child experiences or is targeted by potentially harmful *adult* contact	Conduct Child witnesses, participates in or is a victim of potentially harmful *peer* conduct	Contract Child is party to or exploited by potentially harmful contract
Aggressive	Violent, gory, graphic, racist, hateful or extremist information and communication	Harassment, stalking, hateful behaviour, unwanted or excessive surveillance	Bullying, hateful or hostile communication or peer activity e.g. trolling, exclusion, shaming	Identity theft, fraud, phishing, scams, hacking, blackmail, security risks
Sexual	Pornography (harmful or illegal), sexualization of culture, oppressive body image norms	Sexual harassment, sexual grooming, sextortion, the generation and sharing of child sexual abuse material	Sexual harassment, non-consensual sexual messaging, adverse sexual pressures	Trafficking for purposes of sexual exploitation, streaming (paid-for) child sexual abuse
Values	Mis/disinformation, age-inappropriate marketing or user-generated content	Ideological persuasion or manipulation, radicalisation and extremist recruitment	Potentially harmful user communities e.g. self-harm, anti-vaccine, adverse peer pressures	Gambling, filter bubbles, micro-targeting, dark patterns shaping persuasion or purchase
Cross-cutting	**Privacy violations** (interpersonal, institutional, commercial) **Physical and mental health risks** (e.g., sedentary lifestyle, excessive screen use, isolation, anxiety) **Inequalities and discrimination** (in/exclusion, exploiting vulnerability, algorithmic bias/predictive analytics)			

Fig. 13.1 The CO:RE classification of online risk to children. (Published in Open Access under Creative Commons - Attribution 4.0)

potential risks where both children and parents are fully informed about the potential harms and how to combat these. This may include but is not limited to education on privacy and privacy settings, discussion around how best to report abusive content and developing critical thinking skills to enable children and young people to question and evaluate the true credibility of information they may see online. Emphasis is also put on parental and caregiver guidance in terms of monitoring children's Internet use. In addition to parental advice and education, the UN also heavily advises that all governments and organisations should implement polices and regulations which aim to do more to protect children and young people online (UNICEF 1989).

> "So, I think that better moderating on social media platforms would be better"—Young person 3

One such legislation is the "The Online Safety Act 2023" which has recently been passed by the UK government (GOV UK 2023). The Act was developed to address a wide range of concerns around internet use and online safety, with a particular focus on legislation which aims to mitigate online risk to children, young people and other vulnerable individuals. The Act increases the responsibility of tech companies and service providers by establishing a legal duty of care, requiring them to take and demonstrate that they are taking active and reasonable steps to address harmful content and protect service users. Potentially harmful content listed in the Act includes cyberbullying, hate speech, disinformation, child exploitation and other age-inappropriate content. Online platforms are required to remove illegal content promptly, have effective ways of reporting and removing harmful content and behaviour in place, have tested and robust provisions for age verification to protect children from age-restricted content and to publish regular reports detailing their efforts to reduce harmful content. To ensure tech companies and service providers follow these new requirements, an independent regulator, known as Ofcom, has been put in charge of monitoring online platforms (e.g. social media sites, messaging apps, search engines and online forums) This regulatory body has the power to impose substantial fines on platforms that fail to comply with their duty of care (GOV UK 2023; NSPCC Learning n.d.).

13.5 Conclusion

> "The challenge is to help children and young people enjoy the benefits of going online while maintaining the skills and knowledge to identify and avoid risks" (Jang and Ko 2023)

Overall, as the internet has become increasingly available and young people are spending large amounts of their days accessing online content, the need and opportunity for mental health professionals to have guidance and a wider understanding of the impact it can have are needed (Global Web Index 2018). When developing resources, professionals, educator and youth workers have all expressed the need for guidelines around working with young people/parents to understand how to protect their young person online (Clarke et al. 2017). Parents need to adopt the same boundaries as they would in terms of their offline behaviour. Further to this, a psychologist in a study discussed the need for up-to-date, reliable, evidence-based and culturally relevant resources. As access to the internet grows, so does the need for professionals to keep up to date and have access to relevant information in order to support young people (Clarke et al. 2017).

Various guidelines are provided for professionals including those in healthcare settings. These guidelines and bills provide safety tips, resources and advice; however, there is not a singular set of guidance (NSPCC Learning, no date). As many offer general themes, the UK Safer Internet Centre suggests further insight, including the need for more relevant questions in healthcare assessment to understand young people's use of technology as well as professionals keeping up to date with online trends and risks (UK Safer Internet Centre n.d.). The internet can be both helpful and harmful to young people. All those supporting young people need to understand the young person's internet use and keep up to date with the risks, trends and up-to-date resources. This could help professionals support and give them a better understanding of the young person's mental health by including the importance of online behaviour in determining risk and informing risk formulation.

From exploring these conflicting effects of the internet in this chapter, the authors recognise that children have a right to be autonomous and creative online in the same way they have carte blanche in their public life. Children are required to learn from setbacks; however, it is imperative for adults in close proximity to the child to minimise the potential risks of exploitation. UNICEF is urging all governments to establish coordinated responses including law enforcement to better protect children online. Such policymakers need to include the opinions and perspectives of the young people themselves. Content can be harmful in that it may overly influence them at a tender age to develop unrealistic expectations for themselves or others. Every child deserves to feel safe online and to benefit from the transformational opportunities the internet has brought to society. Below are some tips that may help create a safer space for our children and young people:

- Recognise that provision of a safe space is part of your role.
- Have an open dialogue with young people about anything they may have experienced which has caused them confusion or distress.
- Demonstrate how you can use privacy settings to manage potential cyberattacks.
- Be aware of the new and emerging online harms.
- Understand the child protection statutory guidance about what constitutes abuse and how to respond.
- Understand the individual and environmental factors that predispose youths to the adverse effects of social media.
- Inspire safe and responsible use by not spending excessive amount of time online yourself.
- Advise on the use of parental controls and taking time away from the screen.
- As stated previously, internet use needs to form part of the risk assessment and case formulation.
- All those responsible for protecting young people need to be aware of who and what the young person is accessing and ensure a balanced digital exposure to encouraging creativity and learning.
- Do not use screen time as a reward or an easy option to avoid other more important things.
- Keep screen use to daytime and promote a healthy norm being mindful of effects on their sleep pattern.
- Be mindful of how online behaviour may contribute to a young person's offline behaviour.
- The objective nature of online dialogue can result in burgeoning perfection and mental health issues.

13.6 Future Research

This chapter has reviewed both helpful and harmful aspects of young people accessing the internet and the impact this can have on their mental health. Although there have been vast amounts of research, more is needed to fully understand the effects. The internet continues to grow and as such so should the research. Therefore, the following suggestions for future research are proposed.

Often articles researching young people and internet use focus upon what is seen as harmful compared to what can be helpful. It is acknowledged that accessing the internet can have positive implications such as information on health/well-being, support groups, peer connections, etc. (Gonzales and Hancock 2011; Swist et al. 2015); however, the research is limited.

Social media platforms often have regulated rules and policies which tend to ban content such as hate speech, terrorist content and dissemination of disinformation; the platforms have established algorithms, filters and technology to identify such content and remove it (Stasi 2019). However, even with the regulatory practice and content moderations of the platforms, not all content is recognised and removed. Those using social media often anticipate how algorithms restrict content and have found ways to evade this by using "algospeak" (Steen et al. 2023). Participants using TikTok often adopted "algospeak" when posting content regarding topics that may violate the guidelines of the platform; this means that the content is less likely to be removed (Steen et al. 2023). There is limited research into the ability to avoid content filters and its impact on young people, as the internet continues to be prominent in young people's lives; this needs to be explored further. Exploration into screening young people's internet use within healthcare assessments is also needed. The American Psychological Association have suggested that routinely screening PIU can help to prevent future risk (American Psychological Association 2023). There has also been calls for clinicians to be more aware of online content and what a young person could be accessing (Rider et al. 2021).

Lastly, as highlighted by Internet Matters (Katz and Aiman n.d.-a, -b), more research needs to look into whether all internet safety guidance/advice fits all young people. A survey revealed that Looked-After Children were three times more likely to try to get around filters and seven times more likely to have their personal details stolen. Further to this, those classed as Looked After were more likely to access harmful content. Likewise, young people with mental health, learning or communication difficulties may have struggle to access safety content, and it is suggested that further research and a more thorough analysis of safety education programmes, needs to be looked in to in order to support all young people (Jones et al. 2014).

References

Aichner T, Jacob F. Measuring the degree of corporate social media use. Int J Mark Res. 2015;57(2):257–76. https://doi.org/10.2501/ijmr-2015-018.

American Psychological Association. Health advisory on social media use in adolescence. [online] Apa.org. 2023. Available at: https://www.apa.org/topics/social-media-internet/health-advisory-adolescent-social-media-use.

Bannon S, McGlynn T, McKenzie K, Quayle E. The positive role of Internet use for young people with additional support needs: identity and connectedness. Comput Hum Behav. 2015;53:504–14. https://doi.org/10.1016/j.chb.2014.11.099.

Beard KW, Wolf EM. Modification in the proposed diagnostic criteria for Internet addiction. Cyberpsychol Behav. 2001;4(3):377–83. https://doi.org/10.1089/109493101300210286.

Brenner V. Psychology of computer use: XLVII. Parameters of Internet use, abuse and addiction: the first 90 days of the Internet usage survey. Psychol Rep. 1997;80(3):879–82. https://doi.org/10.2466/pr0.1997.80.3.879.

Buckingham D. Beyond technology : children's learning in the age of digital culture. Cambridge: Polity; 2008.

Burns JM, Davenport TA, Durkin LA, Luscombe GM, Hickie IB. The internet as a setting for mental health service utilisation by young people. Med J Aust. 2010;192(S11):S22. https://doi.org/10.5694/j.1326-5377.2010.tb03688.x.

Cipolletta S, Malighetti C, Cenedese C, Spoto A. How can adolescents benefit from the use of social networks? The iGeneration on Instagram. Int J Environ Res Public Health [online]. 2020;17(19):6952. https://doi.org/10.3390/ijerph17196952.

Clarke AM, Chambers D, Barry MM. Bridging the digital disconnect: exploring the views of professionals on using technology to promote young people's mental health. School Psychol Int [online]. 2017;38(4):380–97. https://doi.org/10.1177/0143034317700937.

Curtis S. How TikTok is changing the way we SPEAK. [online] Mail online. 2022. Available at: https://www.dailymail.co.uk/sciencetech/article-11262889/TikTok-changing-way-SPEAK-phrases-like-quiet-quitting-le-dollar-bean.html. Accessed 6 Jun 2024.

Dubicka B, Theodosiou L. Technology use and the mental health of children and young people. 2020. https://www.rcpsych.ac.uk/docs/default-source/improving-care/better-mhpolicy/college-reports/college-report-cr225.pdf.

Dyer C. Social media content contributed to teenager's death 'in more than a minimal way,' says coroner. BMJ [online]. 2022;379:o2374. https://doi.org/10.1136/bmj.o2374.

Fernandes B, Maia BR, Pontes HM. Adição à internet ou uso problemático da internet? Qual dos termos usar? Psicol USP. 2019;30 https://doi.org/10.1590/0103-6564e190020.

Fitton VA, Ahmedani BK, Harold RD, Shifflet ED. The role of technology on young adolescent development: implications for policy, research and practice. Child Adolesc Soc Work J. 2013;30(5):399–413. https://doi.org/10.1007/s10560-013-0296-2.

Global Web Index. Social. [online]. 2018. Available at: https://www.gwi.com/hubfs/Downloads/Social-H2-2018-report.pdf.

Gonzales AL, Hancock JT. Mirror, Mirror on my Facebook Wall: effects of exposure to Facebook on self-esteem. Cyberpsychol Behav Soc Netw. 2011;14(1–2):79–83.

Goodyear VA, Armour KM, Wood H. Young people and their engagement with health-related social media: new perspectives. Sport Educ Soc, [online]. 2019;24(7):673–88. https://doi.org/10.1080/13573322.2017.1423464.

GOV UK. Online safety act 2023. [online] Legislation.gov.uk. 2023. Available at: https://www.legislation.gov.uk/ukpga/2023/50/enacted.

Gov.uk. Online Harms White Paper. [online] GOV.UK. 2019. Available at: https://www.gov.uk/government/consultations/online-harms-white-paper/online-harms-white-paper.

Greenwood BN, Gopal A. Research note—Tigerblood: newspapers, blogs, and the founding of information technology firms. Inf Syst Res. 2015;26(4):812–28. https://doi.org/10.1287/isre.2015.0603.

Hampton K, Goulet LS, Purcell K. Social networking sites and our lives. [online] Pew Research Center: Internet, Science & Tech; 2011. Available at: https://www.pewresearch.org/internet/2011/06/16/social-networking-sites-and-our-lives/

Hanckel B, Morris A. Finding community and contesting heteronormativity: queer young people's engagement in an Australian online community. J Youth Stud. 2014;17(7):872–86.

Hudson N., David M., Haux T., Kersting F., Macnaboe L., Mcdonough T., Phillips N., Woolfe E., Myers CA. Content and activity that is harmful to children within scope of the Online Safety Bill A Rapid Evidence Assessment Prepared for: Department for Digital, Culture, Media and Sport. 2022. [online] Available at: https://assets.publishing.service.gov.uk/media/63972fc5d3bf7f3f7d1cf430/Content_and_Activity_that_is_Harmful_to_Children_within_Scope_of_the_Online_Safety_Bill__REA__accessible_.pdf. Accessed 8 Apr 24.

Impact of social media and screen use on young people's health – consultation response (RCPCH). 2019. https://www.rcpch.ac.uk/resources/impact-social-media-screen-use-young-peoples-health-consultation-response.

Internet Matters. Social media benefits for young people | Internet matters. [online] Internet matters. n.d.. Available at: https://www.internetmatters.org/resources/social-media-advice-hub/social-media-benefits/.

ITU. 2021. International telecommunication union: keeping children safe in the digital environment: the importance of protection and empowerment. [online] Available from: https://www.itu-cop-guidelines.com/_files/ugd/24bbaa_cf79ba8d5fdb4639af9b9a4237e07ad9.pdf

Jang Y, Ko B. Online safety for children and youth under the 4Cs framework—a focus on digital policies in Australia, Canada, and the UK. Children (Basel). 2023;10(8):1415. https://doi.org/10.3390/children10081415.

Jones L, Mitchell K, Walsh W. A content analysis of youth Internet safety programs: are effective prevention strategies being used? Crimes Against Children Research Center [online]; 2014. Available at: https://scholars.unh.edu/ccrc/41/

Kardefelt-Winther D. How does the time children spend using digital technology impact their mental Well-being, social relationships and physical activity? An evidence-focused literature review. I how does the time children spend using digital technology impact their mental Well-being, social relationships and physical activity? An evidence-focused literature review. 2017. [online] Available at: https://www.unicef-irc.org/publications/pdf/Children-digital-technology-wellbeing.pdf.

Katz A, Aiman E, Asam. Life online for vulnerable young people. n.d.-a. [online] Available at: https://www.internetmatters.org/wp-content/uploads/2021/01/Internet-Matters-Refuge-And-Risk-Report.pdf.

Katz A, Aiman E, Asam. Vulnerable Children in a Digital World in partnership with Internet Matters. n.d.-b. [online] Available at: https://www.internetmatters.org/wp-content/uploads/2019/04/Internet-Matters-Report-Vulnerable-Children-in-a-Digital-World.pdf.

Kelly Y, Zilanawala A, Booker C, Sacker A. Social media use and adolescent mental health: findings from the UK millennium cohort study. EClinicalMedicine, [online]. 2018;6(2589–5370):59–68. https://doi.org/10.1016/j.eclinm.2018.12.005.

Kuhlemeier H, Hemker B. The impact of computer use at home on students' Internet skills. Comput Educ. 2007;49(2):460–80. https://doi.org/10.1016/j.compedu.2005.10.004.

Lavis A, Winter R. Online harms or benefits? An ethnographic analysis of the positives and negatives of peer-support around self-harm on social media. J Child Psychol Psychiatry, and Allied Disciplines, [online] 61(8). 2020;61:842. https://doi.org/10.1111/jcpp.13245.

Leaver T. Coroner finds social media contributed to 14-year-old Molly Russell's death. In: How should parents and platforms react?. Parenting for a digital future; 2022. [online] https://blogs.lse.ac.uk/parenting4digitalfuture/2022/10/05/molly-russell/.

Lee SY, Kwon Y. Twitter as a place where people meet to make suicide pacts. Public Health. 2018;159:21–6. https://doi.org/10.1016/j.puhe.2018.03.001.

Lester D. The use of the Internet for counseling the suicidal individual: possibilities and drawbacks. OMEGA - J Death Dying. 2009;58(3):233–50. https://doi.org/10.2190/om.58.3.e.

Livingstone S, Stoilova M. The 4Cs: classifying online risk to children. [online]; 2021. https://doi.org/10.21241/ssoar.71817.

Livingstone S, Stoilova M, Nandagiri R. Children's data and privacy online growing up in a digital age an evidence review. 2019. [online] Available at: https://eprints.lse.ac.uk/101283/1/Livingstone_childrens_data_and_privacy_online_evidence_review_published.pdf.

Marchant A, Hawton K, Stewart A, Montgomery P, Singaravelu V, Lloyd K, Purdy N, Daine K, John A. A systematic review of the relationship between internet use, self-harm and suicidal behaviour in young people: the good, the bad and the unknown. PLOS One, [online]. 2017;12(8):e0181722. https://doi.org/10.1371/journal.pone.0181722.

McInroy LB, McCloskey RJ, Craig SL, Eaton AD. LGBTQ+ youths' community engagement and resource seeking online versus offline. J Technol Hum Serv. 2019;37(4):315–33. https://doi.org/10.1080/15228835.2019.1617823.

Mok K, Jorm AF, Pirkis J. Suicide-related Internet use: a review. Australian New Zealand J Psychiatry. 2015;49(8):697–705. https://doi.org/10.1177/0004867415569797.

Mosseri, A., 2019. Instagram policy changes on self-harm related content - protecting vulnerable users | Instagram blog. [online] about.instagram.com. Available at: https://about.instagram.com/blog/announcements/supporting-and-protecting-vulnerable-people-on-instagram.

Naito A. Internet suicide in Japan: implications for child and adolescent mental health. Clin Child Psychol Psychiatry. 2007;12(4):583–97. https://doi.org/10.1177/1359104507080990.

National Bullying Helpline. Cyberbullying | Bullying online advice. 2022. [online] www.nationalbullyinghelpline.co.uk. Available at: https://www.nationalbullyinghelpline.co.uk/cyberbullying.html.

Nesi J, Wolff JC, Hunt J. Patterns of social media use among adolescents who are psychiatrically hospitalized. J Am Acad Child Adolesc Psychiatry [online]. 2019;58(6):635–639.e1. https://doi.org/10.1016/j.jaac.2019.03.009.

Newlove-Delgado T, Marcheselli F, Williams T, Mandalia D, Dennes M, McManus S, Savic M, Treloar W, Croft K, Ford T. Mental health of children and young people in England, 2023. Leeds: NHS England; 2023.

NSPCC Learning. The online safety act: what it means for children and professionals. n.d. [online] Available at: https://learning.nspcc.org.uk/news/2023/november/what-online-safety-act-means-children-professionals#:~:text=To%20make%20sure%20companies%20meet.

Ofcom. Children and parents: media use and attitudes report 2019. 2020. [online] Available at: https://www.ofcom.org.uk/__data/assets/pdf_file/0023/190616/children-media-use-attitudes-2019-report.pdf.

Orehek E, Human LJ. Self-expression on social media. Personal Soc Psychol Bull. 2016;43(1):60–70. https://doi.org/10.1177/0146167216675332.

Perez Vallejos E, Dowthwaite L, Creswich H, Portillo V, Koene A, Jirotka M, McCarthy A, McAuley D. The impact of algorithmic decision-making processes on young people's Well-being. Health Informatics J. 2021;27(1):146045822097275. https://doi.org/10.1177/1460458220972750.

Pirdehghan A, Khezmeh E, Panahi S. Social media use and sleep disturbance among adolescents: a cross-sectional study. Iran J Psychiatry [online]. 2021;16(2):137–45. https://doi.org/10.18502/ijps.v16i2.5814.

Przybylski AK, Orben A, Weinstein N. How much is too much? Examining the relationship between digital screen engagement and psychosocial functioning in a confirmatory cohort study. J Am Acad Child Adolesc Psychiatry. 2019;59(9):1080. https://doi.org/10.1016/j.jaac.2019.06.017.

Radovic A, Gmelin T, Stein BD, Miller E. Depressed adolescents' positive and negative use of social media. J Adolesc [online]. 2017;55(55):5–15. https://doi.org/10.1016/j.adolescence.2016.12.002.

Richardson C. How are young people using screens during lockdown? [online] RCPCH insight. 2020. Available at: https://medium.com/rcpch-insight/how-are-young-people-using-screens-during-lockdown-835f9d525cb3.

Rickwood D, Deane FP, Wilson CJ, Ciarrochi J. Young people's help-seeking for mental health problems. Australian e-J Adv Mental Health, [online]. 2005;4(3):218–51. https://doi.org/10.5172/jamh.4.3.218.

Rider EA, Ansari E, Varrin PH, Sparrow J. Mental health and wellbeing of children and adolescents during the covid-19 pandemic. BMJ, [online]. 2021;374(374):n1730. https://doi.org/10.1136/bmj.n1730.

Riehm KE, Feder KA, Tormohlen KN, Crum RM, Young AS, Green KM, Pacek LR, La Flair LN, Mojtabai R. Associations between time spent using social media and internalizing and externalizing problems among US Youth. JAMA Psychiatry, [online]. 2019;76(12):1266–73. https://doi.org/10.1001/jamapsychiatry.2019.2325.

Rosen LD, Lim AF, Felt J, Carrier LM, Cheever NA, Lara-Ruiz JM, Mendoza JS, Rokkum J. Media and technology use predicts ill-being among children, preteens and teenagers independent of the negative health impacts of exercise and eating habits. Comput Human Behavior, [online]. 2014;35(35):364–75. https://doi.org/10.1016/j.chb.2014.01.036.

Royal Society for Public Health (RSPH). #StatusofMind. 2017. [online] Rsph.org.uk. Available at: https://www.rsph.org.uk/our-work/campaigns/status-of-mind.html.

Russell ST, Fish JN. Mental health in lesbian, gay, bisexual, and transgender (LGBT) youth. Annu Rev Clin Psychol, [online]. 2016;12(1):465–87. https://doi.org/10.1146/annurev-clinpsy-021815-093153.

Smith H, Cipolli W. The Instagram/Facebook ban on graphic self-harm imagery: a sentiment analysis and topic modeling approach. Policy Internet. 2021;14:170. https://doi.org/10.1002/poi3.272.

Song H, Holzer A. Online safety laws by country. J Nonprofit Innov, [online]. 2023;3(3) Available at: https://scholarsarchive.byu.edu/joni/vol3/iss3/3. Accessed 6 Jun 2024

Spada MM. An overview of problematic Internet use. Addict Behav. 2014;39(1):3–6. https://doi.org/10.1016/j.addbeh.2013.09.007.

Stasi ML. Social media platforms and content exposure: how to restore users' control. Compet Regul Netw Ind [online]. 2019;20(1):86–110. https://doi.org/10.1177/1783591719847545.

Steen E, Yurechko K, Klug D. You can (not) say what you want: using Algospeak to contest and evade algorithmic content moderation on TikTok. Social Media Soc. 2023;9(3) https://doi.org/10.1177/20563051231194586.

Swist T, Collin P, McCormack J, Third A. Social media and the wellbeing of children and young people: a literature review. [online] Westernsydney.edu.au. 2015. Available at: https://researchdirect.westernsydney.edu.au/islandora/object/uws:36407.

Thorn P, Sala LL, Hetrick S, Rice S, Lamblin M, Robinson J. Motivations and perceived harms and benefits of online communication about self-harm: an interview study with young people. Digital Health, [online]. 2023;9 https://doi.org/10.1177/20552076231176689.

UK Safer Internet Centre. Our internet, our choice report. 2019. [online] Available at: https://saferinternet.org.uk/blog/our-internet-our-choice-report.

UK Safer Internet Centre. Healthcare professionals. n.d.. [online] Available at: https://saferinternet.org.uk/guide-and-resource/healthcare-professionals.

UNICEF. UN convention on the rights of the child (UNCRC). [online] UNICEF. 1989. Available at: https://www.unicef.org.uk/what-we-do/un-convention-child-rights/.

University of Minnesota., Publisher, A. removed at request of original. 6.3 Adolescence: developing independence and identity. 2015. [online] open.lib.umn.edu. Available at: http://open.lib.umn.edu/intropsyc/chapter/6-3-adolescence-developing-independence-and-identity/. Accessed 30 Mar 2021.

United Nations (UN). Child and youth safety online. United Nations; United Nations. 2023. [Online] https://www.un.org/en/global-issues/child-and-youth-safety-online.

Uttal DH, Meadow NG, Tipton E, Hand LL, Alden AR, Warren C, Newcombe NS. The malleability of spatial skills: a meta-analysis of training studies. Psychol Bull. 2013;139(2):352–402.

Vaingankar JA. Social media–driven routes to positive mental health among youth: qualitative enquiry and concept mapping study. JMIR Pediatrics Parenting, [online]. 2022;5(1):1–14. https://doi.org/10.2196/32758.

Vera V. Nonsuicidal self-injury and content moderation on TikTok. Proc Assoc Inf Sci Technol. 2023;60(1):1164–6. Available from: https://doi.org/10.1002/pra2.979.

Weinstein E, Kleiman EM, Franz PJ, Joyce VW, Nash CC, Buonopane RJ, Nock MK. Positive and negative uses of social media among adolescents hospitalized for suicidal behavior. J Adolesc. 2021;87(87):63–73. https://doi.org/10.1016/j.adolescence.2020.12.003.

Yeung K. Algorithmic regulation: a critical interrogation. Regulation Governance. 2017;12(4):505–23. https://doi.org/10.1111/rego.12158.

14 Conclusions

Gemma Trainor and Vanessa Heaslip

14.1 Introduction

Over the past two decades, conversations regarding young people's mental health have increased; there is a noticeable progressive change of culture where it has become more acceptable to speak out about mental health issues and challenges. During the COVID-19 pandemic, mental health of young people declined due to prolonged social isolation, disruption of daily routines, concerns over the health and well-being of family members, financial issues and individual health anxieties in terms of fear of contracting the COVID virus itself. Additionally, a person born in 2006 will have had experienced living in recession and its accompanying austerity measures, war in the Middle east and Europe and a world having to grapple with climate change. This has resulted in young people facing uncertain futures. Young Minds reported that 52% of 16–20-year-olds have self-harmed in the last year (Young Minds 2023) and, globally, one in seven 10–19-year-old olds experience a mental disorder accounting for 13% of the global burden of disease for this age group (UNICEF 2024a, b).

The COVID-19 pandemic brought children and young people's well-being into sharp focus. The commitments outlined in the NHS Long-Term Plan (LTP) in the UK make it clear that achieving parity of esteem is a key priority. Whilst recognising there have been some improvements made, there is still some way to go to meet

G. Trainor (✉)
Mental Health Nursing, Directorate of Nursing and Midwifery, University of Salford, Salford, UK
e-mail: gemma.trainor@outlook.com

V. Heaslip
Directorate of Nursing and Midwifery, University of Salford, Salford, UK
e-mail: V.A.Heaslip@salford.ac.uk

G. Trainor, V. Heaslip (eds.), *Needs of Children and Young People Living with Complex Mental Health Difficulties*,
https://doi.org/10.1007/978-3-031-84532-1_14

the disparity between mental health and physical health. Parity of esteem was enshrined in law by the Health and Social Care Act 2012; however, whilst mental health problems account for 28% of the burden of disease, it only accounts for only 18% of NHS spending (Shafan-Azhar and Treloar 2023), demonstrating there is a long way to go before parity is achieved. Mental and physical health are equally important to a young person's overall health. Chronic physical health conditions can increase the risk of mental illness, and conversely depression increases risk of long-term physical health conditions such as diabetes and heart disease (Mental Health Foundation (MHF) 2024b). As discussed throughout the book, Future in Minds, the Five Year Forward View for Mental Health, the NHS Long Term Plan and the Transformation of Children and Young People's Provision: A Green Paper are key documents that have had national significance in addressing some of the inequities. Good mental health underpins everything in life; in contrast poor mental health leads to significant costs to individuals and societies. As noted in the chapters, there is a link between poverty and inequalities in mental health and well-being, yet we argue it should no longer be the case that someone's mental ill health should be a barrier to achieving a good life. There are currently very few robust treatment trials to guide those supporting young people living with a mental illness as most research is conducted on adults and extrapolated to children and young people. However, throughout the book we have presented various ways of promoting positive mental health and well-being and supporting those living with mental distress, such as:

- Early intervention and prevention
- Tackling stigma and discrimination
- Driving innovation and minimising harm from young people's social media use
- Building resilient communities to make a difference to its residents' well-being
- Ensuring more access to young people's services including 24-h responses
- Giving young people the right support at the right time
- More meaningful involvement of young people, parents/carers in service delivery and research
- Greater collaboration across public, private, government and third sector organisations to reduce the gap between the supply and demand for mental health services
- Assessing young peoples' Internet use to inform case formulation and risk management.
- Ensuring that young people's mental health is everyone's business by strengthening mental health support in wherever young people are

To reach children and young people without access, services need to be provided across a wide range of sectors and delivery platforms including health, social care and education.

14.2 Integrated Care in Young People

Developing integrated approaches to mental health is a key priority in England due to a disconnect from coordinated care working together to address both physical and mental health needs. Systematic reviews of job stress (LaMontagne et al. 2014, 2019) have shown that system-level approaches are the most effective. Globally, this is being achieved through integrated care (Hope et al. 2023). However, currently much of the literature, research and clinical practice models are largely based in the adult population, so it is less clear about how this initiative would address specific needs of children and young people. Endeavours so far are to increase community integration and reduce the need for expensive specialist services. Distinct features of integration require involvement from family, schools and community-based activities which incorporate the changing needs from childhood to adolescence (Wolfe et al. 2020). Wolfe et al. (2020) assert there is a need to encompass vertical integration (between primary and secondary care), horizontal integration (between health, education and social sectors), longitudinal integration (developmentally appropriate integration of health and non-health services), and finally population integration (taking a public health focus including health promotion and prevention measures). A recent systematic review investigated integrated care pathways for young people experiencing medical emergencies related to mental illness in Canada, the USA and Australia (Otis et al. 2023), exploring whether innovations in the acute crisis around integration would result in young people recovering quicker and being well enough to remain out of hospital. The results showed promise in that the triage innovations reduced admissions between 4% and 16%, reduced re-admissions and included things like provision of guided meal supervision for young people with eating disorders. Current practice is that emergency services are required to take a young person in crisis to the emergency paediatric service; therefore, this review reinforces the importance and success of upskilling the paediatric workforce to support these young people.

However, the lack of child and adolescent services (CAMHS) is a global problem (Shaligram et al. 2022) which we assert needs to be addressed. We argue that commissioners and service planners across health, social care, education and the criminal justice system must plan and commission services jointly, pooling resources so that the system works flexibly to provide person-centred care built around the young person, their families and communities. The focus of integrating care is an overarching theme throughout the book and illuminates ways in which it needs to be the business of everyone to take advantage of opportunities to promote, protect and care for our future generation and not just their own health and well-being but in building resilient and healthy communities.

14.3 Lessons and Insights from Chapters

This book forms a natural split with the first half addressing and describing complex mental health issues and how best to support young people and their families. These early chapters have focussed on presenting the global picture of mental illness in young people as well as introducing the concepts of risk and protective factors for children and young people before exploring some complex mental health conditions and comorbidities such as self-harm, eating disorders, psychosis and personality issues. The second half of the book explores coexisting issues which can contribute or perpetuate existing ill health such as a learning disability or neurodiversity or transgenderism as well as examining some wider social and environmental factors that can impact upon young people's mental health and well-being such as social exclusion, discrimination, as well as intersectionality between these, relationship difficulties and Internet use.

The book also provides chapters to support and develop the practitioners' professional practice, covering aspects such as trauma-informed care and how these issues affect not only the young person's fragility but the staff providing interventions contributing important insights into ensuring the experience is not retraumatising. In recognising the importance of trauma-informed care, much has been explained about the role of early childhood adversity (adverse childhood experiences or ACEs) in affecting future mental health. Assessing and responding to risks also provide practitioners with key strategies to manage risk in whatever settings they work. We recognise that working with children and young people in mental distress can also be distressing for the practitioners involved and as such have provided guidance regarding the importance of reflective practice and therapeutic use of self when working with young people and their families. Lastly, the important issue of child protection and safeguarding is also covered to support practitioners to work within national and international safeguarding parameters.

The key take-home messages from this book are:

- That many children and young people experience mental distress and many of these children will not be under the care of mental health services. We believe that promoting good mental health and responding to mental distress are everyone's responsibility in whatever sector you work (health, education, police, criminal justice, charity, social care, statutory services, etc.).
- To recognise that sometimes signs of mental health distress, such as self-harm or aggression, may be a symptom of unmet need as opposed to a condition in itself.
- The more risk factors and reduced protective factors a young person is exposed to, the greater the potential for these to impact on the young person's mental health and well-being. Therefore, a thorough multi-agency risk assessment is fundamental as well as recognising that risk is a constantly changing phenomenon.
- Multi-agency cooperation and communication are vital to ensure there is a holistic and accurate picture of the child, young person and their family; no one agency alone can address all the factors that can contribute to mental distress.

- There is increasing evidence to suggest that those who use social media sites can experience self-objectification (the extent to which your self-worth relies on appearance). Vulnerable young people may seek solace in accessing the dark web which can serve as a mirror exacerbating their problems. Globally there is a call for the regulation of social platforms to comply with age controls and offer youth-friendly versions of content.
- The therapeutic use of self and developing a positive therapeutic alliance as being key ingredients in promoting agency and empowerment. In recognising the importance of trauma-informed care, much has been explained about the role of early childhood adversity in affecting future mental health. Trauma-informed care (TIC) services should create a safe space which requires meaningful service user involvement working with the whole system supporting cross-agency collaboration and integrated communication (Dermody et al. 2018).
- Mental health distress can be linked to critical moments in brain development which can be affected by toxic stress triggered by experiencing adverse childhood experiences.
- The importance of listing to and working with young people, seeing them as an active participant in their care.

Globally, there is a need for a profound cultural change, and children and young people can play an active role in their decision-making and care. Chapter 7 emphasises the impact of feeling marginalised, disadvantaged and disaffected in reinforcing stigma. The authors explain the need to challenge discriminatory practice, raise mental health literacy and ensure these young people have a voice and a meaningful place in society. Inclusive schools are a place where these young people can learn critical skills to bolster their well-being particularly where it is a safe space free from bullying, racism, peer pressure and academic stress. Social and emotional learning approaches require a whole school sign-up to provide an environment to support mental health and reduce risks of bullying and exposing children to unnecessary risks.

Throughout the book there are interspersed case studies which can help the reader analyse and interpret a young person's condition and set of circumstances. They can capture the richness of the young person and families' experiences and some of the contextual factors that may influence their behaviour. They also provide some helpful advice about how best to intervene by setting a real-life context and the perspectives of all those involved. Furthermore, there are also reflective activities which enable the reader the opportunity to stop and consider their current knowledge, skills and professional practice, with targeted activities to assist them in further developing the way in which they support young people and their families.

Young people today have the poorest mental health of any age group in the UK, whereas the reverse was true two decades ago (MHF 2024a). Surveys such as NHS Digital inform (NHS England 2023) how young people from socio-economically deprived backgrounds are more likely to experience a "probable mental disorder" especially if they live in a household that has fallen behind with bills, rents and mortgages, and considering the global austerity measures currently being faced, this is likely to increase. Poor mental health has a lifelong impact, especially upon education attainment, future careers as well as their future choices as highlighted in the Resolution Foundation Report (McCurdy and Murphy 2024). As stated at the outset of the book, half of the mental health problems affecting young people in adulthood have their onset during or before adolescence, emphasising the need to address these problems early to build a mentally healthy society. This book stresses the importance of young people seeing themselves as a part of the solution, as experts in their own world rather than passive recipients of care.

Identifying problems early can be achieved through raising awareness across the existing workforce including frontline services such as police, ambulance staff, pharmacists, and job centre employees and not just health and social care staff. Trauma-informed care services should create a safe space which requires meaningful service user involvement working with the whole system supporting cross-agency collaboration and integrated communication (Dermody et al. 2018). Many of the social determinants of health lie outside the boundaries of the healthcare system, so strategically there is an obvious need to coordinate action across the extant of services within schools, communities and everyone involved in the promotion of mental well-being to improve the lives of young people and their families. Developing a coherent sense of identity is crucial for adolescent mental health where relationships serve as a vital source of support that aid young people to navigate this task.

14.4 The Eye of the Storm

This book has quite rightly kept children and young people at the centre of the agenda. However, due to confirmed high prevalence of self-harm and suicide, this also presents challenges for parents, siblings, peers and all concerned. Parents often describe feelings such as being in the “eye of the storm”. This metaphor describes a temporary period of calm or stability within a larger context of sheer turmoil, confusion and fear of the unknown.

We would like to conclude by introducing you to Sam, who at 15 started to show signs of anxiety and depression, and his family. Sam committed suicide at the age of 15, only 4 months after he had shown signs and symptoms of mental distress. Below is Sam’s mother’s experiences of the care Sam received before he died.

> Every week I would take Sam to his private appointment as he was on a waiting list for CAMHS. I would drive Sam to his weekly appointment and sit in the reception area while he disappeared down a corridor to his therapy session. I was never spoken to or given any advice or feedback on how best to support Sam and keep him safe. After he died I came across a scrappy piece of paper which I now realise was his safety plan—no copy had been given to me school or anyone else involved in supporting Sam as far as I knew. The therapist told me that she could not have conversations like this with parents as she needed to remain impartial. I felt very shut out and was asked to check in on him daily, whatever that was supposed to mean. I appreciate that Sam was entitled to a degree of confidentiality; however he was only 15 years old. I believe that it would have been supportive for Sam and me to have been included in some part of the therapy session. In fact, it would have been good for

> all the family as we may have been part of the solution to Sam's recovery and imperative to our family in navigating the journey through the 'eye of the storm'. Most parents know their children best. I believe there is a good chance Sam would be alive today if he had received integrated care for his mental health; this would involve the psychiatrist and/or his clinical psychologist frequently liaising with and educating his family and school with Sam involved every step of the way.

Grief following suicide is complex and is often one of life's most painful experiences. Sam's brother has since written a book *This Book Could Save Your Life: Breaking the Silence Around the Mental Health Emergency* (West 2022) and is an award-winning mental health campaigner concentrating on mental health awareness. He started a petition to make mental health first aid a compulsory part of teacher training. The book is an excellent read, as it helps understand the wider impact on the family and can help those who support bereaved families and friends. We are eternally grateful for Sam's mum agreeing to share her incredibly painful experiences with us and is a stark reminder that of the significant levels of distress some children and young people can face. We ultimately hope that through this book, you, as a practitioners, wherever you work, will feel more confident in having conversations with children and young people about mental distress as well as feel more empowered and knowledgeable about the range of services available to support them.

References

Dermody A, Gardner C, Davis S, Lambert S, Dermody J, Fein M. Resilience in the face of trauma: implications for service delivery. Irish Probat J. 2018;15:161–78.

Hope S, Stepanova E, Lloyd-Houldey O, Hillier-Brown F, Hargreaves D, Nicholls D, Summerbell C, Viner RM, Dedat Z, Owen EC, Scott S. This needs to be a journey that we're actually on together' – the introduction of integrated care systems for children and young people in England: a qualitative study of the views of local system stakeholders during winter 2021/22. BMC Health Serv Res. 2023;23(1):1448. https://doi.org/10.1186/s12913-023-10442-6.

LaMontagne AD, Martin A, Page KM, Reavley NJ, Noblet AJ, Milner AJ, Keegel T, Smith PM. Workplace mental health: developing an integrated intervention approach. BMC Psychiatry. 2014;14:131. https://doi.org/10.1186/1471-244X-14-131.

LaMontagne AD, Martin A, Page KM, Reavley NJ, Noblet AJ, Milner AJ, Keegel T, Allisey A, Papas A, Witt K, Smith PM. Developing an integrated approach to workplace mental health. In: Hudson HL, Nigam JA, Sauter SL, Chosewood LC, Schill AL, Howard J, editors. Total worker health. American Psychological Association; 2019. p. 211–27. https://doi.org/10.1037/0000149-013.

McCurdy C, Murphy L. We've only just begun: action to improve young people's mental health, education and employment. Resolution Foundation; 2024. February 2024. Available from: https://www.resolutionfoundation.org/app/uploads/2024/02/Weve-only-just-begun.pdf. Accessed 17 Nov 2024

Mental Health Foundation. Children and young people: statistics. 2024a. Available from: https://www.mentalhealth.org.uk/explore-mental-health/statistics/children-young-people-statistics. Accessed 17 Nov 2024.

Mental Health Foundation. Physical and mental health. 2024b. Available from: https://www.mentalhealth.org.uk/explore-mental-health/a-z-topics/physical-health-and-mental-health. Accessed 17 Nov 2024.

NHS England. Mental health of children and young people in England, 2023 – wave 4 follow up to the 2017 survey. 2023. Available from: https://digital.nhs.uk/data-and-information/publications/statistical/mental-health-of-children-and-young-people-in-england/2023-wave-4-follow-up. Accessed 17 Nov 2024.

Otis M, Barber S, Amet M, Nicholls D. Models of integrated care for young people experiencing medical emergencies related to mental illness: a realist systematic review. Eur Child Adolesc Psychiatry. 2023;32(12):2439–52. https://doi.org/10.1007/s00787-022-02085-5.

Shafan-Azhar Z, Treloar N. The state of children and young people's mental health. Centre for Mental Health; 2023. Available from: https://www.centreformentalhealth.org.uk/the-state-of-children-and-young-peoples-mental-health-in-2023/. Accessed 17 Nov 2024.

Shaligram D, Skokauskas N, Aragones E, Azeem MW, Bala A, Bernstein B, Cama S, Canessa L, Silva FD, Engelhard C, Garrido G, Guerrero APS, Hunt J, Jadhav M, Martin SL, Miliauskas C, Nalugya J, Nazeer A, Ong SH, Robertson P, Sassi R, Seker A. International perspective on integrated care models in child and adult mental health. Int Rev Psychiatry. 2022;34(2):101–17. https://doi.org/10.1080/09540261.2022.2059346.

UNICEF. Mental health children and adolescents. 2024a. Available from: https://data.unicef.org/topic/child-health/mental-health/. Accessed 17 Nov 2024.

UNICEF. Child and adolescent mental health The State of Children in the European Union. Policy brief 2. 2024b. Available from: https://www.unicef.org/eu/media/2576/file/Child%20and%20adolescent%20mental%20health%20policy%20brief.pdf. Accessed 17 Nov 2024.

West B. This book could save your life – breaking the silence around the mental health emergency. London: Harper Collins; 2022.

Wolfe I, Satherley RM, Scotney E, Newham J, Lingam R. Integrated care models and child health: a meta-analysis. Pediatrics. 2020;145(1):e20183747. https://doi.org/10.1542/peds.2018-3747.

Young Minds. Mental health statistics. 2023. Available from: https://www.youngminds.org.uk/about-us/media-centre/mental-health-statistics/. Accessed 17 Nov 2024.

GPSR Compliance

The European Union's (EU) General Product Safety Regulation (GPSR) is a set of rules that requires consumer products to be safe and our obligations to ensure this.

If you have any concerns about our products, you can contact us on ProductSafety@springernature.com

In case Publisher is established outside the EU, the EU authorized representative is:

Springer Nature Customer Service Center GmbH
Europaplatz 3
69115 Heidelberg, Germany

Batch number: 10723317

Printed by Printforce, the Netherlands